Clinician's Guide to Pediatric Sleep Disorders

SLEEP DISORDERS

Advisory Board

Clinician's Guide to Pediatric Sleep Disorders

Edited by

Mark A. Richardson
Oregon Health & Science University
Portland, Oregon, U.S.A.

Norman R. Friedman
University of Colorado Health Sciences Center
Denver, Colorado, U.S.A.

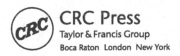

CRC Press
Taylor & Francis Group
Boca Raton London New York

CRC Press is an imprint of the
Taylor & Francis Group, an **informa** business

CRC Press
Taylor & Francis Group
6000 Broken Sound Parkway NW, Suite 300
Boca Raton, FL 33487-2742

© 2007 by Taylor & Francis Group, LLC
CRC Press is an imprint of Taylor & Francis Group, an Informa business

First issued in paperback 2019

No claim to original U.S. Government works

ISBN 13: 978-0-367-45347-3 (pbk)
ISBN 13: 978-0-8493-9819-3 (hbk)

Library of Congress Cataloging-in-Publication Data

Clinician's guide to pediatric sleep disorders / edited by Mark A. Richardson, Norman R. Friedman.
    p. ; cm. -- (Sleep disorders ; 1)
    Includes bibliographical references and index.
    ISBN-13: 978-0-8493-9819-3 (hardcover : alk. paper)
    ISBN-10: 0-8493-9819-3 (hardcover : alk. paper)
    1. Sleep disorders in children. 2. Children--Sleep. I. Richardson, Mark A. II. Friedman, Norman R. III.
Series: Sleep disorders (New York, N.Y.) ; 1.
    [DNLM: 1. Sleep Disorders. 2. Child. 3. Sleep Apnea, Obstructive. WM 188 C6415 2006]

RJ506.S55C45552 2006
618.92'8498--dc22   2006048590

Visit the Taylor & Francis Web site at
http://www.taylorandfrancis.com

and the CRC Press Web site at
http://www.crcpress.com

Preface

Sleep medicine is still in its infancy. Few medical schools have a department of sleep medicine. Dedicated pediatric sleep programs are even less common. Book stores do not have a designated place to shelve textbooks on the subject. Sleep medicine's borders are ill-defined. Many sleep problems require expertise from a variety of specialties. The specialty spans multiple disciplines including neurology, otolaryngology, psychiatry, and pulmonary. Pediatric sleep disorders encompass a variety of medical conditions; however, the most common diagnosis is sleep-disordered breathing.

Sleep-disordered breathing is a spectrum of disrupted sleep patterns from primary snoring to obstructive sleep apnea. Obstructive sleep apnea exists when the child attempts to breathe but the breath is aborted/interrupted by obstruction in the upper airway. In the 1980s, obstructive sleep apnea was rarely recognized in children and children were presenting to the hospital with severe manifestations of obstructive sleep apnea—heart failure, pulmonary hypertension and failure to thrive. Over the last few decades, obstructive sleep apnea is no longer a "zebra" diagnosis. Nowadays, the most common indication for an adenotonsillectomy is obstructed breathing rather than recurrent infections. In 2002, the American Academy of Pediatrics published guidelines to assist clinicians in the diagnosis and management of obstructive sleep apnea for children. Increasingly, research is demonstrating neurobehavioral and neurocognitive consequences in children who have the mildest forms of sleep-disordered breathing, primary snoring. Sleep-disordered breathing has also been associated with poor school performance and a decreased quality of life.

Although sleep-disordered breathing is the most common pediatric sleep disorder, clinicians should be aware of more obscure sleep disorders which affect a child's health. As an infant, one will sleep most of the time. Subsequently, any condition that affects sleep could interfere with future development. As one ages, inadequate sleep disrupts one's quality of life. With the development of the light bulb, our society was transformed from one where sleep was considered natural to one where it was a luxury. Unfortunately, many people support Thomas Edison's beliefs regarding sleep: "Anything which tends to slow work down is a waste. We are always hearing people talk about 'loss of sleep' as a calamity. They better call it loss of time, vitality and opportunities." Another myth is that sleep is a passive process. Multiple biological process occur only during sleep. Therefore, disruption of sleep interrupts body homeostasis.

This book provides comprehensive coverage of sleep-disordered breathing but does not neglect other conditions. The primary aim of this book is to educate primary care practitioners so that they may accurately diagnose and treat pediatric sleep disorders. The text is a practical guide to provide the fundamental essentials to recognizing the sleep disorder and to initiate treatment. We have recruited a collection of pediatric specialists—anesthesiologists, neurologists, otolaryngologists, pulmonologists, and psychiatrists to achieve our goal of reaching across disciplines to raise the awareness of pediatric sleep disorders. The authors are renowned in their fields. By providing practical knowledge to the reader, the authors enable the clinician to educate a child's family on their disorder. Since the major pediatric sleep disorder is sleep-disordered breathing, multiple chapters are dedicated to this disorder. Children with sleep-disordered breathing have variable presenting symptoms which may bring them to the attention of a variety of medical specialists: neurologists → sleepiness, otolaryngologists → tonsil hypertrophy, pediatrics → failure to thrive, psychiatry → behavioral, pulmonary → breathing, and urologists → enuresis. Other chapters will enlighten the reader on sleep disorders from infancy through adolescence. Both behavioral and physiologic sleep topics are addressed by the leaders in the field. By reading *Clinician's Guide to Pediatric Sleep Disorders*, one will become more aware of the consequences of sleep-disordered breathing as well as other common pediatric sleep disorders. The text is a valuable reference for any individual who cares for children.

Mark A. Richardson
Norman R. Friedman

Contents

Contributors

Steven H. Abman Department of Pediatrics, The Children's Hospital, University of Colorado, Denver, Colorado, U.S.A.

Charles M. Bower Department of Pediatric Otolaryngology, Arkansas Children's Hospital, Little Rock, Arkansas, U.S.A.

Karla M. Dzienkowski Restless Legs Syndrome Foundation, Rochester, Minnesota, U.S.A.

Helene A. Emsellem The Center for Sleep and Wake Disorders, Chevy Chase, Maryland, and George Washington School of Medicine, Washington, D.C., U.S.A.

Norman R. Friedman Department of Otolaryngology/Head and Neck Surgery, University of Colorado Health Sciences Center and The Children's Hospital, Denver, Colorado, U.S.A.

Nira A. Goldstein Division of Pediatric Otolaryngology, Department of Otolaryngology, State University of New York, Downstate Medical Center, Brooklyn, New York, U.S.A.

David Gozal Departments of Pediatrics, Pharmacology and Toxicology, Psychology, and Brain Sciences, Kosair Children's Hospital Research Institute, University of Louisville School of Medicine, Louisville, Kentucky, U.S.A.

Ann C. Halbower Pediatric Sleep Disorders Program, Division of Pediatric Pulmonology, Johns Hopkins University School of Medicine, Baltimore, Maryland, U.S.A.

Jerome E. Hester Lucille Packard Children's Hospital, Stanford University Hospital, Palo Alto, California, U.S.A.

Kyle P. Johnson   Division of Child and Adolescent Psychiatry, Departments of Psychiatry and Pediatrics, Oregon Health & Science University, Portland, Oregon, U.S.A.

James Kelly   Department of Surgery, University of New Mexico, Albuquerque, New Mexico, U.S.A.

Anna S. Kenny   Pediatric Respiratory Medicine, Rush University Medical Center, Chicago, Illinois, U.S.A.

Leila Kheirandish-Gozal   Division of Pediatric Sleep Medicine, Department of Pediatrics, University of Louisville School of Medicine, Louisville, Kentucky, U.S.A.

Jeffrey Koh   Department of Anesthesia and Perioperative Medicine and Pediatrics, Oregon Health & Science University, Portland, Oregon, U.S.A.

Rees L. Lee   Pediatric Pulmonary Medicine, Department of Pediatrics, Naval Medical Center, Portsmouth, Virginia, U.S.A.

Holger Link   Pediatric Sleep Lab, Pediatrics and Pulmonary Medicine, Oregon Health & Science University, Portland, Oregon, U.S.A.

Maria Cecilia Lopes   Stanford Sleep Disorders Clinic, Stanford University, Palo Alto, California, U.S.A., and Department of Psychobiology, Federal University of Sao Paulo, Sao Paulo, Brazil

Lisa J. Meltzer   Division of Pulmonary Medicine, Department of Pediatrics, University of Pennsylvania and The Children's Hospital of Philadelphia, Philadelphia, Pennsylvania, U.S.A.

Ron B. Mitchell   Department of Otolaryngology and Pediatrics, Saint Louis University School of Medicine, Cardinal Glennon Children's Medical Center, St. Louis, Missouri.

Gregory S. Montgomery   Department of Pediatrics, Riley Hospital for Children, Indiana University, Indianapolis, Indiana, U.S.A.

Karen E. Murtagh   The Center for Sleep and Wake Disorders, Chevy Chase, Maryland, U.S.A.

Sara I. Pai   Department of Otolaryngology/Head and Neck Surgery, Johns Hopkins University School of Medicine, Baltimore, Maryland, U.S.A.

Rafael Pelayo   Stanford Sleep Disorders Clinic, Stanford University, Palo Alto, California, U.S.A.

Jonathan Perkins   Otolaryngology-Head and Neck Surgery, University of Washington and Children's Hospital and Regional Medical Center, Seattle, Washington, U.S.A.

Daniel Picchietti   University of Illinois and Carle Clinic Association, Urbana, Illinois, U.S.A.

Nelson B. Powell   Lucille Packard Children's Hospital, Stanford University Hospital, Palo Alto, California, U.S.A.

R. Mark Ray   Department of Pediatric Otolaryngology, Arkansas Children's Hospital, Little Rock, Arkansas, U.S.A.

Mark A. Richardson   Department of Otolaryngology/Head & Neck Surgery, Oregon Health & Science University, Portland, Oregon, U.S.A.

Robert R. Riley   Lucille Packard Children's Hospital, Stanford University Hospital, Palo Alto, California, U.S.A.

Richard M. Rosenfeld   Division of Pediatric Otolaryngology, Department of Otolaryngology, State University of New York, Downstate Medical Center, Brooklyn, New York, U.S.A.

Veronica C. Swanson   Department of Anesthesia and Perioperative Medicine and Pediatrics, Oregon Health & Science University, Portland, Oregon, U.S.A.

David E. Tunkel   Department of Otolaryngology/Head and Neck Surgery, Johns Hopkins University School of Medicine, Baltimore, Maryland, U.S.A.

Debra E. Weese-Mayer   Pediatric Respiratory Medicine, Rush University Medical Center, Chicago, Illinois, U.S.A.

1

Pediatric Sleep Disorders

Charles M. Bower and R. Mark Ray

Department of Pediatric Otolaryngology, Arkansas Children's Hospital, Little Rock, Arkansas, U.S.A.

CHAPTER HIGHLIGHTS

- Sleep laboratories are critically important to ascertain the control of breathing in infants and children. They can separate obstructive sleep-disordered breathing (SDB) from non-apneic disorders such as periodic limb movements, narcolepsy, and other parasomnias.
- SDB is a continuum of disorders, from primary snoring to upper airway resistance syndrome and true obstructive sleep apnea (OSA).
- High risk populations benefit from being evaluated in a sleep laboratory to determine the exact nature and severity of a sleep disorder, if it is present.

INTRODUCTION

Pediatric sleep medicine has evolved dramatically over the last 30 years into an important, multidisciplinary specialty for the diagnosis and treatment of pediatric sleep disorders. Treatment of sleep disorders provides significant relief for infants and children with a variety of sleep-related medical and behavioral problems. This broad area of medicine encompasses the management of early sleep problems such as central apnea, acute life-threatening events (ALTEs), and sudden infant death syndrome (SIDS) as well as very prevalent problems such as obstructive sleep apnea syndrome (OSAS) and sleep onset insomnia in infants and children, in addition to unusual disorders such as narcolepsy and central apnea in children and teenagers. The specialty has grown dramatically over the last several years with an increasing number of sleep disorders centers dedicated to the diagnostic evaluation, testing, and treatment of affected patients.

Interest in sleep dates back thousands of years. It has been addressed by authors over the millennia with specific attention given to the importance of sleep and dreaming and their effect on all aspects of life. Sleep has long been recognized as being critically important to the health and well-being of individuals (1,2). Over the past 100 years, our understanding of sleep physiology and normal sleep structure has increased dramatically. Stages 1 through 4 of sleep have been described and characterized. The discovery of rapid eye movement (REM) sleep and the recognition that it is associated with dreaming has been very important in the understanding of sleep (3,4). Further research by Dement and Kleitman expanded the understanding of REM and nonREM sleep with a description of sleep cycles (5).

Development of sleep labs in the 1960s led to the rapid advancement of sleep medicine. Reports in 1965 by Gestaut, Tesinauri, and Deron, as well as Jung and Kuhlo, led to further research on the important cardiovascular consequences of sleep apnea (6,7). Further research has documented not only the significant life threatening cardiovascular consequences of OSA, but also revealed important daytime behavioral difficulties associated with it. These behavioral consequences include poor attention, hyperactivity, abnormal behavior, and poor school performance, all of which are particularly important in child development (8,9). Treatment of sleep apnea in children tends to result in significant improvement in behavioral disturbances (10–12). The risk of behavioral consequences is important in relatively mild sleep apnea, including upper airway resistance syndrome (UARS) and possibly even primary snoring (13).

SLEEP DISORDERS CENTERS

The American Sleep Disorders Association (ASDA) was formed in the 1970s and has become an important forum for research and scholarly discussion. The ASDA and the more recently organized American Academy of Sleep Medicine have provided important leadership for the work of dedicated clinicians and support for continuing researchers. This has led to an understanding of the important place sleep medicine has in the management of patients across the world. Multiple-accredited sleep labs and sleep centers for the diagnosis and treatment of sleep disorders have opened in many places in recent years. The first accredited pediatric sleep lab was established in 1987. Pediatric sleep medicine continues to evolve, with over a dozen fully accredited pediatric sleep centers in the United States. The recognition by the American Academy of Pediatrics of the importance of sleep medicine led to the development of a policy statement on pediatric sleep apnea in 2002 (14). It emphasizes the importance of early evaluation and treatment of pediatric sleep disorders. It identifies the role of pediatric polysomnography (PSG) in the diagnosis of pediatric obstructive sleep-disordered breathing (SDB) and suggests treatment strategies to improve the quality of care for these patients.

Pediatric sleep medicine covers a broad clinical spectrum of abnormalities. Sleep labs and centers assess the control of breathing during sleep in infants and children. This includes evaluation and treatment of SIDS, central apnea, and other infant sleep disorders. Sleep onset insomnia and the behavioral aspects of sleep onset and maintenance remain important and challenging aspects of sleep medicine. Of particular interest to sleep labs, because of its high prevalence, is obstructive sleep-disordered breathing. This ranges from mild snoring to upper airway resistance to severe and even life-threatening OSAS in children and adults. The diagnosis of SDB is suspected clinically and in many cases confirmed in the sleep lab. Consistently reliable surgical treatments such as adenotonsillectomy, uvulopalatopharyngoplasty (15), and advanced techniques such as mandibular and maxillary advancement are available through many sleep centers (16,17). Nonsurgical treatment of sleep apnea includes medications, oxygen, or continuous positive airway pressure in some children. Treatment of pediatric sleep apnea has been shown to improve daytime behavior, including academic performance, which can lead to substantial improvement in children's lives (13).

Sleep labs are also important for the diagnosis of nonsleep apnea nighttime disorders such as restless leg syndrome and periodic limb movement disorders, which are important contributors to disrupted sleep. Daytime sleepiness can also be assessed by pediatric sleep centers. Narcolepsy can be diagnosed as early as young childhood, and an accurate diagnosis can lead to an early treatment and improvement in the patient's abilities to cope with this lifelong disorder. Many patients have mild forms of excessive sleepiness including idiopathic hypersomnia, which also benefits from medical management. Finally, parasomnias including night terrors and nightmares, circadian rhythm disorders, insomnia, and insufficient sleep are problems that a pediatric sleep center is well-equipped to evaluate and treat.

OBSTRUCTIVE SLEEP APNEA SYNDROME

OSA in children is a "disorder of breathing during sleep characterized by prolonged partial upper airway obstruction and/or intermittent complete obstruction (obstructive apnea) that disrupts normal ventilation and sleep patterns" (18). OSA has been recognized for many generations. Most authors cite the early account of pediatric sleep apnea by Dickens in his description of Joe, who was a "fat and red-faced boy, in the state of somnolency" (19). William Osler described childhood OSAS in his 1892 textbook with great clarity. "At night the child's sleep is greatly disturbed; the respirations are loud and snorting, and there are sometimes prolonged pauses, followed by deep, noisy inspirations" (20). After Osler first described OSA in children, little was published in the medical literature until 1965 when Noonan described reversible cor pulmonale in children as a result of adenotonsillar hypertrophy (21). Ten years later, the first series of childhood OSA was reported by Guilleminault et al. (22). Early on, sleep apnea was recognized only in the face of severe cardiovascular sequelae. Since the time of Guilleminault's article, our understanding of OSAS has increased dramatically. It is now recognized that SDB exists across a spectrum of severity. This ranges from isolated snoring, without significant cardiovascular or behavioral consequences in most children, to UARS characterized by true obstructive events that cannot be easily quantified but result in arousals and sleep disruption. This can lead to significant daytime behavior problems. True severe obstructive sleep apnea with hypoxia, hypercarbia, and cardiovascular sequelae exists on the far end of the spectrum. However, to this date, there is no true consensus on definitions of obstructive sleep apnea parameters and very little information is available regarding the natural history, prevalence, pathophysiology, diagnosis, and management of OSA in children (14). It is also important to recognize the different clinical pattern of OSAS in children compared with adults (Table 1).

It is estimated that approximately 7% to 10% of children snore habitually and 20% or more snore on an intermittent basis (8,23). The prevalence of childhood sleep apnea is estimated to be around two percent. This translates into a figure of more than 500,000 children with OSA in the United States (8,24). OSA tends to peak in prevalence at approximately four to five years of age, at which point adenotonsillar hypertrophy is most prominent (9). There is a second peak in late adolescence. Gender distribution is equal in young children as opposed to the male predominance seen in adults (25). Despite the relatively high prevalence of sleep pathology in children, diagnosis and treatment are frequently delayed for years (26).

Table 1   Differences Between Child and Adult Obstructive Sleep Apnea Syndrome

Criteria	Adult	Child
Snoring	With pauses	Continuous
EDS	Common	Rare
Obesity	Common	Rare
FTT	No	Rare
Mouth breathing	No	Common
Gender	M:F 10:1	M:F 1:1
ATH	Uncommon	Most common
Pattern	Obstructive apnea	Hypoventilation
Surgery	Minority	T and A in most
CPAP	Common	Minority

Abbreviations: ATH, adenotonsillar hypertrophy; CPAP, continuous positive airway pressure; EDS, excessive daytime sleepiness; FTT, failure to thrive; OSAS, obstructive sleep apnea syndrome.

Primary snoring, which is very common, occurs when no consequences of snoring exist; however, recent data suggest that cognitive and behavioral sequelae may occur in patients with this diagnosis (27). These findings underscore the current need for developing universally accepted criteria for identifying OSA in all of its forms.

Upper airway resistance syndrome is a more recently described abnormal sleep pattern in which significant intrathoracic negative pressure during inspiration leads to electroencephalographic arousals and sleep fragmentation (10). There is usually no significant decrease in airflow or O_2 saturation. Biphasic abdominal respiratory pattern, paradoxical breathing with paradoxical ribcage movement, and snoring are usually seen with UARS. A definitive diagnosis can be made through esophageal pressure manometry, though standard PSG may fail to reveal the severity of the problem. Treatment is as beneficial for patients with UARS as for those with more classically defined OSAS.

In OSAS, periods of hypoxia associated with frequent bouts of partial or complete upper airway obstruction are noted throughout the night. Obstructions in children are usually more common in REM sleep than non-REM sleep due to the fact that muscle tone reaches a nadir during this stage. PSG plays an important role in the evaluation of select pediatric patients with OSA. Indications for PSG will be discussed later in this chapter. A directed history and physical are effective in identifying most pediatric patients with OSA who will benefit from treatment, although severity of disease correlates poorly with clinical parameters. Chronic mouth breathing, loud snoring, and frequent repositioning during sleep in association with adenotonsillar hypertrophy are hallmark findings in most affected children.

The clinical consequences of OSAS are myriad. Recent literature continues to define the importance of SDB on medical and behavioral abnormalities in children. OSAS is associated with snoring and difficult breathing to the point where the parents are afraid. Patients have restless sleep and frequent nocturnal arousals. While almost all children with OSAS snore and most snore loudly, this is not universal. Children with partial airway obstruction may have significant disruption of sleep and hypoxia with fairly minimal noise. This tends to be more common in very young children and those with marked tonsil hypertrophy. Snoring is usually exacerbated by upper respiratory tract infections, allergies, or other causes of nasal obstruction. Snoring may also be worsened by acute bouts of tonsillitis, upper airway infections, and mononucleosis. While snoring is an important indicator of the need to evaluate for OSA, the absence of snoring in patients with compelling physical findings should not preclude further evaluation. Nocturnal enuresis has also been linked to OSA (28). Children are often difficult to arouse in the morning and morning headaches may occur.

Daytime behavior may be significantly affected by OSAS (8,29–31). Children with significant OSAS have been documented as having true daytime sleepiness, in some cases, hyperactivity, inattention, and aggressive behavior.

Emotional problems, impairment of school performance, and decreased intellectual performance have been documented in some small studies. Growth hormone release may be impaired by OSA, causing somatic growth abnormalities. This is a fairly common feature of advanced OSA (32). Sleep apnea may be associated with either markedly underweight or overweight children. Failure to thrive, though infrequently observed, is more likely to affect infants and young children with OSA.

A comprehensive head and neck examination should be performed in all children with the potential for OSA. Evaluation of the nose for the size of the nasal passageways, septal deformity, turbinate hypertrophy, anatomic obstruction or evidence of rhinorrhea pathologic exudates, sinus infection, or polyps is important. Examination of the mouth should include assessment of the tonsil size (1+, small to 4+, nearly touching), size of the uvula, tonsil pillars, tongue base, oropharyngeal, and palatal shape and size. The tongue should be depressed to visualize the inferior poles of the tonsils. Facial structure is important. Adenoid faces characterized by a long narrow facial structure are often seen in children with OSAS. Midface hypoplasia and retrognathia can be detected (Table 2). Evaluation of the neck to rule out obstructive masses or deviation of the airway is necessary. Evaluation of the patient for stertor (nasopharynx, oropharynx, and hypopharynx), stridor (cartilaginous airway), or evidence of other

Table 2   Predisposing Factors for Childhood Obstructive Sleep Apnea Syndrome

Nasal obstruction	Laryngeal obstruction
Allergic/nonallergic rhinitis	Laryngeal papilloma/other tumors
Foreign body	Laryngeal web
Polyps	Subglottic stenosis
Adenoid hypertrophy	Laryngomalacia
Pharyngeal flap surgery	Laryngeal hemangioma
Sinusitis	Vocal cord paralysis
Septal deviation	Previous airway surgery/scar/stenosis
Nasal stenosis/hypoplasia	Irritative/social
Choanal atresia	Cigarette smoke exposure
Pyriform aperture stenosis	Pollution
Oropharyngeal obstruction	Increased indoor allergen load
Tonsil hypertrophy	Sleep deprivation
Lingual tonsil hypertrophy	Pharmacologic
Cleft palate repair	Sedation (chloral hydrate/morphine)
Obesity (increased fat/soft tissue)	Anesthesia
Macroglossia	Antihistamines (sedating)
Micrognathia	
Retrognathia	
Short neck	
Tissue infiltration	
Sarcoidosis of the tonsils/adenoids	

Table 3 Syndromes/Diseases Associated with Obstructive Sleep Apnea Syndrome in Children

Achondroplasia	Arthrogyposis multiplex congenital
Apert's syndrome	Beckwith-Wiedemann syndrome
Conradi–Hunermann syndrome	Crouzon syndrome
Down's syndrome	Fragile X syndrome
Goldenhar sequence	Hemifacial microsomia
Hallermann–Streiff syndrome	Hurler's syndrome
Hunter's syndrome	Kleeblattschadel deformity
Klippel–Feil syndrome	Marfan syndrome
Larsen's syndrome	Mucolipidosis
Prader–Willi syndrome	Pfeiffer's syndrome
Pierre Robin Sequence	Rubinstein-Taybi syndrome
Stickler syndrome	Shy–Drager syndrome
Riley–Day syndrome	6q deletion syndrome
Treacher Collins syndrome	Velocardiofacial (Shprintzen's) syndrome
Cerebral palsy	Arnold–Chiari malformation
Hydrocephalus	Hypothyroidism
Meningomyelocele	Myotonic dystrophy
Laryngeal neurofibroma	Sickle cell disease
Morbid obesity	Syringobulbia/myelia
Lymphoproliferative disorders	Gastroesophageal reflux
Vascular rings	Goiter
Hypotonia	Temperomandibular dysfunction
Fetal hydantoin syndrome	Fetal alcohol syndrome
Polio	Head injury

pulmonary disease is also important. OSA is noted with increased frequency in children with a variety of syndromes (Table 3).

DIAGNOSIS

Polysomnogram parameters in normal children have been defined by both Carol Marcus and Nadav Traeger (33,34) (Table 4). Normal children do not have any significant evidence of OSA. Obstructive hypopneas are infrequent. Desaturations, hypercarbia, and nocturnal arousals are also quite infrequent in normal children.

Abnormal PSG criteria for pediatric patients remain poorly defined and are debated in the literature. An obstructive apnea or hypopnea can be defined by duration in seconds or by the number of breath cycles involved (35). Typically, a duration of more than 10 seconds in older children or more than 6 seconds or 1.5 to 2 breaths for younger children is appropriate. An apnea/hypopnea index of more than five has been considered abnormal in the past (Table 5). It is now recognized that lower indices associated with arousals and sleep

Table 4 Pediatric Normative Sleep Data

No obstruction >10 sec		
Central apnea index	0.08	0.0–6.0
Obstructive apnea index	0.01	0.0–0.1
Obstructive hypopnea index	0.3	0.0–3.4
Respiratory disturbance index	0.1–0.4	0.0–4.0
Baseline O_2	97	95–98
Minimum O_2 saturation	92–96%	81–95%
Maximal change in saturation	$4 \pm 2\%$	
$CO_2 >55$ mmHg	0.5% sleep time	
PLM index	1.3	0.0–9.5

Abbreviation: PLM, periodic limb movement.
Source: Adapted from Refs. 33, 34.

fragmentation have important daytime consequences (36). Obstructive events are more common during REM sleep. An elevated number of obstructive events during REM sleep or REM index greater than five is associated with daytime sequelae of OSA. An arousal index of more than 12 or evidence of frequent stage shifts during sleep are also correlated with a positive outcome after the intervention for OSA in our lab. Frequent desaturations less than 90%, a baseline below 94%, or persistent hypercarbia are measures of inadequate ventilation, which may be related to obstruction or primary pulmonary disease. Dysfunctional sleep architecture and frequent arousals in children impair sleep quality and increase the degree of daytime dysfunction. Both obstructive and nonobstructive events disrupt normal sleep architecture (37,38). Debate continues on the relevance of these parameters in terms of pediatric symptoms. Further discussion is available in Chapter 12.

The gold standard for diagnosing sleep apnea syndrome in children remains overnight PSG (14). PSG is the best test for quantifying the degree of obstructive events in children with presumed OSA. Overnight PSG can help identify the degree of risk of the patient's disease and provide information to assist in

Table 5 Abnormal Values on Pediatric Polysomnography

AI > 1
AHI > 5 (REM index > 5)
CO_2 50 mmHg $> 10\%$ sleep time
CO_2 45 mmHg $> 60\%$ sleep time
Minimum O_2 saturation $< 92\%$ (95%)
Elevated arousal index > 15
Increased sleep stage shifts

Abbreviations: AI, apnea index; REM, rapid eye movement; AHI, apnea hypopnea index.

management. Common treatment modalities include oxygen, continuous positive airway pressure (CPAP), bi-level positive airway pressure (BiPAP), and surgical intervention. Perioperative risk can also be estimated by PSG (14).

In our sleep center, not all children undergo PSG. Those with obstructive symptoms, daytime symptoms, and compelling physical findings such as 3 to 4+ tonsils or nearly obstructing adenoids undergo surgical management as primary treatment without documentation of disease by PSG. The benefit of surgery in clinically diagnosed patients has recently been documented (39). PSG is recommended in situations in which this data is likely to help with medical management. Liberal use of PSG is recommended for patients with serious underlying medical conditions such as severe asthma, cerebral palsy, or other neuromuscular diseases. PSG is also recommended before intervention for most children of less than two years; for those with craniofacial syndromes such as Down's syndrome; those in which nonsurgical therapy is likely to be indicated; and borderline cases in which the presence or severity of OSA is unclear. Alternative studies are often used to diagnose OSAS. Simple overnight pulse oximetry, if abnormal, suggests obstructive sleep-disordered breathing, which may warrant further intervention or diagnosis. Limited and nonattended sleep studies can be performed in a hospital ward or in an outpatient setting. Most limited sleep studies include at least four channels for recording, including heart rate, respiratory rate, airflow, and oxy-hemoglobin saturation. Nonmonitored studies may be difficult to score because of the lack of EEG staging. Sleep audio/video tapes seem to correlate well with presence of OSA, and can provide the ability to document trends in the degree of snoring and obstruction in children on an outpatient basis. Obtaining a short segment of sleep videotape is recommended frequently in our sleep clinic. The role of these diagnostic modalities will be further discussed in Chapter 6.

Radiographs, including a lateral neck film, can be helpful in evaluating adenoid size. Cine magnetic resonance imaging and CT scans have been recommended to document the site of obstruction in patients with difficult-to-manage OSAS.

Treatment will be addressed in detail in other chapters in this book. The majority of children with OSA have a very favorable response to tonsillectomy and adenoidectomy (40). Other airway surgery, which may be recommended, includes uvulopalatopharyngoplasty, septoplasty, hyoid advancement/expansion, tongue reduction, tongue suspension, lingual tonsillectomy, genioglossoplasty, maxillo-mandibular advancement, and tracheostomy (41). All of these procedures have been described in children and have various benefits depending upon the specific pathology and degree of OSA. Recent research emphasis has been on decreasing postoperative morbidity through improved surgical techniques and expanding the surgical options available for patients that have failed conventional treatment. Nonsurgical management includes weight loss in obese patients; management of allergic or nonallergic rhinosinusitis with intranasal steroids, antihistamines and decongestants; antibiotics for the treatment of acute tonsillitis; and systemic steroids for acute adenotonsillitis related to Epstein–Barr virus. Low-flow oxygen not only helps maintain oxygenation but actually stents the airway open in young children with mild obstructive breathing. CPAP and BiPAP can be used in children of any age. These modalities are recommended if a surgical option is not available, tracheotomy is not desired, and the patient tolerates the intervention. Patients with chronic lung disease and neuromuscular disease are more likely to benefit from noninvasive ventilation by CPAP or BiPAP. Optimal methods of delivering and titrating positive pressure are being investigated.

A variety of high-risk cases will be addressed in Chapter 7. Children with Down's syndrome have a very high probability of developing OSA. Even asymptomatic patients may have obstructive sleep apnea. Recent data suggest that a screening PSG should be performed on all children with Down's syndrome at the age of three or four (42). Children with cerebral palsy or other neuromuscular diseases are quite likely to have severe OSA with relatively poor tongue tone (43). Sleep studies are recommended in these children because of the increased risk of surgical management. Craniofacial abnormalities such as Robin Sequence, Crouzon syndrome, and Treacher Collins syndrome have a high probability of developing OSA. Because of the abnormalities of facial bone structure, pharyngeal surgery is less likely to be effective. Craniofacial skeletal surgery, tracheotomy, CPAP, or BiPAP need to be considered in these patients.

Fortunately, outcome of OSA remains excellent in children. Over 90% of children undergoing tonsillectomy and adenoidectomy for OSA will have a favorable outcome. Resolution of snoring and improvement in daytime behavior and cognition, normal arousability, and the absence of morning headaches are common postoperative improvements. A positive outcome is documented not only by PSG but by multiple quality-of-life trials (44–46). Long-term outcome seems to be quite favorable for most children with OSA.

NARCOLEPSY

Excessive daytime sleepiness may be caused by problems other than OSA. Increasingly, narcolepsy is diagnosed in children. Patients as young as seven to eight years of age are being identified. Narcolepsy is caused by a deficiency of hypocretin. It usually presents as excessive daytime sleepiness in children, but may not have the typical tetrad of cataplexy, hypnogogic hallucinations, and sleep paralysis that is characteristic in adults (47,48). Children rarely present with a primary complaint of cataplexy or sleep paralysis. Some degree of sleep disturbance including restlessness is more common. Children may snore, but OSA is not necessarily present. OSAS needs to be ruled out by PSG. Often a family history of narcolepsy or excessive daytime sleepiness is present. Narcolepsy has a strong inherited component related to HLA-DR15 (DR2). In children with excessive daytime sleepiness that cannot be explained by obstructive apnea or poor sleep hygiene, overnight PSG as well as a mean latency sleep test (MSLT) should be obtained (49). If the PSG is normal, patients undergo an MSLT, in which they are allowed to take four or five 20-minute naps. A diagnosis of narcolepsy is made when patients fall asleep quickly (mean sleep latency of under five minutes) and have sleep onset REM on at least two of the five naps (50). An increasing number of children are now diagnosed with narcolepsy. This trend is likely related to the easy access to pediatric sleep labs and the availability of genetic testing (51). The patients who fall asleep quickly but do not have sleep onset REM may have idiopathic hypersomnia, a mild form of daytime sleepiness, which may not be associated with cataplexy and hypnogogic hallucinations.

Once diagnosed, narcolepsy treatment includes medical, behavioral, and social management. Patients benefit from a consistent night sleep but may also benefit from daytime naps. These naps can oftentimes be worked into school schedules at lunchtime or during break times. The addition of stimulants has markedly improved the quality of life for many patients with narcolepsy (52). In the past, amphetamines and other stimulants were used as first-line treatment. More recently, Modafinil has been approved for the treatment of narcolepsy. It is effective and has minimal risk of side effects or abuse (53). Modafinil, starting at 200 mg going up to 400 mg per day, provides adequate palliation for most children with narcolepsy (54). The addition of other medications is appropriate in patients with more severe symptoms. Unfortunately, no cure for narcolepsy exists. New data suggest additional treatment options, including the use of auto-immune treatment or the stimulation of hypocretin-producing cells that may have a positive effect. Replacement of hypocretin-producing cells by transplantation is a future possibility (55). Narcolepsy and other disorders of excessive daytime sleepiness will be further discussed in Chapter 20.

PARASOMNIAS

Parasomnias include nightmares, night terrors, sleep-walking, and other manifestations of abnormal sleep. Nightmares and night terrors have been described in medical and lay literature for centuries, and interpreted in many different manners. Religious, spiritual, and psychological significance has been ascribed to them. Nearly 15% of children have parasomnias (56). They are more common in 9- to 10-year-old boys and are associated with other medical and behavioral problems. Nightmares are very common in children, but occur throughout life and may be reactive sleep states due to daytime anxiety, stress, and inadequate sleep, among a variety of other causes (57). They occur throughout the night and are associated with arousal and a recall of the nightmare. Night terrors classically occur during Stage 4 sleep and therefore shortly after sleep onset. They are associated with the sudden onset of screaming, agitation, and a terrified look. They are not typically associated with arousals; in fact, patients may be difficult to arouse from sleep. The events may last a few minutes up to 15 to 20 minutes. In contrast to nightmares, when patients are aroused, they have no recall of the night terror. Classically, they have an onset at two to three years of age and may last for several years. Fortunately, night terrors typically resolve as patients grow and mature. Precipitating factors include sleep deprivation, fever, psychological distress, and seizures. Recent data suggest that parasomnias may be triggered by OSAS, even mild snoring (58). An appropriately utilized PSG plays an important role in documenting OSAS in children with parasomnias. If OSAS is present, treatment and resolution of the obstructive component of SDB may dramatically improve the parasomnia.

Nightmares are best addressed by reducing daytime stressors. A comfortable sleep environment, adequate sleep, and a routine sleep pattern are helpful. As described previously, night terrors may be treated by a variety of means. If they are infrequent, simple safety precautions are appropriate. Making sure that children cannot endanger themselves or others during an event is very appropriate. In children who have frequent and severe night terrors occurring more than two to three times per week, anticipatory arousals can be implemented. Waking up the children 1.5 to 2 hours after bedtime, shortly before the anticipated night terror, on a regular basis for two weeks can break the cycle of night terrors. Many children with frequent events do well with sedative medications, which decrease the frequency of night terrors (59). Clonazepam at a dose of .01 to .03 mg/kg q h.s. is very effective for suppressing night terrors. Clonazepam can be used at increasing doses until the night terrors are suppressed. Medication is usually continued for six months to a year or more. Occasional withdrawal of medication is done to determine if the events have resolved. Rarely, other medications are required for parasomnias.

DISORDERS OF SLEEP ONSET

Similar to adults, disorders of sleep onset and sleep maintenance are quite common in children (60). Disorders of sleep onset can be categorized into sleep association disorders and limit-setting sleep disorder. In sleep onset association, the child learns to fall asleep only under certain circumstances such as in mom's lap, while feeding, or while rocking. Children expect similar circumstances every time they go to sleep. During arousals at night when parents are not available, children cry out, which creates significant frustration in the family. This is somewhat more common in children who have other medical problems such as frequent ear infections, wheezing, or other difficulties. Treatment involves withdrawal of parental assistance or other undesirable associations at bedtime. Introduction of an appropriate sleep association item or transitional items such as a blanket or a stuffed animal is helpful in most cases. Positive reinforcement for remaining in bed is very important. Advocates of both gradual versus sudden withdrawal of associated sleep items exist. Parental consistency is very important in re-establishing independent sleep.

Limit-setting sleep disorders usually occur in older children. They occur most commonly during preschool when parents have not established a routine bedtime. These disorders associated with difficulty falling asleep or bedtime resistance. They are frequently exacerbated by the child's oppositional behavior. Treatment includes prescribed and consistent bedtimes with parent attention directed toward bedtime routine. Consistent bedtime routine and positive reinforcement for good behavior are very important.

Practices contributing to healthy sleep hygiene include consistent bedtime routines and wake-up times. It is important to avoid caffeine, and children should not be sent to bed hungry. Daily exercise and outside time are important. The bedroom should be quiet and dark and the environment comfortable. Televisions in the bedroom are not recommended. The bed should not be used for behavioral modification during the daytime.

Older children and teenagers can develop circadian rhythm disturbances such as delayed sleep phase. Most teenagers have difficulty settling in the evening. If allowed to, they may stay up well into the night. This causes marked problems related to insufficient sleep and difficulty waking up in the morning. Patients with delayed sleep phase are best treated by appropriate limit-setting and consistency in bedtime routine. Good sleep hygiene measures as described earlier remain very important in routine sleep. See Chapter 18 for a further discussion of adolescent sleep disorders.

Acute Life-Threatening Event and Sudden Infant Death Syndrome

ALTE and SIDS remain poorly defined and are potentially fatal disorders of infant sleep (61). Infants and children frequently have immature respiratory control and are prone to develop apnea from relatively minor insults. Eighty-five percent of SIDS cases occur in children between two and four months of age and 95% in infants before six months of age. SIDS virtually always occurs between midnight and 9:00 a.m., and the risk increases with birth order. Males are somewhat more predisposed than females, and in the United States the incidence is higher among African Americans and native Americans. Though SIDS remains an unexplained death, certain factors have a positive correlation with risk. These are listed in Table 6.

Though the pathologic mechanism of SIDS is not known, a variety of causes have been proposed. Hypoxia may occur because of children's immature respiratory control. This may be a more important issue in the prone sleeping position. Presumably, re-breathing of CO_2 with resulting CO_2 narcosis or respiratory obstruction due to mandibular and tongue retrodisplacement contribute to the disorder. Nasal or oral obstruction against an object and other causes have been implicated. Prevention of SIDS should be addressed with all newborn families. The most important precaution seems to be bedding arrangements. A child should sleep in a warm, but not hot room with adequate ventilation. Patients should have safe bedding with minimal covers and certainly no heavy blankets. Cribs which meet safety standards are readily available and should be used. Comforters, pillows, beanbag cushions, and other potentially obstructing

Table 6   Sudden Infant Death Syndrome Risk Factors

Infant
  Prematurity <37 wk and < 2500 gm
  Apgar scores utes <6 at 5 min
  Intensive neonatal care requirement
  Neonatal respiratory abnormalities
  Bronchopulmonary dysplasia
  Anemia
  Twins
  Previous ALTE
  Sibling with SIDS
Maternal
  Anemia
  Smoking
  Alcohol and drug abuse
  Maternal age < 20 yr
Other
  Prone sleeping position
  Soft bedding
  Race
  Ethnicity
  Socioeconomic status
  Cultural influences
  Lack of breast feeding

Abbreviations: ALTE, acute life-threatening event; SIDS, sudden infant death syndrome.

objects should be avoided in the bed. It is recommended that babies be breastfed as long as possible. Mothers should avoid alcohol, tobacco, or drugs during pregnancy and breastfeeding. Smoking should be strictly prohibited in the house. Supine position (on the back to sleep) seems to be associated with an improved outcome in the United States, although the importance of the campaign remains under debate (62). Further information on this topic will be discussed in Chapter 17.

SUMMARY

In summary, infant and pediatric sleep disorders are extremely prevalent. Data suggest that sleep disorders are infrequently addressed by pediatricians and family physicians. When sleep disorders are brought to the attention of medical personnel by families, they may not be diagnosed or treated appropriately. Increased knowledge and understanding of sleep disorders and effective treatment options for affected children are vital. The discipline of sleep medicine is expanding to meet this goal.

All practitioners should be willing and ready to discuss sleep disorders with their patients and families. Simple and leading questions regarding the quality of sleep, troubles with sleep onset or maintenance, problems with daytime sleepiness or behavioral problems may suggest that further and more detailed investigation is appropriate. Sleep labs and specific sleep disorder centers are available in most regions to address problems more difficult to manage. PSG is becoming increasingly available. The development of standardized diagnosis and treatment parameters for pediatric OSAS, UARS, and other sleep diseases are important for data interpretation and for consistent treatment application. Advances in pediatric sleep medicine should allow all children to have a good night's sleep.

REFERENCES

1. Thorpy M. History of sleep and man. In: Thorpy M, Yager J, eds. The Encyclopedia of Sleep and Sleep Disorders. New York: Facts on File, 1991.
2. Kryger M. Sleep apnea: from the needles of Dionysius to continuous positive airway pressure. Arch Intern Med 1983; 143:2301–2308.
3. Aserinski E, Kleitman N. Two types of ocular motility occurring in sleep. J Appl Physiol 1955; 8:11–18.
4. Aserinski E, Kleitman N. Regularly occurring periods of eye motility, and concomitant phenomena, during sleep. Science 1953; 118:273–274.
5. Dement WC, Kleitman N. Cyclic variations in EEG during sleep and their relation to eye movements, body motility, and dreaming. Electroencephalogr Clin Neurophysiol 1957; 9:673–690.
6. Gestaut H, Tesinauri C, Deron B. Etude Polygraphique des manifestations épisodiques (hypniques et respiratoires) du syndrome de Pickwick. Rev Neurol 1965; 112:568–579.
7. Jung R, Kuhlo W. Neurophysiological studies of abnormal night sleep and the Pickwickian syndrome. Prog Brain Res 1965; 18:140–159.
8. Ali NJ, Pitson D, Stradling JR. Natural history of snoring and related behaviour problems between the ages of 4 and 7 years. Arch Dis Child 1994; 71:74–76.
9. Guilleminault C, Korobkin R, Winkle R. A review of 50 children with obstructive sleep apnea syndrome. Lung 1981; 159:275–287.
10. Guilleminault C, Winkle R, Korobkin R, Simmons B. Children and nocturnal snoring: evaluation of the effects of sleep related respiratory resistive load and daytime functioning. Eur J Pediatr 1982; 139:165–171.
11. Stradling JR, Thomas G, Warley AR, Williams P, Freeland A. Effect of adenotonsillectomy on nocturnal hypoxaemia, sleep disturbance, and symptoms in snoring children. Lancet 1990; 335:249–253.
12. Weissbluth M, Davis AT, Poncher J, Reiff J. Signs of airway obstruction during sleep and behavioral, developmental, and academic problems. J Dev Behav Pediatr 1983; 4:119–121.
13. Gozal D. Sleep-disordered breathing and school performance in children. Pediatrics 1998; 102:616–620.
14. Clinical practice guideline: diagnosis and management of childhood obstructive sleep apnea syndrome. Pediatrics 2002; 109:704–712.

15. Wiet GJ, Bower C, Seibert R, Griebel M. Surgical correction of obstructive sleep apnea in the complicated pediatric patient documented by polysomnography. Int J Pediatr Otorhinolaryngol 1997; 41:133–143.

16. Guilleminault C, Li KK. Maxillomandibular expansion for the treatment of sleep-disordered breathing: preliminary result. Laryngoscope 2004; 114:893–896.

17. Denny AD, Talisman R, Hanson PR, Recinos RF. Mandibular distraction osteogenesis in very young patients to correct airway obstruction. Plast Reconstr Surg 2001; 108:302–311.

18. American Thoracic Society. Standards and indications for cardiopulmonary sleep studies in children. Am J Respir Crit Care Med 1996; 153:866–878.

19. Dickens C. The Posthumous Papers of the Pickwick Club. London: Chapman & Hall; 1836.

20. Osler W. Chronic tonsillitis. In: Osler W, ed. The Principles and Practice of Medicine. New York: Appleton and Co., 1892:335–339.

21. Noonan J. Reversible cor pulmonale due to hypertrophied tonsils and adenoids: studies in two cases. Circulation 1965; 32:164.

22. Guilleminault C, Eldridge FL, Simmons FB, Dement WC. Sleep apnea in eight children. Pediatrics 1976; 58:23–30.

23. Gislason T, Benediktsdottir B. Snoring, apneic episodes, and nocturnal hypoxemia among children 6 months to 6 years old: an epidemiologic study of lower limit of prevalence. Chest 1995; 107:963–966.

24. Leach J, Olson J, Hermann J, Manning S. Polysomnographic and clinical findings in children with obstructive sleep apnea. Arch Otolaryngol Head Neck Surg 1992; 118:741–744.

25. Loughlin GM. Obstructive sleep apnea in children. Adv Pediatr 1992; 39:307–336.

26. Richards W, Ferdman RM. Prolonged morbidity due to delays in the diagnosis and treatment of obstructive sleep apnea in children. Clin Pediatr (Phila) 2000; 39:103–108.

27. Chng SY, Goh DY, Wang XS, Tan TN, Ong NB. Snoring and atopic disease: a strong association. Pediatr Pulmonol 2004; 38:210–216.

28. Brooks LJ, Topol HI. Enuresis in children with sleep apnea. J Pediatr 2003; 142:515–518.

29. Ali NJ, Pitson DJ, Stradling JR. Snoring, sleep disturbance, and behaviour in 4–5 year olds. Arch Dis Child 1993; 68:360–366.

30. Ali NJ, Pitson D, Stradling JR. Sleep-disordered breathing: effects of adenotonsillectomy on behaviour and psychological functioning. Eur J Pediatr 1996; 155:56–62.

31. Chervin RD, Archbold KH, Dillon JE, et al. Inattention, hyperactivity, and symptoms of sleep-disordered breathing. Pediatrics 2002; 109:449–456.

32. Nieminen P, Lopponen T, Tolonen U, Lanning P, Knip M, Lopponen H. Growth and biochemical markers of growth in children with snoring and obstructive sleep apnea. Pediatrics 2002; 109:e55.

33. Marcus CL, Omlin KJ, Basinki DJ, et al. Normal polysomnographic values for children and adolescents. Am Rev Respir Dis 1992; 146:1235–1239.

34. Traeger N, Schultz B, Pollock AN, Mason T, Marcus CL, Arens R. Polysomnographic values in children 2–9 years old: additional data and review of the literature. Pediatr Pulmonol 2005; 40:22–30.

35. American thoracic society. Standards and indications for cardiopulmonary sleep studies in children. Am J Respir Crit Care Med 1996; 153:866–878.

36. Bao G, Guilleminault C. Upper airway resistance syndrome—one decade later. Curr Opin Pulm Med 2004; 10:461–467.
37. Tauman R, O'Brien LM, Holbrook CR, Gozal D. Sleep pressure score: a new index of sleep disruption in snoring children. Sleep 2004; 27:274–278.
38. O'Brien LM, Tauman R, Gozal D. Sleep pressure correlates of cognitive and behavioral morbidity in snoring children. Sleep 2004; 27:279–282.
39. Goldstein NA, Pugazhendhi V, Rao SM, et al. Clinical assessment of pediatric obstructive sleep apnea. Pediatrics 2004; 114:33–43.
40. Schechter MS. Technical report: diagnosis and management of childhood obstructive sleep apnea syndrome. Pediatrics 2002; 109:e69.
41. Bower CM, Gungor A. Pediatric obstructive sleep apnea syndrome. Otolaryngol Clin North Am 2000; 33:49–75.
42. De Miguel-Diez J, Villa-Asensi JR, Alvarez-Sala JL. Prevalence of sleep-disordered breathing in children with Down syndrome: polygraphic findings in 108 children. Sleep 2003; 26:1006–1009.
43. Cohen SR, Simms C, Burstein FD, Thomsen J. Alternatives to tracheostomy in infants and children with obstructive sleep apnea. J Pediatr Surg 1999; 34:182–186; discussion 187.
44. Tran KD, Nguyen CD, Weedon J, Goldstein NA. Child behavior and quality of life in pediatric obstructive sleep apnea. Arch Otolaryngol Head Neck Surg 2005; 131:52–57.
45. Crabtree VM, Varni JW, Gozal D. Health-related quality of life and depressive symptoms in children with suspected sleep-disordered breathing. Sleep 2004; 27: 1131-1138.
46. Mitchell RB, Kelly J. Outcome of adenotonsillectomy for severe obstructive sleep apnea in children. Int J Pediatr Otorhinolaryngol 2004; 68:1375–1379.
47. Young D, Zorick F, Wittig R, Roehrs T, Roth T. Narcolepsy in a pediatric population. Am J Dis Child 1988; 142:210–213.
48. Dahl RE, Holttum J, Trubnick L. A clinical picture of child and adolescent narcolepsy. J Am Acad Child Adolesc Psychiatry 1994; 33:834–841.
49. Littner MR, Kushida C, Wise M, et al. Practice parameters for clinical use of the multiple sleep latency test and the maintenance of wakefulness test. Sleep 2005; 28:113–121.
50. Thorpy MJ. The clinical use of the multiple sleep latency test: the standards of practice committee of the American Sleep Disorders Association. Sleep 1992; 15:268–276.
51. Han F, Chen E, Wei H, et al. Childhood narcolepsy in North China. Sleep 2001; 24:321–324.
52. Guilleminault C, Pelayo R. Narcolepsy in children: a practical guide to its diagnosis, treatment and follow-up. Paediatr Drugs 2000; 2:1–9.
53. Banerjee D, Vitiello MV, Grunstein RR. Pharmacotherapy for excessive daytime sleepiness. Sleep Med Rev 2004; 8:339–354.
54. Ivanenko A, Tauman R, Gozal D. Modafinil in the treatment of excessive daytime sleepiness in children. Sleep Med 2003; 4:579–582.
55. Mignot E. A year in review—basic science, narcolepsy, and sleep in neurologic diseases. Sleep 2004; 27:1209–1212.
56. Agargun MY, Cilli AS, Sener S, et al. The prevalence of parasomnias in preadolescent school-aged children: a Turkish sample. Sleep 2004; 27:701–705.

57. Sheldon SH. Parasomnias in childhood. Pediatr Clin North Am 2004; 51:vi, 69–88.
58. Guilleminault C, Palombini L, Pelayo R, Chervin RD. Sleepwalking and sleep terrors in prepubertal children: what triggers them? Pediatrics 2003; 111:e17–e25.
59. Wills L, Garcia J. Parasomnias: epidemiology and management. CNS Drugs 2002; 16:803–810.
60. Hoban TF. Sleep and its disorders in children. Semin Neurol 2004; 24:327–340.
61. Daley KC. Update on sudden infant death syndrome. Curr Opin Pediatr 2004; 16:227–232.
62. Tong EK, England L, Glantz SA. Changing conclusions on secondhand smoke in a sudden infant death syndrome: review funded by the tobacco industry. Pediatrics 2005; 115:e356–e366.

2

Pediatric Obstructive Sleep Apnea

Jonathan Perkins

*Otolaryngology-Head and Neck Surgery, University of Washington and Children's
Hospital and Regional Medical Center, Seattle, Washington, U.S.A.*

CHAPTER HIGHLIGHTS

- Sleep physiology and anatomy in children are significantly different than in adults. The combination of increased upper airway resistance and diminished functional residual capacity combined with the high percentage of rapid eye movement (REM) sleep, during which muscle tone and ventilatory drive diminish, increases the likelihood of sleep-disordered breathing (SDB).
- Sites of obstruction contributing to SDB change with age. Younger children are more dependent on an adequate nasal airway. Older children exhibit more problems with the retropalatal pharyngeal region.
- Adenotonsillectomy is a first line treatment for SDB in children and can be effective in the absence of adenotonsillar hypertrophy. This occurs probably on the basis of creating decreased upper airway collapsibility.

INTRODUCTION

The average child sleeps half of every day, making sleep a major part of childhood. Most respiratory illnesses, such as upper airway obstruction and chronic lung disease, are worse during sleep. Since sleep is such a large part of childhood and it is a time when respiration can be compromised, recognizing SDB is important. SDB is still an often unrecognized condition (1). It is estimated that obstructive sleep apnea (OSA) occurs in 2% to 3% of children (2). Milder forms of SDB are more frequent and occur in up to 10% to 30% of children aged three to six years (3). Despite the frequency of disordered breathing during sleep, many of the consequences of pediatric sleep disorders are unknown.

This chapter will attempt to highlight the underlying physiology of pediatric sleep, the known consequences of SDB, and how these conditions are diagnosed and treated.

PEDIATRIC BREATHING PHYSIOLOGY DURING SLEEP

Increased Upper Airway Resistance

Breathing during sleep is more difficult than when awake. In children, there are several reasons for this (Table 1). Upper airway resistance is increased and functional residual capacity is decreased during sleep (4). A high percentage of pediatric sleep is REM sleep, where muscle tone and ventilatory drive decrease (5). Any structural blockage of the upper airway further increases upper airway resistance, further increasing the work of breathing.

Thoracic Anatomy and Development

Airway structure in children significantly impacts breathing during sleep. In infancy, inward chest movement with inspiration results from chest wall compliance being less than lung compliance. As the child grows older, chest wall compliance decreases and paradoxical chest wall motion diminishes. Intercostal muscle activity is decreased in REM sleep, decreasing chest wall function. Chest wall rib position changes in childhood. During infancy, the ribs are horizontal but develop a more vertical position in childhood and adolescence, allowing greater chest expansion. With greater rib mobility, muscles of respiration have increased mass. The combination of increased chest wall compliance, changing rib position, and minimal respiratory muscle mass, means that in childhood there are multiple thoracic factors that potentially affect ventilatory capacity in sleep.

Upper Airway Anatomy and Development

The upper airway changes dramatically in childhood. In infancy, the larynx is directly behind the soft palate to enable better feeding. Due to this position,

Table 1   Factors that Potentially Alter Breathing in Sleep

General	Thoracic	Upper airway
Increased airway resistance	Chest wall compliance	Lymphoid tissue hyperplasia
Decreased functional capacity	Rib position	Upper airway collapse
Decreased respiratory drive	Respiratory muscle mass	
Decreased muscle tone		

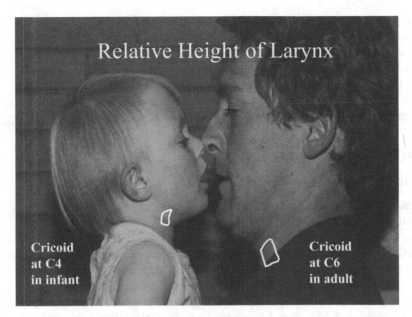

Figure 1 Relative height of a child's larynx compared to an adult. *Source*: Courtesy of Michael Saunders.

any compromise to the nasal airway will result in significant breathing difficulties, especially during sleep. Frequently infants have nasal congestion or nasopharyngeal obstruction, adversely impacting breathing during sleep (6). In older children, the larynx descends in the pharynx, allowing easy air passage in the oropharyngeal and nasal airway (Fig. 1). Analysis of children with SDB shows that after laryngeal descent the retropalatal airway does not enlarge and is a key area of airway narrowing (7,8). From two to eight years of age, pharyngeal lymphoid tissue enlarges (i.e., tonsil, adenoid, or Waldeyer's ring) and is largest in comparison to the airway between three and six years of age (9). This tissue narrows the upper airway and can partially occlude the nasopharyngeal and oropharyngeal airways when the pharyngeal musculature relaxes during sleep (10). Traditionally, it has been thought that during this same period the mandibular–maxillary complex grows at a much slower rate, but abnormal upper airway neuromotor tone is another factor (11).

Upper Airway Collapsibility

While a narrowed upper airway can result from disproportionate growth rates of lymphoid tissue and the mandibular–maxillary complex, evidence suggests that the upper airway is more collapsible in children with OSA compared to children without OSA (12,13). During REM sleep, muscle tone is decreased, decreasing the efficiency of the muscles of respiration and increasing the possibility of upper airway collapse. Compounding decreased muscle tone and increased airway collapsibility are elevated arousal thresholds in sleeping children (14). Unlike adults, where disordered sleep with hypoxemia causes arousal and sleep architecture fragmentation, in children arousal occurs primarily with hypercapnia (15). These factors, a high arousal threshold, increased REM sleep, and frequent upper airway collapse, predispose children to sleep with disordered breathing.

OBSTRUCTIVE SLEEP APNEA

Apnea in Children

Apnea is the cessation of air movement during breathing. In sleep, children frequently have central apnea. This often occurs during REM sleep and is significant if longer than 20 seconds or associated with an age-specific bradycardia (16). Obstructive apnea occurs less commonly. Studies of normal children have shown that obstructive apneas are less than 1/hr [i.e., apnea–hypopnea index (AHI) <1] (17). Recently, Dr Marcus reviewed the raw data from her initial study and reported that the mean AHI was 0.2 ± 0.6. The statistically significant AHI (i.e., mean ± 2 SD) was 1.5 events/hr (18). Obstructive hypopneas, a decrease in airflow during breathing, are fairly frequent during childhood sleep and their effect on ventilation is similar to an obstructive apnea.

Pediatric Sleep-Disordered Breathing (Table 2)

OSA is a type of SDB (19). Central apneas, which frequently occur in normal infants and toddlers, are in the spectrum of SDB. The incidence of central apnea diminishes over time and is less common in adulthood. On the other end of the spectrum is OSA. In between these two extremes are primary snoring and upper airway resistance syndrome (13). Both primary snoring and upper airway resistance syndrome are very common in children due to enlargement of pharyngeal lymphoid tissue (i.e., tonsil and adenoid) and the tendency toward upper airway collapse.

Demographics

SDB can occur throughout childhood. It is most common between two and eight years of age. As has been previously mentioned, the prevalence is estimated at

Table 2   Spectrum of Pediatric Sleep-Disordered Breathing

Central apnea
Primary snoring
Upper airway resistance syndrome
Obstructive sleep apnea

---

approximately 2% of the population. However, these estimates did not include polysomnography (PSG) testing and frequently used adult sleep study criteria to diagnose SDB. At this time, there has not been a demographic study of SDB in children in the United States based in PSG measures. What is known of SDB in children is that there is an equal incidence between sexes and there are distinct differences in sleep apnea by age.

Neonates can have significant airway obstruction from congenital airway anomalies. Most commonly, significant airway problems are associated with craniofacial abnormalities that reduce the size of the mandible and/or maxilla. This commonly occurs in the oropharyngeal airway with Pierre Robin sequence, in which there is a cleft palate, glossoptosis, and retrognathia. The nasal airway can be blocked partially or completely in neonates. This can be from nasal septal deviation, an intranasal mass (i.e., encephalocele), or choanal atresia. Bilateral nasal obstruction in the neonate causes severe airway embarrassment and necessitates urgent airway intervention, because neonates and infants are obligate nasal breathers. Congenital anomalies can also involve the larynx. Most commonly, prolapse of the superior laryngeal structures over the vocal cords (i.e., laryngomalacia) causes inspiratory stridor. Occasionally, the airway is compromised by unilateral or bilateral vocal cord paralysis.

During infancy, airway compromise can occur through both congenital and acquired processes. Partial nasal obstruction from any cause can induce SDB. Nasal inflammation from infection or gastroesophageal reflux is a common cause of mucosal hypertrophy and increased mucous production, resulting in a narrowed nasal airway. A more unusual cause of nasal obstruction is a nasolacrimal duct cyst. The nasopharynx and oropharynx can be narrowed from adenoid or tonsillar hyperplasia or other space-occupying lesion (i.e., macroglossia). The lower airway can be narrowed from congenital and/or acquired subglottic stenosis. External compression of the trachea from vascular structures can also cause significant airway compromise during sleep.

Toddlers and adolescents frequently have OSA. Most commonly, this is due to tonsilloadenoid hypertrophy. However, other factors can contribute to OSA in these age groups. As in younger patients, nasal airway compromise can adversely affect breathing during sleep. Allergic rhinitis often causes turbinate hypertrophy and is associated with OSA. Obesity can also adversely affect sleep quality, as it does in adults.

Etiology of Obstructive Sleep Apnea

Pediatric OSA is related to fixed and dynamic narrowing of the airway in several sites that vary with patient age (11). The most common source of airway narrowing is tonsil and adenoid hypertrophy. Additionally, any craniofacial anomaly, such micrognathia, can narrow the upper airway. Lower airway abnormalities such as laryngomalacia or tracheomalacia also adversely impact airway patency. Rapid air movement through an airway narrowed by any of these conditions induces airway collapse and obstruction. Neuromuscular conditions such as pharyngeal muscular hypotonia and/or muscular incoordination related to cerebral palsy can disturb respiratory function during sleep, through dynamic airway narrowing. In this manner there is compromise of airway patency and/or ventilation. When arousal is deficient, as seen in neurodevelopmentally delayed patients, there can be significant SDB.

Symptoms and Signs of Sleep-Disordered Breathing in Children (Table 3)

The most common symptom of SDB in children is snoring (20). Several reports have shown that parental report of the characteristics of their children's sleep is unreliable, and OSA can be overlooked (21,22). However, most commonly there is a report of increasing loudness of snoring on a nightly basis without evidence of upper respiratory infection or lower airway inflammation. This can be associated with apnea events or struggling to breathe. Often, there is a very restless sleeping pattern as the patient is frequently aroused from sleep due to partial upper airway obstruction. During the daytime, there can be significant changes in behavior and issues related to attention span. On physical examination, the child with SDB may appear healthy and have only enlarged tonsil and adenoid tissue. However, subtle signs of SDB may relate to failure to thrive and delayed growth.

Consequences of Obstructive Sleep Apnea in Childhood

There is a significant association between SDB and problem behaviors in children such as hyperactivity disorder and excessive sleepiness (23–25). Older elementary age children with poor academic performance have a high incidence of SDB (24,26,27). Treatment of the SDB resulted in improvement of academic performance (26). Subsequent work demonstrates an increased risk of daytime sleepiness and problem behaviors associated with SDB in five-year-old children (28). In addition, children with SDB are prone to diastolic hypertension (29). In severe OSA cor pulmonale can occur, though today this is rare (30). Untreated SDB and sleep apnea can result in failure to thrive in infancy and in later

Table 3 Symptoms of Pediatric Sleep-Disordered Breathing

Snoring
Apnea
Restless sleep
Hyperactivity
Tiredness
Poor school performance
Enuresis

childhood, decreased growth (31). Commonly, children have a growth spurt after treatment of OSA. The exact mechanism of diminished growth in children with OSA is unknown, but there is an increase in an insulin-like growth factor following tonsillectomy/adenoidectomy (31,32). The quality of life of children who have SDB and OSA has improved with treatment (33,34). Further evaluation of the consequences of OSA in children is ongoing and will help us understand the indications for appropriate intervention in affected individuals.

Diagnostic and Treatment Options of Obstructive Sleep Apnea in Children (Tables 4 and 5)

Proper diagnostic testing for children having symptoms of SDB is debated (3,35). Frequently, a questionnaire completed by parents is used to analyze the symptoms associated with SDB. This is coupled with a historical evaluation and physical examination and is usually sufficient for determining the diagnosis of SDB. Some centers have used nap sleep studies to assess the severity of the sleep disturbance, but this is not felt to be optimal (36). Full-night PSG has been regarded as the gold standard for diagnosing sleep-disturbed breathing in children, but this is debated, as clinical measures of OSA do not always correlate with PSG measures (3,37). The exact role of PSG in the evaluation of children with SDB is currently being determined.

Adenotonsillectomy is the first-line treatment for SDB in children (16). The efficacy of this procedure is related to the size of tonsil and adenoid tissue and the presence of neuromuscular dysfunction (11). However, even if patients have SDB without tonsillar enlargement, their quality of life and breathing is significantly improved following adenotonsillectomy, even if the postoperative polysomnogram is not normal (34). It is thought that adenotonsillectomy decreases upper airway collapsibility (38). When adenotonsillectomy cannot be performed or has already been performed and there is still significant SDB, supplemental oxygen is frequently given to reduce the hypoxia (39,40). Also, continuous positive airway pressure (CPAP) can be used in children who have evidence of upper airway collapse that is not amenable to surgical intervention. This device is most commonly used in children with neurodevelopmental delays and muscular hypertonia. When nasal airway compromise is present, recognition of the type of nasal pathology and treatment of it is essential and may significantly improve OSA. When CPAP therapy is necessary and the nasal airway is narrow, careful treatment to improve nasal patency will maximize CPAP

Table 4 Diagnosis of Pediatric Sleep-Disordered Breathing

Clinical history
Physical exam
Polysomnography

Table 5   Treatment of Pediatric Sleep-Disordered Breathing

Airway enlargement
Tonsillectomy adenoidectomy
Continuous positive airway pressure
Craniofacial surgery
Bypass upper airway
Tracheotomy

efficacy. There have been reports on using craniofacial surgery to enlarge the upper airway (41,42). In patients with a small mandible, anterior mandibular advancement enlarges the oropharyngeal airway. This is especially effective when the patient has isolated micrognathia (43,44). Mid-face and maxillary advancement have been performed to enlarge the nasopharyngeal airway. This improves the airway patency, but the effect of combined mandibulomaxillary surgery on PSG measures is unknown. The final option for treatment of severe SDB in children is a tracheotomy, which bypasses the compromised upper airway, enabling good ventilation.

REFERENCES

1. Marcus CL. Pediatric sleep medicine comes into its own. Pediatrics 2004; 113(5):1393–1394.
2. Redline S, Tishler PV, Schluchter M, Aylor J, Clark K, Graham G. Risk factors for sleep-disordered breathing in children. Associations with obesity, race, and respiratory problems. Am J Respir Crit Care Med 1999; 159(5 Pt 1): 1527–1532.
3. Carroll JL. Obstructive sleep-disordered breathing in children: new controversies, new directions. Clin Chest Med 2003; 24(2):261–282.
4. Hudgel DW, Devadatta P. Decrease in functional residual capacity during sleep in normal humans. J Appl Physiol 1984; 57(5):1319–1322.
5. Douglas NJ, White DP, Weil JV, et al. Hypoxic ventilatory response decreases during sleep in normal men. Am Rev Respir Dis 1982; 125(3):286–289.
6. Miller MJ, Martin RJ, Carlo WA, Fouke JM, Strohl KP, Fanaroff AA. Oral breathing in newborn infants. J Pediatr 1985; 107(3):465–469.
7. Arens R, McDonough JM, Corbin AM, et al. Upper airway size analysis by magnetic resonance imaging of children with obstructive sleep apnea syndrome. Am J Respir Crit Care Med 2003; 167(1):65–70.
8. Fregosi RF, Quan SF, Kaemingk KL, et al. Sleep-disordered breathing, pharyngeal size and soft tissue anatomy in children. J Appl Physiol 2003; 95(5):2030–2038.
9. Jeans WD, Fernando DC, Maw AR, Leighton BC. A longitudinal study of the growth of the nasopharynx and its contents in normal children. Br J Radiol 1981; 54(638):117–121.
10. Smith PL, Wise RA, Gold AR, Schwartz AR, Permutt S. Upper airway pressure-flow relationships in obstructive sleep apnea. J Appl Physiol 1988; 64(2):789–795.
11. Marcus CL. Pathophysiology of childhood obstructive sleep apnea: current concepts. Respir Physiol 2000; 119(2–3):143–154.

12. Isono S, Shimada A, Utsugi M, Konno A, Nishino T. Comparison of static mechanical properties of the passive pharynx between normal children and children with sleep-disordered breathing. Am J Respir Crit Care Med 1998; 157(4 Pt 1):1204–1212.
13. Gold AR, Marcus CL, Dipalo F, Gold MS. Upper airway collapsibility during sleep in upper airway resistance syndrome. Chest 2002; 121(5):1531–1540.
14. McNamara F, Issa FG, Sullivan CE. Arousal pattern following central and obstructive breathing abnormalities in infants and children. J Appl Physiol 1996; 81(6): 2651–2657.
15. Marcus CL, Lutz J, Carroll JL, Bamford O. Arousal and ventilatory responses during sleep in children with obstructive sleep apnea. J Appl Physiol 1998; 84(6):1926–1936.
16. Marcus CL. Sleep-disordered breathing in children. Am J Respir Crit Care Med 2001; 164(1):16–30.
17. Marcus CL, Omlin KJ, Basinki DJ, et al. Normal polysomnographic values for children and adolescents. Am Rev Respir Dis 1992; 146(5 Pt 1):1235–1239.
18. Witmans MB, Keens TG, Davidson Ward SL, Marcus CL. Obstructive hypopneas in children and adolescents: normal values. Am J Respir Crit Care Med 2003; 168(12):1540.
19. Anstead M, Phillips B. The spectrum of sleep-disordered breathing. Respir Care Clin N Am 1999; 5(3):363–77, viii.
20. Wang RC, Elkins TP, Keech D, Wauquier A, Hubbard D. Accuracy of clinical evaluation in pediatric obstructive sleep apnea. Otolaryngol Head Neck Surg 1998; 118(1):69–73.
21. Suen JS, Arnold JE, Brooks LJ. Adenotonsillectomy for treatment of obstructive sleep apnea in children. Arch Otolaryngol Head Neck Surg 1995; 121(5): 525–530.
22. Carroll JL, McColley SA, Marcus CL, Curtis S, Loughlin GM. Inability of clinical history to distinguish primary snoring from obstructive sleep apnea syndrome in children. Chest 1995; 108(3):610–618.
23. Bass JL, Corwin M, Gozal D, et al. The effect of chronic or intermittent hypoxia on cognition in childhood: a review of the evidence. Pediatrics 2004; 114(3):805–816.
24. O'Brien LM, Holbrook CR, Mervis CB, et al. Sleep and neurobehavioral characteristics of 5- to 7-year-old children with parentally reported symptoms of attention-deficit/hyperactivity disorder. Pediatrics 2003; 111(3):554–563.
25. Chervin RD, Archbold KH, Dillon JE, et al. Inattention, hyperactivity, and symptoms of sleep-disordered breathing. Pediatrics 2002; 109(3):449–456.
26. Gozal D. Sleep-disordered breathing and school performance in children. Pediatrics 1998; 102(3 Pt 1):616–620.
27. Kaemingk KL, Pasvogel AE, Goodwin JL, et al. Learning in children and sleep disordered breathing: findings of the Tucson Children's Assessment of Sleep Apnea (tuCASA) prospective cohort study. J Int Neuropsychol Soc 2003; 9(7):1016–1026.
28. Shin C, Kim J, Lee S, Ahn Y, Joo S. Sleep habits, excessive daytime sleepiness and school performance in high school students. Psychiat Clin Neurosci 2003; 57(4):451–453.
29. Marcus CL, Greene MG, Carroll JL. Blood pressure in children with obstructive sleep apnea. Am J Respir Crit Care Med 1998; 157(4 Pt 1):1098–1103.
30. Brouillette RT, Fernbach SK, Hunt CE. Obstructive sleep apnea in infants and children. J Pediatr 1982; 100(1):31–40.

31. Marcus CL, Carroll JL, Koerner CB, Hamer A, Lutz J, Loughlin GM. Determinants of growth in children with the obstructive sleep apnea syndrome. J Pediatr 1994; 125(4):556–562.

32. Bar A, Tarasiuk A, Segev Y, Phillip M, Tal A. The effect of adenotonsillectomy on serum insulin-like growth factor-I and growth in children with obstructive sleep apnea syndrome. J Pediatr 1999; 135(1):76–80.

33. Goldstein NA, Fatima M, Campbell TF, Rosenfeld RM. Child behavior and quality of life before and after tonsillectomy and adenoidectomy. Arch Otolaryngol Head Neck Surg 2002; 128(7):770–775.

34. Stewart MG, Glaze DG, Friedman EM, Smith EO, Bautista M. Quality of life and sleep study findings after adenotonsillectomy in children with obstructive sleep apnea. Arch Otolaryngol Head Neck Surg 2005; 131(4):308–314.

35. Goldstein NA, Pugazhendhi V, Rao SM, et al. Clinical assessment of pediatric obstructive sleep apnea. Pediatrics 2004; 114(1):33–43.

36. American Thoracic Society. Cardiorespiratory sleep studies in children. Establishment of normative data and polysomnographic predictors of morbidity. Am J Respir Crit Care Med 1999; 160(4):1381–1387.

37. Melendres C, Lutz JM, Rubin ED, Marcus CL. Daytime sleepiness and hyperactivity in children with suspected sleep disordered breathing. Pediatrics 2004; 114:768–775.

38. Marcus CL, Katz ES, Lutz J, Black CA, Galster P, Carson KA. Upper airway dynamic responses in children with the obstructive sleep apnea syndrome. Pediatr Res 2005; 57(1):99–107.

39. McNamara F, Sullivan CE. Treatment of obstructive sleep apnea syndrome in children. Sleep 2000; 23(suppl 4):S142–S146.

40. Palombini L, Pelayo R, Guilleminault C. Efficacy of automated continuous positive airway pressure in children with sleep-related breathing disorders in an attended setting. Pediatrics 2004; 113(5):e412–e417.

41. Cohen SR. Surgical treatment of obstructive sleep apnea in neurologically compromised patients. Plast Reconstr Surg 1997; 99(3):638–646.

42. Cohen SR, Simms C, Burstein FD, Thomsen J. Alternatives to tracheostomy in infants and children with obstructive sleep apnea. J Pediatr Surg 1999; 34(1):182–186; discussion 187.

43. Sidman JD. Distraction osteogenesis of the mandible for airway obstruction in children. Laryngoscope 2001; 111(7):1137–1146.

44. Mandell DL, Yellon RF, Bradley JP, Izadi K, Gordon CB. Mandibular distraction for micrognathia and severe upper airway obstruction. Arch Otolaryngol Head Neck Surg 2004; 130(3):344–348.

3

Nonobstructive Sleep Patterns in Children

Rees L. Lee

Pediatric Pulmonary Medicine, Department of Pediatrics, Naval Medical Center*, Portsmouth, Virginia, U.S.A.

CHAPTER HIGHLIGHTS

- Control of breathing involves the integration of peripheral and central chemoreceptor afferent signals by the respiratory control centers within the medulla and subsequent efferent signals to the respiratory muscles. Periodic breathing and central apnea are manifestations of a disorder in the respiratory control pathways.
- Periodic breathing is common in infants but the prevalence declines rapidly in the first two years of life.
- Central apnea is the simultaneous cessation of airflow and respiratory effort lasting more than 20 seconds or of any duration associated with significant oxygen desaturation or bradycardia. It is an uncommon occurrence at any age and the presence of three or more episodes per hour should be investigated. The differential diagnosis for central apnea is extensive and the workup should be tailored to the particular patient.

---

*The views expressed in this chapter are those of the author and do not reflect the official policy or position of the Department of the Navy, Department of Defense, or the U.S. Government.

- Treatment of central apnea must be individualized for each patient on the basis of the underlying pathology. For example, methylxanthines are effective in the treatment of apnea of prematurity. They have no role in the treatment of congenital central hypoventilation syndrome, a rare disorder for which affected persons usually require some form of mechanical ventilation.

INTRODUCTION

The unconscious drive to breathe is often taken for granted. Most parents put their children to sleep without giving it a second thought. Yet, the survival of their child depends on the complex interactions between sensory afferents, the central nervous system (CNS), and motor efferents to maintain the rhythmic chest movements during sleep. Disruption or disease in any arm of this system will lead to centrally mediated disordered breathing patterns, hypoventilation, apnea, and at the extreme, respiratory failure. This chapter will review the physiologic mechanisms controlling breathing, sleep patterns that result from the dysfunction of these control mechanisms, and disease states in which these patterns can be observed.

CONTROL OF BREATHING

The act of breathing is a complex choreography involving the CNS, peripheral nervous system, and the respiratory muscles. While voluntary breathing is initiated from the cerebral cortex, the automatic breathing during sleep requires the body to first determine the need for a breath on the basis of input from peripheral and central chemoreceptors. The peripheral chemoreceptors lie primarily within the carotid bodies and respond to hypoxia and, to a lesser extent, to hypercapnia/acidosis. The central chemoreceptors appear to be widely distributed within the medulla and lower brain. These central chemoreceptors respond to the acidosis within the cerebrospinal fluid resulting from hypercapnia. Input from both the peripheral and central chemoreceptors feeds into the respiratory centers within the medulla (especially, the nucleus of the solitary tract) and influence the rhythm of the breathing pattern.

Rhythmicity is a key aspect of the respiratory pattern. The source of this rhythm is unknown but an area of the ventral lateral medulla called the pre-Bötzinger complex exhibits bursting qualities, which suggests that it may act as the respiratory pacemaker (1). Output from the medulla is relayed to the respiratory muscles via the phrenic nerve, thoracic intercostal nerves as well as upper airway motor neurons. Finally, chest wall movement is dependent on sufficient muscular strength to contract the diaphragm and accessory respiratory muscles. A disruption at any point within these respiratory control pathways can manifest as a disordered breathing pattern such as periodic breathing or central sleep apnea/hypopnea.

The respiratory control pathways described earlier are underdeveloped in the fetus and neonate. Fetal breathing movements are observed by ultrasound at 11 weeks gestation and play a crucial role in intrauterine lung development. Breathing at this stage appears mediated by the spinal cord as transection of the cord at C1 does not appear to affect these respiratory movements. With advancing gestational age, the pattern of fetal breathing transitions from continuous irregular movements to a characteristic pattern in which there is cessation of breathing during nonrapid eye movement (non-REM) sleep. By the third trimester, the presence of breathing movements only during rapid eye movement (REM) sleep is well entrenched and suggests the development of CNS inhibitory pathways. The factors involved in the transition back to a continuous breathing pattern necessary for extrauterine life have not been fully delineated.

During the fetal period, the predominance of CNS inhibition within the immature respiratory control pathways is manifested by a restricted sensitivity to hypercapnia. A limited hypercapneic response first appears at approximately 24 weeks gestational age and becomes more robust as the fetus approaches term (2). Term babies and adults with a normal hypercapneic response increase the tidal volume and frequency of breaths when exposed to hypercapnia. By contrast, preterm neonates have a blunted CO_2 response and do not show increases in respiratory frequency. Additionally, preterm neonates show a paradoxical depression of respiratory movements in response to hypoxia. Acute hypoxia causes a brief (1–2-minute) ventilatory increase in preterm neonates followed by respiratory depression (3). This depression in ventilation disappears with increased age. The immature responses of the preterm neonatal respiratory control system are partly responsible for the increases in periodic breathing and apnea noted in these patients (4).

SLEEP PATTERNS OF DISORDERED BREATHING CONTROL

Periodic Breathing

Periodic breathing describes an alternating pattern of respirations followed by a respiratory pause (Fig. 1). The criteria for scoring a periodic breathing episode are listed in Table 1. The exact cause of periodic breathing is not completely understood. The hypocapneic alkalosis induced with hyperventilation may decrease the ventilatory drive and result in a period of central apnea. As the pCO_2 rises, respiratory efforts are again seen as another cycle of this "seasaw" pattern of respirations begins. One hypothesis as to the etiology of periodic breathing suggests that enhanced baseline sensitivity of the peripheral arterial chemoreceptors is important. The peripheral chemoreceptors respond to acute hypoxemia and CO_2/pH changes quickly. In preterm infants, the peripheral chemoreceptors show evidence of elevated activity. Because of the the rapid response to changes in O_2 and CO_2 tension, the enhanced sensitivity of these peripheral chemoreceptors makes periodicity in the breathing pattern more

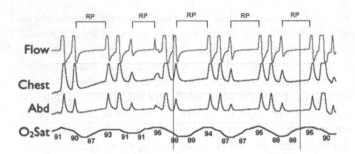

Figure 1 Periodic breathing. A pattern of at least three episodes of respirations followed by a central respiratory pause (RP) is called periodic breathing. In this polysomnogram, the central RPs show the characteristic lack of movement in both the abdominal (Abd) and chest wall leads as well as a lack of air flow. Though not a consistent finding in all patients, the periodic breathing episodes in this patient were associated with oxygen desaturations. Periodic breathing is commonly observed in infants but is less common in older children and adults (see Fig. 2).

likely (5). Similarly, persons who ascend to high altitudes can also show a periodic breathing pattern because of the decrease in O_2 tension and the enhanced peripheral chemoreceptor sensitivity which results. This periodic breathing often disappears as the chemoreceptor set point is reset when the person becomes acclimated. Cheyne–Stokes respirations are a form of periodic breathing usually seen in patients with heart failure and chronic hypoxemia.

A periodic breathing pattern during sleep is common in healthy neonates. At birth, approximately 80% of infants have some occasional periodic breathing averaging no more than two episodes per hour and accounting for no more than 4% of the total sleep time (6). The percentage of children with periodic breathing

Table 1 Polysomnographic Criteria for Periodic Breathing and Central Apnea

---

Periodic breathing
    Child <2 yr: ≥3 episodes of central RPs lasting ≥3 sec interrupted by respirations
        lasting <20 sec
    Child >2 yr: ≥3 episodes of central RPs in which ≥2 breaths are missed interrupted
        by respirations lasting <20 sec
    Consider further evaluation if ≥5% of total sleep time
Central apnea
    Absence of both airflow and respiratory effort lasting ≥20 sec or any duration associated
        with oxygen desaturation ≥4% below baseline or associated with bradycardia
    Consider further evaluation if ≥3 episodes per hr

Abbreviation: RPs, respiratory pauses.
Source: Adapted from Refs. 8, 28.

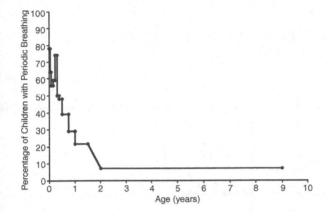

Figure 2 Prevalence of periodic breathing during childhood. The prevalence of periodic breathing during sleep decreases dramatically in the first two years of life. *Source*: Adapted from Refs. 6, 7, 29.

declines with age (Fig. 2). Less than 10% of children over two years old show periodic breathing patterns (7). In children with periodic breathing, an underlying pathologic process including CNS abnormalities should be ruled out if the periodic breathing exceeds 5% of the total sleep time.

Central Sleep Apnea

Central sleep apnea describes the cessation of both airflow and respiratory effort (Fig. 3). For comparison, obstructive sleep apnea (OSA) involves the cessation of airflow with the continuation of respiratory efforts. Central apnea can be scored in a sleep study if the apnea lasts 20 seconds or longer. Alternatively, the absence of both airflow and respiratory effort of any duration can be scored as central apnea if it is associated with an oxygen desaturation equal to or greater than 4% compared to baseline or associated with bradycardia (Table 1) (8).

While central apnea can certainly result from abnormalities of the respiratory centers of the CNS, central apneic and hypopneic events can be seen in normal children as well as being caused by pathologies outside the CNS respiratory centers such as in neuromuscular diseases. Central apneas can be seen in all age groups but the frequency of these events, even in term infants, is low. Most children have well less than one central apneic event per hour (6,7), and three or more events per hour should be considered abnormal and worthy of further investigation.

CLINICAL PRESENTATION

The diagnosis of central apnea and periodic breathing may be difficult based on simply history and physical examination alone. Many infants will show no

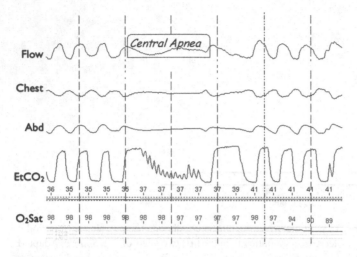

Figure 3   Central apnea. Central apnea is the simultaneous cessation of air flow and respiratory effort. Air flow is measured by a nasal thermistor (Flow) and the absence of flow is characteristic of an apneic event. The lack of abdominal (Abd) and chest movements in this patient demonstrates the absence of respiratory effort and defines the apneic event as central apnea. By contrast, obstructive apnea is characterized by continued respiratory movements without the presence of significant air flow.

symptoms in the doctor's office, though a history of an abnormal respiratory pattern may be provided by the parent. In the preterm child, abnormal respiratory patterns may be observed by the neonatal intensive care unit (NICU) team. Some of these children are initially admitted to the hospital with an acute life-threatening event and it is only during further evaluation that an abnormal sleep pattern is suspected. Older children and adults may complain of daytime hypersomnolence, restless sleep, and nighttime arousals similar to that experienced by persons with OSA (Table 2). Classically, children with central apnea do not

Table 2   Comparison of Signs and Symptoms Observed in Central Apnea and Obstructive Sleep Apnea

Sign or symptom	Central sleep apnea	Obstructive sleep apnea
Duskiness with sleep	Yes	Variable
Daytime sleepiness	Yes	Yes
Restless sleep	Yes	Yes
Snoring	No	Yes
Nocturnal choking	No	Yes
Nocturnal dyspnea	Variable	No
Morning headache	Variable	Variable

snore. However, as both OSA and central apnea can occur in the same child, the presence or absence of snoring is not a completely reliable finding. In the end, if the physician suspects the possibility of a disordered sleep pattern, a sleep study should be ordered.

DISEASES ASSOCIATED WITH ABNORMAL RESPIRATORY CONTROL

Central sleep apnea and periodic breathing are part of the symptom complex of a variety of diseases (Table 3). The evaluation and workup of a child with central apnea should be individualized based on the likely etiologies.

Table 3 Differential Diagnosis of Central Apnea

Normal child
  High-altitude periodic breathing
Congenital
  Apnea of prematurity (often has mixed central and obstructive apnea components)
  Mild alveolar hypoventilation
  CCHS (Ondine's Curse)
  Late-onset central hypoventilation with hypothalamic dysfunction
Congenital CNS anomalies
  Chiari malformation
  Myelomenigocele
  Prader–Willi
  Riley–Day syndrome
  Shy–Drager syndrome
Acquired
  Brainstem, cervical spinal cord, or phrenic nerve trauma
  Infection: encephalitis, cervical transverse myelitis
  Brainstem or cervical spinal cord tumor
  Hydrocephalus
  Brainstem infarct
  Asphyxia
  Drug-induced (long-acting opiates)
Neuromuscular diseases
  Botulism
  Spinal muscular atrophy
  Guillain–Barre syndrome
  Amyotrophic lateral sclerosis
  Poliomyelitis
  Myasthenia gravis
  Muscular dystrophies
  Metabolic disorders (acid maltase deficiency, hypophosphatemia, hypermagnesemia, Leigh's disease, pyruvate dehydrogenase deficiency, carnitine deficiency)

Abbreviations: CCHS, congenital central hypoventilation syndrome; CNS, central nervous system.

High Altitude Periodic Breathing

Taken to a sufficient altitude, everyone will show periodic breathing when they sleep. Most people who ascend from sea level to 4000 m (13,000 ft) will exhibit this pattern, but certain individuals appear predisposed to developing periodic breathing at lower altitudes because of the increased chemoresponsiveness to hypoxia. The hypoxic ventilatory response of these people induces hyperventilation in response to the decreased oxygen tension at high altitude. The body's response to the hyperventilation-induced drop in CO_2 tension is a period of apnea during which the CO_2 level rises. When the CO_2 level exceeds the apnea threshold, the hypoxic ventilatory response again induces hyperventilation and the cycle starts anew. Affected individuals have a disrupted sleep pattern with frequent arousals and restlessness. Periodic breathing in infants brought to altitude may become more pronounced and have greater swings in oxygen saturations (9). There are no specific treatments. Infants born at high-altitude may require a short period on home oxygen therapy to avoid significant desaturations. Older children and adults rarely need oxygen, but a slow ascent will minimize the sleep disruption. The abnormal sleep usually improves as the chemoreceptors reset and the person acclimates to altitude. There is no clear association between high-altitude periodic breathing and other diseases of high altitude such as acute mountain sickness, high-altitude pulmonary edema, or high-altitude cerebral edema (10,11).

Apnea of Prematurity

Preterm children have many respiratory challenges including immaturity of the respiratory control pathways. As described at the beginning of this chapter, preterm neonates show a blunted hypercapneic response and ventilatory depression in the presence of hypoxia. Ultimately, the most significant manifestation of this respiratory control immaturity is apnea.

Symptomatic apnea occurs in 84% of infants less than 1000 g and 25% of those less than 2500 g (11). The apnea pattern is commonly a mixed central and obstructive apnea. While respiratory control immaturity accounts for the majority of infants with apnea, symptomatic apneic episodes require consideration of other etiologies including CNS abnormalities (such as intracranial hemorrhage or brain malformations), bacterial or viral infection, anemia, hypoglycemia, electrolyte imbalances, and sedating medications. The role of gastroesophageal reflux disease (GERD) as a cause of apnea in preterm infants is controversial. GERD may induce apnea via activation of the laryngeal reflex, which is exaggerated in preterm infants. Activation of the laryngeal reflex by chemical irritation can result in prolonged apnea (3). The chemical irritation of the larynx by a GERD episode may be sufficient to induce apnea, but a clear causal relationship between GERD and apnea has yet to be demonstrated in the clinical setting.

Treatment of apnea in preterm children should be first aimed at any underlying causes. In the absence of a defined etiology, continuous positive airway pressure at 5 to 6 cm H_2O or even high-flow nasal cannula therapy may be effective by splinting open the upper airway and preventing the obstructive component of longer apneic episodes. Such therapy may also enhance the oxygenation status by increasing the functional residual capacity (FRC). The onset of oxygen desaturation and bradycardia is delayed in babies with a higher FRC (3). Methylxanthines have been used for years as an effective treatment of apnea of prematurity. A review by the Cochrane Collaboration concluded that infants with recurrent apnea treated with methylxanthines had fewer treatment failures [relative risk (RR) 0.43] and less need for intermittent positive pressure ventilation (RR 0.34) than controls. The most commonly used methylxanthines are theophylline and caffeine. Caffeine has a superior side-effect profile and its use is becoming more common (12).

Congenital Central Hypoventilation Syndrome

Congenital central hypoventilation syndrome (CCHS) is an extremely rare entity in which affected children show severe hypoventilation, particularly during sleep, in the absence of any identifiable neurologic, pulmonary, or cardiac disease process (13,14). Only about 300 cases in the U.S. have been diagnosed but this may be an underestimate. Despite the small numbers, this small cohort of children has provided the opportunity to make great inroads into the understanding of the body's respiratory control pathways. Children with CCHS lack the normal ventilatory response to hypercarbia and hypoxia. During sleep these children can develop severe hypercarbia and hypoxemia. In the wake state, they continue to have absent hypercarbic and hypoxic responses and have a blunted sensation of dyspnea. However, they do maintain conscious control of breathing. Therefore, it is during sleep that children with CCHS are most at risk.

CCHS children typically present shortly after birth with cyanosis upon falling asleep. There is no change in breathing frequency despite the presence of hypoxia and hypercarbia. During quiet sleep there is progressive hypoxia and hypercapnia without significant changes in respiratory rate or effort. This pattern may partially normalize during active sleep.

CCHS is a diagnosis of exclusion and an extensive search for other etiologies must be conducted (Table 4). Primary neuromuscular, cardiac, pulmonary, and metabolic diseases must be thoroughly investigated and ruled out. After ruling out other organic causes and confirming the diagnosis with a sleep study in a pediatric sleep physiology laboratory, the vast majority of children with CCHS require the placement of a tracheostomy to allow mechanical ventilation. Many children, especially infants, require ventilation at least part of the time even when awake. Titrating the ventilator to attain an end tidal CO_2 of 30–35 mmHg and an O_2 saturation $\geq 95\%$ has been recommended. Children who are slightly hyperventilated at night have improved spontaneous ventilation during the day (15). Respiratory stimulants are not effective in treating CCHS. Diaphragm pacing via phrenic nerve stimulation may be an alternative for the older child. Such children may be able to have the tracheostomy removed, but

Table 4 Tests to Consider in Workup of Congenital Central Hypoventilation Syndrome

Chest X-ray and fluoroscopy of the diaphragm
Bronchoscopy
EKG, echocardiogram, and Holter monitoring
Neurology consultation
Muscle biopsy (if myopathy likely)
MRI of brain and brainstem
Urine and serum studies to rule out inborn errors of metabolism, especially carnitine
   deficiency
Ophthalmology evaluation
Rectal biopsy (rule out Hirschsprung's disease)
Polysomnogram (sleep study)
PHOX2b mutation analysis

Abbreviations: EKG, electrocardiogram; MRI, magnetic resonance imaging.

almost half of these patients still require additional ventilatory assistance at night using bi-level positive pressure (BiPAP). For patients requiring only nighttime ventilation, mask BiPAP with close home monitoring may be an alternative to the tracheostomy. In fact, most children can be transitioned to other ventilation modalities and even discontinue mechanical ventilation altogether when awake. In a survey of 196 CCHS patients (aged 0.4–38 years), only 10% required 24-hour ventilation and 39% of the patients had never had a tracheostomy or been decanulated (16).

The exact abnormality resulting in the CCHS phenotype is unknown. Abnormalities in the central chemoreceptors and/or the integration of inputs from the central and peripheral chemoreceptors have been suggested as the cause of the disordered breathing (17). However, CCHS patients often present with comorbid disease processes, which suggest a more generalized disorder of the autonomic nervous system (ANS) possibly caused by deficient neural crest cell migration. Approximately 15–20% of CCHS patients present with Hirschsprung's disease, but other ANS-related abnormalities occurring in some patients include baseline bradycardia with decreased heart rate variability, vasovagal syncope, pupillary abnormalities, altered sweating and temperature regulation, esophageal dysmotility, and constipation (even in the absence of Hirschsprung's disease).

Researchers examining the genetics of CCHS have concentrated on genes involved in the development and regulation of the ANS. The homeobox domain transcription factor *PHOX2b* appears to play a key role in the formation of the ANS pathways, and mutations in this gene have been found in the majority of CCHS patients. In a CCHS cohort from the United States, 65 of 67 patients (97%) had a polyalanine expansion of exon 3 within *PHOX2b* (18). The frequency of this mutation was lower in studies conducted outside the United States, but still accounted for a significant portion of the patients. *PHOX2b* mutation analysis should be considered in the diagnosis of CCHS. Chapter 16 discusses CCHS in greater detail.

Disorders of the Central Nervous System

Integration of central and peripheral chemoreceptor inputs takes place within the medullary respiratory centers of the brainstem. Congenital or acquired abnormalities of the CNS can alter the function of these respiratory centers and result in disordered breathing patterns including central apnea/hypopnea. A study of 14 children with a variety of CNS neoplasms showed that only two (14%) had central apnea on polysomnogram. However, both these children had tumors involving the brainstem medulla (19), reinforcing the importance of this area in respiratory control. It is therefore prudent to obtain a sleep study in any child who presents with a brainstem tumor to investigate for central sleep apnea/hypopnea. Patients with elevated end tidal CO_2 or hypoxia may require nighttime ventilatory support.

Disruption of the normal anatomical relationships within the brainstem can result in disordered respiratory control. This occurs in Chiari malformations, which result from the herniation of cerebellar appendages through the foramen magnum. Two primary types have been described. Type I presents primarily in older children and adults but can occur as young as infancy. In Chiari malformation type I (CM-I), the cerebellar tonsils herniate through the foramen magnum and are often associated with a syrinx (20). While CM-I can be asymptomatic, presenting symptoms classically involve occipital headaches associated with coughing or exertion. These headaches generally last from a few seconds to a few minutes and can radiate down the posterior neck and shoulders. A wide variety of other neurological symptoms can occur including drop attacks, sensory and motor deficits, dysphagia, hoarseness, tinnitus, seizures, nystagmus, and abnormal reflexes (both hypo- and hyper-reflexia). Apneic events have also been described. In a small study of 11 patients with CM-I, three (27%) had apnea as the presenting complaint (21). However, the incidence of central apnea in CM-I patients is likely much higher. Sleep studies conducted in CM-I patients (regardless of presenting symptom) show 72% with apneic or hypopneic events (22). Periodic breathing has also been reported but is not common (23).

Chiari malformation Type II (CM-II) is usually diagnosed shortly after birth, as it is always associated with a myelomeningocele. In CM-II, there is caudal displacement of the cerebellar vermis and brainstem. Hydrocephalus is common and must be treated. The increased intracranial pressure from untreated hydrocephalus may worsen the cerebellar and brainstem herniation of the CM-II lesion. Respiratory complications are common and potentially fatal. Inspiratory stridor requires prompt evaluation for vocal paralysis and manifests as obstructive apnea. Babies with CM-II demonstrate a unique and dramatic form of apnea associated with painful or startling experiences in which the child has a complete cessation of respiratory movements resulting in cyanosis (24). This prolonged expiratory apnea with cyanosis (PEAC) can lead to bradycardia and death. Nonfatal events can be mistaken for prolonged breath-holding spells. Though less common, older children with CM-II present with symptoms similar to CM-I and similar to CM-I can develop syringomyelia.

Children with symptoms suggestive of a Chiari malformation require magnetic resonance imaging (MRI) of the posterior fossa and brainstem. Additional imaging of the spine should be considered to investigate for spinal abnormalities such as syringomyelia. Children with Chiari malformations should be referred to a neurologist or neurosurgeon for management.

In CM-I, the presence of apnea is an absolute indication for surgery, as well as is a history of syncope, the presence of vocal paralysis, or swallowing dysfunction resulting in aspiration (20). In patients without absolute indications for surgery, medical management of headache and other symptoms is often successful. Refractory patients should be referred for surgical intervention. No single surgical approach is used, but most rely on osseous decompression and dural grafting. More aggressive decompression and intradural dissection are performed in patients with a syrinx present (25). Asymptomatic CM-I patients can be managed expectantly. In a survey of members of the Pediatric Section of the American Association of Neurological Surgeons, only 9% performed surgery on asymptomatic patients (26). For patients with CM-II, the presence of a hydrocephalus requires immediate shunting to avoid worsening of the cerebellar herniation, followed by decompression surgery.

The outcome for CM-I is excellent with 80–90% having complete resolution of symptoms or cessation of symptom progression. The outcomes for patients with CM-II are not nearly as good, with up to 15% dying by three years of age and one-third having neurological deficits. Even after surgical intervention, CM-II patients remain at risk for severe apneic events and PEAC is a common cause of death (27).

REFERENCES

1. Feldman J, Mitchell G, Nattie E. Breathing: rhythmicity, plasticity, chemosensitivity. Annu Rev Neurosci 2003; 26:239–266.
2. Connors G, Hunse C, Carmichael L, Natale R, Richardson B. Control of fetal breathing in the human fetus between 24 and 34 weeks gestation. Am J Obstet Gynecol 1989; 160:932–938.
3. Martin R, Abu-Shaweesh J, Baird T. Apnoea of prematurity. Paediatr Respir Rev 2004; 5(suppl A): S377–S382.
4. Abu-Shaweesh J. Maturation of respiratory reflex responses in the fetus and neonate. Semin Neonatol 2004; 9:169–180.
5. Gauda E, McLemore G, Tolosa J, Marston-Nelson J, Kwak D. Maturation of peripheral arterial chemoreceptors in relation to neonatal apnoea. Semin Neonatol 2004; 9:181–194.
6. Kelly D, Stellwagen L, Kaitz E, Shannon D. Apnea and periodic breathing in normal full-term infants during the first twelve months. Pediatr Pulmonol 1985; 1:215–219.

7. Traeger N, Schultz B, Pollock A, Mason T, Marcus C, Arens R. Polysomnographic values in children 2–9 years old: additional data and review of the literature. Pediatr Pulmonol 2005; 40:22–30.
8. American Thoracic Society. Standards and indications for cardiopulmonary sleep studies in children. Am J Respir Crit Care Med 1996; 153:866–878.
9. Parkins K, Poets C, O'Brien L, Stebbens V, Southall D. Effect of exposure to 15% oxygen on breathing patterns and oxygen saturation in infants: interventional study. Br Med J 1998; 316:887–891.
10. West J. The physiologic basis of high-altitude diseases. Ann Intern Med 2004; 141:789–800.
11. Hauri P, Sateia M, eds. International Classification of Sleep Disorders (ICSD-2). Diagnostic and Coding Manual. 2nd edn. Westchester, IL: American Academy of Sleep Medicine, 2005.
12. Steer P, Henderson-Smart D. Caffeine vs theophylline treatment for apnea in preterm infants. In: Cochrane Neonatal Group, ed. The Cochrane Library. Chichester, UK: John Wiley and Sons, Ltd, 2004.
13. Weese-Mayer D, Shannon D, Keens T, Silvestri J. Idiopathic congenital central hypo-ventilation syndrome: diagnosis and management. Am J Respir Crit Care Med 1999; 160:368–373.
14. Chen M, Keens T. Congenital central hypoventilation syndrome: not just another rare disorder. Paediatr Respir Rev 2004; 5:182–189.
15. Gozal D, Keens T. Passive nighttime hypocapnic hyperventilation improves daytime eucapnia in mechanically ventilated children. Am J Respir Crit Care Med 1998; 157:A779.
16. Vanderlaan M, Holbrook C, Wang M, Tuell A, Gozal D. Epidemiologic survey of 196 patients with congenital central hypoventilation syndrome. Pediatr Pulmonol 2004; 37:217–229.
17. Spengler C, Gozal D, Shca S. Chemoreceptive mechanisms elucidated by studies of congenital central hypoventilation syndrome. Respir Physiol 2001; 129:247–255.
18. Weese-Mayer D, Berry-Kravis E. Genetics of congenital central hypoventilation syndrome: lessons from a seemingly orphan disease. Am J Respir Crit Care Med 2004; 170:16–21.
19. Rosen G, Bendel A, Neglia J, Moertel C, Mahowald M. Sleep in children with neo-plasms of the central nervous system: case review of 14 children. Pediatrics 2003; 112:46–54.
20. Yassari R, Frim D. Evaluation and management of the Chiari malformation type I for the primary care pediatrician. Pediatr Clin North Am 2004; 51:477–490.
21. Dure L, Percy A, Cheek W, Laurent J. Chiari type I malformation in children. J Pediatr 1989; 115:573–576.
22. Botelho R, Bittencourt L, Rotta J, Tufik S. Polysomnographic respiratory findings in patients with Arnold-Chiari type I malformation and basilar invagination, with or without syringomyelia: preliminary report of a series of cases. Neurosurg Rev 2000; 23:151–155.
23. Hershberger M, Chidekel A. Arnold-Chiari malformation type I and sleep-disordered breathing: an uncommon manifestation of an important pediatric problem. J Pediatr Health Care 2003; 17:190–197.
24. Stevenson K. Chiari Type II malformation: past, present, and future. Neurosurg Focus 2004; 16(2):article 5.

25. Alden T, Ojemann J, Park T. Surgical treatment of Chiari I malformation: indications and approaches. Neurosurg Focus 2001; 11(1):article 2.
26. Haroun R, Guarnieri M, Meadow J, Kraut M, Carson B. Current opinions for the treatment of syringomyelia and chiari malformations: survey of the Pediatric Section of the American Association of Neurological Surgeons. Pediatr Neurosurg 2000; 33(6):311–317.
27. Cochrane D, Adderley R, White C, Norman M, Steinbok P. Apnea in patients with myelomeningocele. Pediatr Neurosurg 1990–1991; 16(4–5):232–239.
28. Uliel S, Tauman R, Greenfeld M, Sivan Y. Normal polysomnographic respiratory values in children and adolescents. Chest 2004; 125:872–878.
29. Kelly D, Riordan L, Smith M. Apnea and periodic breathing in healthy full-term infants, 12–18 months of age. Pediatr Pulmonol 1992; 13:169–171.

4

Behavioral Insomnia of Childhood: The Diagnosis and Treatment of Bedtime Problems and Night Wakings

Lisa J. Meltzer

Division of Pulmonary Medicine, Department of Pediatrics,
University of Pennsylvania and The Children's Hospital of Philadelphia,
Philadelphia, Pennsylvania, U.S.A.

CHAPTER HIGHLIGHTS

- Behavioral insomnia of childhood is a common disorder that results in prolonged sleep onset, increased night wakings, and overall shorter total sleep time.
- There are three diagnostic categories that fall under behavioral insomnia of childhood: sleep-onset association type (the inability to fall asleep without the assistance of another person, object, or situation, resulting in frequent and prolonged night wakings), limit-setting type (delayed bedtime due to bedtime struggles and/or resistance), and combined type.
- Behavioral insomnia of childhood can result in increased daytime sleepiness, decreased emotion regulation, and greater marital strain.
- The four main areas that need to be addressed are the child's bedtime and sleep schedule, the bedtime routine, teaching children to fall asleep independently, and parental consistency.
- With consistent behavioral interventions, behavioral insomnia of childhood is easily treated.

INTRODUCTION

One of the most common complaints of parents of infants and toddlers is that their child either has difficulty going to bed (e.g., crying, struggling, and refusing to stay in bed) or wakes multiple times per night. These nightly struggles can leave parents tired, frustrated, and very stressed. However, for many families, bedtime refusal and night wakings can be easily remedied with consistent parental behaviors that encourage children to fall asleep independently at bedtime. This chapter provides an overview of the diagnostic criteria for behavioral insomnia of childhood, the impact of this disorder on the child and family, how to evaluate these problems, and practical treatment suggestions for practitioners and parents.

DIAGNOSTIC CRITERIA

Behavioral insomnia of childhood occurs in approximately 10–30% of infants and toddlers (1–3). The essential feature of behavioral insomnia of childhood, as defined by the revised International Classification of Sleep Disorders (ICSD-2), is difficulty falling asleep and/or staying asleep in a child. In addition, these difficulties are related to an identified behavior in the parent or child, a pattern that fits the sleep-onset association type or limit-setting type (Table 1) (4).

Table 1 Diagnostic Criteria for Behavioral Insomnia of Childhood

---

A. A child's symptoms meet the criteria for insomnia based on reports of parents or other adult caregivers
B. The child shows a pattern consistent with either the sleep-onset association type or limit-setting type of insomnia described below.
  1. Sleep-onset association type includes each of the following:
     a. Falling asleep is an extended process that requires special conditions
     b. Sleep-onset associations are highly problematic or demanding
     c. In the absence of the associated conditions, sleep onset is significantly delayed or sleep is otherwise disrupted
     d. Nighttime awakenings require caregiver intervention for the child to return to sleep
  2. Limit-setting type includes each of the following:
     a. The individual has difficulty initiating or maintaining sleep
     b. The individual stalls or refuses to go to bed at an appropriate time or refuses to return to bed following a nighttime awakening
     c. The caregiver demonstrates insufficient or inappropriate limit setting to establish appropriate sleeping behavior in the child
C. The sleep disturbance is not better explained by another sleep disorder, medical or neurological disorder, mental disorder, or medication use

---

Source: International Classification of Sleep Disorders, 2nd ed. (ICSD-2).

Sleep-Onset Association Type

Sleep-onset associations are certain conditions that are necessary for a child to fall asleep at bedtime and then return to sleep with each normal arousal during the night. Positive sleep associations are conditions that the children can provide for themselves (e.g., thumb sucking or cuddly object), whereas negative sleep associations require the assistance of another person (e.g., bottle or rocking). Negative sleep associations can also include external stimulation (e.g., watching television, in a car seat on top of the washing machine) or different settings (e.g., parents' bed or driving in the car). As all children typically arouse two to six times per night, any condition present at bedtime will be required again during normal arousals (1). Simply stated, a child who requires a parent to nurse or rock him to sleep at bedtime will also require a parent to nurse or rock him back to sleep following each naturally occurring nighttime arousal. When the sleep association is present, the child will fall asleep quickly. If the sleep association is not available, the child may experience frequent and prolonged night wakings.

Sleep-onset association type typically occurs in children aged six months to three years. Sleeping through the night is a developmental skill that occurs between three and six months of age, so prior to this, a diagnosis of behavioral insomnia of childhood would not be appropriate. For infants and toddler, frequent and persistent night wakings will likely continue without intervention. However, negative sleep associations generally decrease over time as different situations and behaviors that lead to negative sleep associations (e.g., bottle feeding or nursing) occur less frequently (5). In general, the prevalence of night wakings significantly decreases after three years of age; however, for children with developmental disorders (e.g., autism), sleep-onset association disorder may continue into adulthood.

Limit-Setting Type

Limit-setting sleep disorder presents as bedtime stalling or refusal to go to bed at an appropriate time. When limits are set, children typically fall asleep quickly and easily. Although bedtime resistance is found in 10–30% of toddlers and preschoolers, approximately 15% of parents of children ages 4 to 10 years also reported problematic bedtime behaviors. Bedtime refusal includes refusing to get ready for bed, go to bed, or stay in bed, whereas bedtime stalling is typically an attempt to delay bedtime. Stalling techniques include curtain calls (e.g., repeated requests for a drink, trips to the bathroom, or one more goodnight kiss) or additional activities at bedtime (e.g., watching one more television show or reading one more chapter). Once children fall asleep, their sleep quality is normal and they have few arousals. However, children with limit-setting sleep disorder have a shorter total sleep time (~30–60 minutes less per night).

Limit-setting sleep disorder is related to the development of a child. Toddlers and preschoolers, who are learning to become more independent during daytime, will frequently assert their newfound independence at bedtime. In addition, limit-setting sleep disorder can occur during naptime. As children grow older, parental involvement typically decreases at bedtime, reducing the opportunity for problematic limit-setting behaviors.

In limit-setting sleep disorder, there are two primary behavioral patterns seen in parents. First, there are parents who place few, if any, limits on the child's sleep behaviors. For example, parents may allow children to set their own bedtime or allow children to fall asleep watching the television in their bedroom, prolonging the child's sleep onset. Second, there are parents who set unpredictable and inconsistent limits, sending children a mixed message, which results in maintaining or increasing unwanted behaviors. For example, parents who "give in" on some evenings to a child's tantrum for an additional six bedtime books, although standing firm on only reading one book on other evenings, will only see a continuation of tantrum behaviors. One way to determine whether parental behavior is contributing to the child's insomnia is to ask whether the child has difficulty falling asleep for others (e.g., babysitter or day care) or the child falls asleep quickly at the desired bedtime, but in an undesired location (e.g., in front of the television or in the parents' bed).

Behavioral Insomnia of Childhood: Combined Type

The ICSD-2 includes a diagnostic category which recognizes that a child may be experiencing both sleep-onset association type and limit-setting type (4). For example, children who have difficulty initiating or maintaining sleep may initially stall at bedtime with frequent requests for "one more hug" (limit-setting type), then are unable to go to sleep until a parent lies with them (sleep-onset association type), and then wake multiple times during night, unable to return to sleep without a parent present.

IMPACT OF BEHAVIORAL INSOMNIA OF CHILDHOOD

Behavioral insomnia of childhood impacts not only the functioning and behavior of the child, but also the entire household. For children, shortened total sleep time and frequent night wakings result in daytime fatigue and irritability. It is important to explain to parents that for toddlers and preschoolers, fatigue often manifests as hyperactivity. Parents may claim that their child has "endless energy," especially at bedtime, when really the child is overtired. Limit-setting difficulties at bedtime are also seen during the day, with an increase in the daytime behavior problems.

Sleep problems in children also negatively impact parents and caregivers. For parents who disagree about how to handle a child's bedtime routine, marital tension may result. This conflict can increase inconsistencies at both bedtime and during the night, perpetuating the child's sleep difficulties. For children with multiple night wakings, parents are also having multiple night wakings, resulting in increased daytime sleepiness in caregivers. These sleep disruptions may result in poor concentration at work, drowsy driving, or negative mood. Some parents may even develop negative feelings toward a child who is difficult at bedtime or causes disruption to the parent's sleep. To avoid the unpleasantness of bedtime, parents often prolong the bedtime routine, which only delays the child's sleep-onset time, perpetuating the negative cycle.

ASSESSMENT

Behavioral insomnia of childhood frequently occurs along with other pediatric sleep disorders. For example, a child who has obstructive sleep apnea may be unable to fall asleep without a parent present at bedtime. Although the sleep apnea may be treated medically, the child will continue to be unable to initiate sleep without a parent present, thus the frequency of night wakings and levels of daytime sleepiness may not improve without the treatment of the sleep-onset association. Therefore, along with questions about symptoms of physiological sleep disorder (e.g., snoring and breathing pauses), a comprehensive evaluation of the child's sleep patterns and routines is essential.

Assessment of sleeping patterns

To assess a child's sleep routine, it is often easiest to guide parents through a "typical" day, starting at dinnertime. Along with questions about nighttime symptoms of physiological sleep disorders (e.g., obstructive sleep apnea), the following questions can be used to assess sleep patterns:

1. What time is dinner?
2. What happens between dinner and bedtime?
3. What occurs during the bedtime routine (e.g., bath, snack, stories) and how long does the routine take from start to end?
4. What time does the child go to bed, who is present, and how long does it take the child to fall asleep?
5. How frequently and at what time does the child wake during the night, and what happens?
6. What time does the child wake in the morning? Is it spontaneous or do you have to wake the child?
7. What time and how long are the child's naps during the day? Are there other scheduled or routine activities during the day?

An assessment for sleep disorders should include questions about the child's sleep schedule (e.g., bedtime and wake time on weekdays and weekends, sleep-onset latency), bedtime routines (e.g., stories, stalling behaviors), nocturnal behaviors (e.g., snoring, pauses in breathing, night wakings, and sleep terrors), daytime behaviors (e.g., naps, fatigue, meals, caffeine, and medications), and mood and functioning (e.g., irritability, hyperactivity, and difficulty concentrating). In addition, it is important to ask about significant life events (e.g., parental divorce, moving, new school, and new sibling), as these events can have a significant impact on a child's sleep (6).

Along with a thorough sleep history, sleep diaries are useful for tracking a child's sleep patterns over time (e.g., one to two weeks) and can be helpful in diagnosing behavioral insomnia of childhood. A typical diary asks parents to record what time the child went to bed, how long it took the child to fall asleep, the frequency and duration of night wakings, what time the child wakes in the morning, total sleep time, and the duration and timing of naps. For parents who may be poor historians or non-compliant with a sleep diary, sleep can also be measured through actigraphy. The actigraph is the size of a small wristwatch and contains a motion sensor that provides valid estimates of sleep onset, sleep offset, sleep disruptions, and total sleep time (7). Although a nocturnal polysomnography is warranted if an underlying sleep disrupter is suspected (e.g., sleep-disordered breathing, periodic limb movements of sleep), this approach does not provide information about the child's sleep routine, sleep-onset associations, or the behavior of either the child or parent at bedtime.

TREATMENT

Empirical studies have demonstrated that behavioral treatments for both sleep-onset association type and limit-setting type are highly effective (6,10). Although there are many different approaches to the treatment of behavioral insomnia of childhood, there are several basic treatment principles that apply to all children with this disorder. First, children need a consistent, age-appropriate bedtime and sleep schedule. Second, the bedtime routine should be short and sweet, always moving in the direction of the bedroom. Third, children must learn to fall asleep independently at bedtime. Finally, parents must be consistent every single night in order for these treatment approaches to be successful.

Bedtime/Sleep Schedule

Children need to have a consistent, age-appropriate bedtime every single night. Although some children are "night owls," showing a preference for later bedtimes at an early age, for most young children, an appropriate bedtime is between 7:00 pm and 8:30 pm. When bedtime is later, children often become overtired and are unable to fall asleep. In addition, bedtimes should not vary for weekdays and weekends, as an inconsistent bedtime can make it more difficult for children to fall asleep.

Naps are an essential part of a child's sleep schedule. It is a common, but incorrect, belief that if children skip their nap, they will fall asleep easier at bedtime. In fact, the opposite is true, as children who miss their naps will become overtired, making it difficult to settle at bedtime. Most children continue to nap until at least three years of age, with 26% continuing to nap until the age of five years (8). Like bedtime, naps should occur at the same time every day. However, for children who find it difficult to fall asleep at the appropriate bedtime, nap schedules should be evaluated to ensure that the child's nap is not interfering with sleep onset. For example, naps should not end past 3:00 pm or 4:00 pm if the child has an early bedtime.

Bedtime fading can be used to help advance a child's bedtime, with the first step setting bedtime to the actual time the child falls asleep. Once a child is quickly falling asleep at bedtime, parents can advance their child's bedtime by 15 minutes every two to three nights. This approach helps to alleviate many of the bedtime struggles that occur for children who naturally want to fall asleep later.

Bedtime Routine

A consistent bedtime routine is essential. Routines are a key feature of everyday life for children. When children know what to expect, they are better able to move from one activity to another. Bedtime routines can begin as early as three months, establishing a habit of consistency at bedtime that includes a quiet activity (e.g., song, book) at the end of the routine in the child's own room. For young children, verbal reminders (e.g., five minutes until bedtime, one minute until bedtime) help prepare them to transition and will decrease the number of protests and arguments that may arise. The bedtime routine itself should be short and sweet, no more than 20 to 30 minutes, and should always move toward the child's bedroom. For example, a preschooler's typical routine may include a snack in the kitchen, a bath and brushing teeth in the bathroom, putting on pajamas and reading two stories in the child's room, and then turning the lights off and saying good night. To help with consistency, a bedtime chart is often helpful for both the child and the parent.

Bedtime chart

Children are very resourceful when they do not want to go to bed. They will find the one thing that will prolong their bedtime (and increase parental attention). Favorite requests are "Just one more hug, Mommy, I love you!" or "Please, Daddy, just one more book." A bedtime chart is helpful for keeping everyone on track at bedtime. For toddlers and preschoolers, parents can use a picture chart to indicate each of the routine activities (e.g., snack, bath, two books, and bed). When each activity is completed, the child or parent can check it off. This prevents bedtime stalling and requests for additional attention.

Falling Asleep Independently

For behavioral insomnia of childhood, one of the key features is that the child is unable to fall asleep without parental intervention. For sleep-onset association type, this could include being rocked or nursed to sleep, whereas for limit-setting type, parents are required to respond to bedtime stalling behaviors. Children should be placed in the crib or go to bed when they are drowsy but awake, and then fall asleep on their own. For children with frequent night wakings, once they learn to fall asleep independently at bedtime, this skill typically generalizes to night wakings in about two weeks, with a child learning to return to sleep following normal arousals. The following are behavioral approaches that have been successfully used to teach children to fall asleep independently at bedtime.

Extinction

More commonly known as "cry it out," extinction is a behavioral technique based on operant condition: a theory that states those behaviors that are reinforced will increase in frequency, whereas behaviors that are ignored will decrease over time until they are extinguished. Applying this to children who are unable to fall asleep without being rocked, they should be placed in the crib drowsy but awake, and then their parents should ignore their cries until they are asleep. If parents are consistent and do not "give in" and respond to the child's cries at bedtime, within three to five nights, the child will be falling asleep on his/her own at bedtime. Studies have shown extinction to be an effective treatment for sleep-onset association disorder (9,10), with treatment gains maintained over time (11).

However, compliance with the approach is poor (12,13). Most parents are unable to tolerate their child's cries, and after a certain time, they will respond to their child. This is problematic because children learn that if they simply cry long enough, they will get the response they are seeking (e.g., attention, rocking, or nursing). There are three things practitioners can tell parents to help prepare them for this treatment approach. First, a child's crying will get worse before it gets better due to an extinction burst (see box). Second, children may cry so hard they throw up. Parents should have a second set of sheets on the crib or bed, and if the child does throw up, the parent should quickly change the sheets and the child's pajamas and return the child to bed. Third, there is no long-term psychological harm caused by letting a child "cry it out." Parents should be reassured that the child (and the parent) will be happier and more alert during the day once bedtime issues and night wakings have been resolved and that the child's cries at bedtime are from exhaustion and frustration at not sleeping, rather than from anger toward the parent.

> **Extinction burst**
>
> An extinction burst is an increase and intensification of a symptom that is to be expected on the second day (or night) of any behavioral intervention. In the case of "crying it out," children will typically cry 45 minutes the first night and up to 90 minutes on the second. If parents are unprepared for this increase in crying, they may become frustrated and respond to the child, which, in the long run, will only prolong the child's cries at bedtime.

Graduated Extinction

Because so many parents are unable to tolerate extinction, graduated extinction has also been demonstrated to be a successful treatment of sleep-onset associ-ation disorder (14–16). Graduated extinction involves putting a child to bed drowsy but awake, and then ignoring his/her cries or requests for progressively longer periods of time (e.g., 1, 2, 5, and 10 minutes). Although it may take longer than extinction (several days to a few weeks), most parents are able to tolerate their children's cries when they have the ability to check on him/her, resulting in better compliance with this treatment approach. Graduated extinction is the most commonly recommended intervention for sleep problems in popular parenting books (17,18).

Checking Method

When checking on a child at bedtime, visits should be brief and boring. The goal of these checks is to reassure the parent that the child's foot is not stuck in the crib or the child truly needs attention (e.g., diaper change). Parents should have minimal interaction with their child during visits, with brief verbal responses, "Mommy loves you, go to sleep." The amount of time between checks should be determined by the child's temperament and the parent's tolerance (18). For a child who becomes more upset each time the parent does a check, parents should be advised to check less frequently. For parents who are unable to tolerate their child's cries, they should check as frequently as they desire (e.g., every 30 seconds). However, parents should be reminded that the goal is for the child to fall asleep when the parent is not in the room, so the fewer checks the better.

Fading of Parental Presence

For parents unable to tolerate extinction or graduated extinction, a more gradual approach is to fade the involvement of parents at bedtime (19). The first area is to decrease a parent's physical contact with the child at bedtime. So, for a mom who nurses her child to sleep, the first step is to move nursing earlier in the bedtime routine and simply rock the child to sleep. Once that is successful, the child should be placed in the crib and the parent should rub his/her head or arm until they fall asleep. The second area is to decrease parental presence in the room. A parent who is lying with a child should first sit on the child's bed for several nights, and then sit on the child's floor for several nights, and then continue moving out of the room two feet every two nights. The third area to decrease parental involvement is the amount of time between bedtime checks, which should be consistently increased every few nights (e.g., 5, 10, and 20 minutes).

Positive Routines

The goal of this intervention is to create a positive and enjoyable bedtime for both the child and the parents. Positive routines involve creating a bedtime routine that includes one or two of the child's favorite, but calm, activities. If the child throws a tantrum, the routine ends and the child is to go to bed immediately. The benefits of this intervention are that it prevents crying, reduces bedtime struggles, and alleviates parental anxiety (14,20). However, the primary drawback is that it requires a consistent parental response and positive verbal reinforcement when the child participates with the routine, and the immediate consequence of going to bed if the child misbehaves. Overall, compared to extinction, positive routines are easier for parents to comply with.

Consistency

Parental consistency is central to the success of behavioral treatments for behavioral insomnia of childhood. Returning to behavioral theory, a consistent response is the fastest way of successfully changing a behavior, whereas an inconsistent response is the surest way to extend the life of a certain behavior. An example of a consistent response for adults is a paycheck. If people know that they are going to get paid every two weeks, they will continue to show up for work every day. An example of an inconsistent response for adults occurs when playing slot machines. As people do not know which pull of the lever will result in winning, they will continue to play for an extended period of time. These same ideas apply to setting bedtimes, creating bedtime routines, and teaching children to fall asleep and return to sleep independently. For example, if a child receives a bottle for some night wakings, and not for others, he/she will continue to wake with each normal arousal, demanding attention in the hope that his/her parents will give them a bottle. Alternatively, if a parent lies with a child on some nights to stop a tantrum, the child will only extend the tantrum longer on other nights, expecting the final result of a parent coming in to lie with him/her.

PRACTICAL SUGGESTIONS FOR PARENTAL LIMIT-SETTING

Although it is age-appropriate for young children to "test the limits" and push the boundaries of what is appropriate behavior, it is a parent's job to set the limits and consistently enforce rules for appropriate behavior (21,22). Without rewards and consequences, children are unable to learn the difference between appropriate and inappropriate behaviors. Although many parents may be successful in setting limits during the day, at bedtime parents may find it more difficult to enforce rules, as their primary goal is to get the child to fall asleep. In addition, as both the child and parent become overtired, it is more difficult to be consistent with behavior management. The following are suggestions for limit-setting at bedtime, but most can also be applied to managing daytime behaviors.

Positive Reinforcement

As children constantly seek parental attention, it is important to pay attention when a child is behaving appropriately or "catch 'em being good!" In terms of bedtime, parents should be encouraged to notice when a child is following the routine (e.g., "I like the way you brushed your teeth"). Positive reinforcements should also be used to reward appropriate behaviors (e.g., staying in bed once the lights are turned off) and can include verbal praise, activities (e.g., going to the park, watching a favorite TV show the next day), or small material gifts (e.g., stickers or pennies). For rewards to be effective, there needs to be a target behavior (e.g., staying in bed) and the reward needs to be presented immediately. Once the behavior is established, rewards can be presented at a more irregular interval (e.g., every three or four days) to keep the child interested.

One positive reinforcement approach for use at bedtime with preschool aged children is the "sleep fairy," which can often be an effective way to prevent bedtime resistance (23). Once children fall asleep, the sleep fairy will leave a small prize (e.g., a sticker or a nickel) under their pillow. Sticker charts are also effective for positive reinforcement, with children earning stickers every day for the targeted behavior (e.g., putting on their pajamas without a fight) and with the child able to redeem the stickers (after five to seven days) for a larger reward (e.g., ice cream or trip to the park).

Ignoring Complaints, Protests, and Inappropriate Behaviors

Although parents increase their focus on positive behaviors, they should also decrease their attention on negative behaviors, including complaints, protests, and inappropriate behaviors (5). When parents focus on a child's temper tantrum or engage in a power struggle with the child, they are providing attention to the child for the wrong reasons. However, the message children receive is that mommy and daddy will pay attention to them for tantrums, increasing the frequency of these negative and unwanted behaviors. In addition, children are able to reach their ultimate goal, prolonging the bedtime routine and delaying bedtime. Parents should be cautioned about this and taught that it is okay to ignore a child's protests at bedtime. In addition, parents should remain calm and firmly stick to a consistent routine, regardless of the child's complaints.

Choices and Commands

It is important to provide children with choices, especially when working toward a goal (e.g., bedtime), as this provides children with a sense of control over the situation. However, in order for parents to remain in control of the situation, these choices should be limited in number (no more than two) and scope (22). For example, five minutes before parents want to start the bedtime routine, they can ask "do you want to start your bedtime routine now or in five minutes?" This helps to avoid many of the arguments that arise with bedtime. In addition, parents should not ask questions when they really want to give a command. For example, instead of asking "do you want to brush your teeth?" which might elicit a "no" response, a parent should simply state, "time to brush your teeth."

Resources for parents

- In 2002, in conjunction with a task force of pediatric sleep experts from the National Sleep Foundation, Johnson & Johnson published resource materials for healthcare practitioners and parents. The evidence-based guidelines for practitioners, "Babies and Sleep: Best Sleep Practices for Newborns, Infants and Toddlers from the National Sleep Foundation," and pamphlets that can be distributed to parents titled "Sleep, Your Baby, and You" can be obtained by calling 1-866-565-2229.

- The following are commonly used parenting books on children's sleep and behavior management:
    Healthy Sleep Habits, Happy Child. Marc Weissbluth (24)
    *Sleeping Through the Night: How Infants Toddlers, and Their Parents
      Can Get a Good Night's Sleep.* Revised ed. Jodi A. Mindell (18)
    Solve Your Child's Sleep Problems. Richard Ferber (17)
    *SOS! Help for Parents: A Practical Guide for Handling Common
      Everyday Behavior Problems.* Lynn Clark (21)
    Your Defiant Child: Eight Steps to Better Behavior. Russell Barkley (22)

PROGNOSIS FOR BEHAVIORAL INSOMNIA OF CHILDHOOD

With parents who consistently follow through with behavioral recommendations, the prognosis is very good for behavioral insomnia of childhood (5). For sleep-onset association type, children who are taught to fall asleep independently will have a significant decrease in the frequency and duration of night wakings within approximately two weeks. For limit-setting type, consistently applied limits will result in decreased struggles at bedtime, an earlier bedtime, faster sleep-onset latency, and overall greater total sleep time.

Contrary to popular belief, children will not simply outgrow behavioral insomnia of childhood. Thus, families who are unable to follow the recommendations given by a pediatrician or other medical provider should be referred to a behavioral specialist who can design a behavioral intervention that will help the family be successful in treating behavioral insomnia of childhood.

REFERENCES

1. Goodlin-Jones BL, Burnham MM, Gaylor EE, Anders TF. Night waking, sleep–wake organization, and self-soothing in the first year of life. J Dev Behav Pediatr 2001; 22(4):226–233.
2. Burnham MM, Goodlin-Jones BL, Gaylor EE, Anders TF. Nighttime sleep–wake patterns and self-soothing from birth to one year of age: a longitudinal intervention study. J Child Psychol Psychiat 2002; 43(6):713–725.
3. Armstrong KL, Quinn RA, Dadds MR. The sleep patterns of normal children. Med J Aust 1994; 161(3):202–206.
4. American Academy of Sleep Medicine. International Classification of Sleep Disorders. 2nd ed. Diagnostic and Coding Manual. Westchester, IL: American Academy of Sleep Medicine, 2005.
5. Mindell JA, Owens JA. A Clinical Guide to Pediatric Sleep: Diagnosis and Management of Sleep Problems. Philadelphia, PA: Lippincott, Williams & Wilkins, 2003.
6. Mindell JA, Owens JA, Carskadon MA. Developmental features of sleep. Child Adolesc Psychiatr Clin N Am 1999; 8(4):695–725.
7. Sadeh A, Acebo C. The role of actigraphy in sleep medicine. Sleep Med Rev 2002; 6(2):113–124.
8. National Sleep Foundation. Sleep in America Poll, 2004.
9. Mindell JA. Empirically supported treatments in pediatric psychology: bedtime refusal and night wakings in young children. J Pediatr Psychol 1999; 24(6):465–481.
10. Kuhn BR, Elliott AJ. Treatment efficacy in behavioral pediatric sleep medicine. J Psychosom Res 2003; 54(6):587–597.
11. France KG. Behavior characteristics and security in sleep-disturbed infants treated with extinction. J Pediatr Psychol 1992; 17(4):467–475.
12. Rickert VI, Johnson CM. Reducing nocturnal awakening and crying episodes in infants and young children: a comparison between scheduled awakenings and systematic ignoring. Pediatrics 1988; 81(2):203–212.
13. Richman N. A community survey of characteristics of one- to two- year-olds with sleep disruptions. J Am Acad Child Adolesc Psychiatry 1985; 20(2):281–291.
14. Adams LA, Rickert VI. Reducing bedtime tantrums: comparison between positive routines and graduated extinction. Pediatrics 1989; 84(5):756–761.
15. Hiscock H, Wake M. Randomised controlled trial of behavioural infant sleep intervention to improve infant sleep and maternal mood. BMJ 2002; 324(7345):1062–1065.
16. Reid MJ, Walter AL, O'leary SG. Treatment of young children's bedtime refusal and nighttime wakings: a comparison of "standard" and graduated ignoring procedures. J Abnorm Child Psychol 1999; 27(1):5–16.
17. Ferber R. Solve Your Child's Sleep Problems. New York: Simon & Schuster, 1985.
18. Mindell JA. Sleeping Through the Night: How Infants, Toddlers, and Their Parents Can Get a Good Night's Sleep. Revised ed. New York: Harper Collins, 2005.
19. Lewin DS. Childhood insomnias: limit setting and sleep onset association disorder. diagnostic issues, behavioral treatment, and future directions. In: Perlis ML, Lichstein KL, eds. Treating Sleep Disorders: Principles and Practice of Behavioral Sleep Medicine. New York: Jossey-Bass, 2003:365–392.
20. Milan MA, Mitchell ZP, Berger MI, Pierson DF. Positive routines: a rapid alternative to extinction for elimination of bedtime tantrum behavior. Child Behav Ther 1981; 3:13–25.

21. Clark L. SOS! Help for Parents. 2nd ed. Bowling Green, KY: Parents Press, 1996.
22. Barkley RA. Your Defiant Child: Eight Steps to Better Behavior. New York: Guilford Press, 1998.
23. Burke RV, Kuhn BR, Peterson JL. Brief report: a "storybook" ending to children's bedtime problems—the use of a rewarding social story to reduce bedtime resistance and frequent night waking. J Pediatr Psychol 2004; 29(5):389–396.
24. Welssbluth M. Healthy Sleep Habits, Happy Child. Revised ed. New York: Ballantine Books, 2003.

5

Sleep Apnea in Children
History and Physical Exam

Mark A. Richardson

Department of Otolaryngology/Head & Neck Surgery, Oregon Health & Science University, Portland, Oregon, U.S.A.

CHAPTER HIGHLIGHTS

- Polysomnography (PSG) is the "gold standard" for diagnosis of sleep disordered breathing (SDB). An accurate history and physical exam can identify patients at risk for sleep disorders and possible complications of surgery.
- High risk populations include the obese, children with Down's syndrome, and children with craniofacial disorders and neuromuscular conditions.
- A history of airway obstruction during the night and daytime, snoring, and behavioral disorders should suggest SDB. The added factor of being a high risk surgical candidate would justify obtaining a PSG.

INTRODUCTION

Primary snoring (PS)—defined as snoring without obstructive apnea, arousals from sleep, or gas exchange abnormalities—and obstructive sleep apnea (OSA) represent a spectrum of disorders indicating increased upper airway resistance to airflow. Snoring is identified in 6% to18% of children (1) and varies by age. OSA is less common, with an estimated prevalence of 2% (2). These entities fit into a larger categorization of SDB and include upper airway resistance syndrome (UARS). Although our ability to categorize the degree or effect of this resistance on sleep quality is limited, history and physical cues often identify a predisposed population group worthy of further investigation and treatment. Anatomic narrowing, muscle or tissue weakness, and neurologic disorders are the primary causes of OSA and SDB, with a large number of other factors contributing to this problem in the population as a whole (3). Large tonsils and adenoids are the most common contributors to PS or OSA; it is, therefore, of critical importance to determine the site and cause of obstruction.

The outcomes of surgical management are significantly better in children than in adults (1). A thorough review of the medical history and a physical exam can help highlight the surgical procedure most likely to be effective and those patients most at risk for complications. There have been no studies to prove the utility of their history and physical findings in distinguishing between patients with PS and with OSA (4).

It should be noted that a small percentage of patients with OSA may have physiologic changes, such as cardiomegaly and pulmonary hypertension, due to the transient but repeated hypoxia that occurs during sleep and that accompanies the disease. The need for additional diagnostic testing can be suggested by the results of a polysomnogram (PSN), as well as the history, physical exam, and special circumstances surrounding any individual patient.

HISTORY

OSA is unusual in children who do not snore: thus, snoring is the most common complaint in this population. Other nighttime symptoms include mouth breathing, diaphoresis, restlessness, enuresis, awakenings, apneas, and other parasomnias. A well-delineated history of interrupted breathing at night does have a high degree of correlation with OSA (5). Daytime symptoms include mouth breathing, hyponasal speech, a variety of behavioral disturbances, and somnolence (6,7). Poor growth and failure to thrive are also more common in children with SDB (Table 1) (8).

In general, symptoms of obstruction that occur during the day will likely produce symptoms at night as well. A history of difficulty with swallowing due to enlarged tonsils, pharyngeal speech, or nasal obstruction should lead to questions about sleep and the possibility of apnea. There may often be brief episodes of nighttime breathing difficulty associated with acute upper respiratory infections that cause lymphoid enlargement. These episodes are usually self-limiting and resolve spontaneously. Supportive care during the episode is usually all that is needed. In some cases, however, once lymphoid hyperplasia occurs, prolonged symptomatic obstruction can take place. Establishing the chronicity and consistency of symptoms is critical in decision-making.

There seem to be increased rates of OSA in African American children (9), and Asian children may also be predisposed to OSA. No sex differences exist in prepubertal children, although once adolescence has been reached, there seems to be a predominance of males, as there is in the adult population.

Table 1 History

Day
Mouth breathing
Hyponasal speech
Audible breathing noise
A variety of behavioral disturbances
Hypersomnolence
Night
Mouth breathing
Snoring
Diaphoresis
Restlessness
Enuresis
Apneas
Awakenings
Nightmares
Somnambulism
General
Poor growth—failure to thrive

Peak prevalence in children occurs at two to eight years, correlating with natural lymphatic tissue growth and atrophy. It should be noted that children under three years have an increased risk of complications with adenotonsillectomy. As a result, these and other high-risk patients may need in-hospital postoperative management.

It is now apparent that a number of behavioral disturbances can be and often are associated with SDB. Questioning about school performance and attention-deficit hyperactivity disorder symptoms may suggest the possibility of sleep disturbance in a snoring child (10).

Although there is no direct link to gastroesophageal reflux disease, there is certainly overlap between these two common conditions. Questioning for reflux symptoms may be useful in beginning non-surgical treatment.

Snoring is an inspiratory noise that parents sometimes refer to as "labored" breathing. There is often a description of chest wall movement and positional changes during sleep. Enuresis is a common complaint, perhaps associated with frequent partial arousals or changes in sleep state. It may resolve after resolution of the obstruction or sleep disturbance.

In all cases, it is important to ascertain the phase of respiration during which the noise occurs as well as the quality of sound. Staccato, irregular breathing during inspiration is characteristic of snoring from upper airway obstruction. The physical exam can help pinpoint the site of obstruction and potential remediation.

QUESTIONNAIRES

A variety of questionnaires now exist, exhibiting a high correlation with SDB where certain scores are achieved. Studies by Chervin (11) and Rosenfeld (12) utilizing the PSQ and OSA 18 have shown strong positive associations with OSA and "yes" answers on the form filled out by parents.

The OSA-18 is a validated quality-of-life (QOL) measure for children with varying levels of SDB. The survey consists of eighteen items grouped into five domains: sleep disturbance (four items), physical suffering (four items), emotional distress (three items), daytime problems (four items), and caregiver concerns (four items). Items are scored on a 7-point ordinal scale (see Appendix A).

The overall survey score is calculated as a mean of the 18 items, which correlates well with respiratory disturbance index and adenoid size. Although not diagnostic of SDB, it may be helpful in estimating the severity of the problem (12).

Chervin's Pediatric Sleep Questionnaire (PSQ) is another measure used to scale snoring, SDB, sleepiness, and behavioral problems. When the 22-item SDB scale is used, it can approximate a screen for polysomnographically determined OSA and UARS (sensitivity 0.81, specificity 0.87) (see Appendix B) (11).

Although neither survey is diagnostic to the same degree that PSN is, both are useful in diagnosing SDB, estimating the effect on QOL, and identifying the behavioral issues that may accompany SDB.

PHYSICAL EXAM

Body mass index (BMI) can be calculated for children to give a BMI/age percentile. Fortunately, these are well-established norms for children that can be plotted as part of any new patient exam. Not all patients with a BMI/age of >95th percentile will have sleep apnea, but overweight children do have a higher prevalence of disease. As opposed to adults, many children with OSA are at the lower end of the growth normograms (height and weight/age).

OVERALL CRANIOFACIAL APPEARANCE

A general sense of normal or abnormal cranial development is important, as is determining the potential existence of maxillary or mandibular hypoplasia. Abnormal occlusal relationships may help in pointing out aberrant facial growth or suggest chronic nasal obstruction.

An anterior nasal exam can identify septal deviations or other masses. The effect of allergy and its contribution to obstructive sleep disorders is not well documented; however, allergic rhinitis does contribute to nasal obstruction, and remediation may be of benefit in some individuals.

The oral exam will alert the examiner to structural abnormalities present there. Macroglossia, palatal abnormalities, and enlarged tonsils can easily be seen.

A Mallampati score can be calculated in the following manner: viewing the pharynx with the mouth open at rest, there should be no phonation and no protrusion of the tongue.

Scores are designated as follows (Fig. 1):

1. Entire tonsil or fossae visible
2. Upper half of tonsil fossae visible
3. Soft and hard palate visible
4. Only hard palate visible

Although Mallampati scores are not currently well correlated with OSA in children, they are a general index for anatomic crowding associated with difficult intubation. Macroglossia is a relative term but can be suggested by a high score. It is likely that a high score will also suggest a potential for OSA.

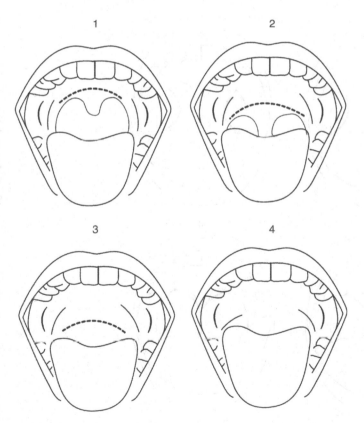

Figure 1 Mallampati scores.

As part of the oral exam, a tonsillar size index can be created as well by using a scale of 0 to 4+ (Fig. 2).

1. 0, Tonsils removed or entirely within the tonsil fossa.
2. 1+, Tonsils occupy <25% of the lateral dimension of the oropharynx as measured between the anterior tonsillar pillars.
3. 2+, Tonsils occupy <50% of the lateral dimension of the oropharynx as measured between the anterior tonsillar pillars.
4. 3+, Tonsils occupy <75% of the lateral dimension of the oropharynx as measured between the anterior tonsillar pillars.
5. 4+, Tonsils occupy 75% or more of the lateral dimension of the oropharynx.

Although the presence of enlarged tonsils does not equal sleep apnea in an individual, tonsillar enlargement (3+ or greater) may be predictive of a successful outcome of adenotonsillar removal for reduction of obstruction. Conversely, small tonsils (1+ or less) should suggest the need for additional examinations to

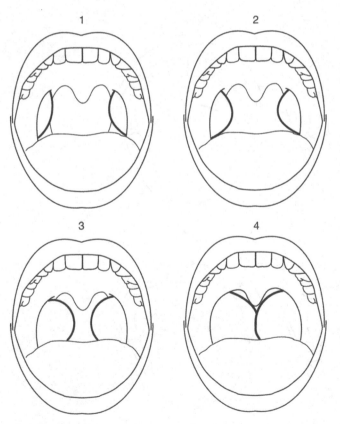

Figure 2   Tonsillar size index.

identify the site of obstruction and, if none is apparent, additional measures to quantify and qualify the sleep disturbance present.

Friedman (13) has developed a scale combining tongue palate position, BMI, and tonsil size. His scale has been shown to have prognostic value in surgery for SDB in adults.

The palate and uvula can contribute to noisy breathing during sleep. Anatomic inspection for abnormalities in uvular length, palatal shape, and development should be performed. Bifid uvulas, submucous clefting, and the presence of a zona pellucida should raise concerns about postoperative complications from adenoidectomy.

FLEXIBLE FIBEROPTIC EXAM

Although an adequate exam of the oral cavity and the anterior nose can be accomplished through routine means, the posterior nasal cavity, nasopharynx, hypopharynx, and laryngeal exam require special equipment. In children especially, the flexible fiberoptic scope can identify other anatomic factors in these areas that contribute to the airway obstruction.

Adenoids are best examined in this fashion and can be easily seen obstructing the choanae of the nasal cavity if they do contribute to nasal or nasopharyngeal obstruction. A lateral nasopharyngeal radiograph may also suggest adenoid hypertrophy.

Adenoids can usually be examined easily, using the appropriate equipment and technique. Accompanied by video, the examination can also be an effective teaching tool for parents. A 50/50 mixture of oxymetazoline and xylocaine 2% is instilled in the nasal cavity via pressurized spray or dropper. (Two percent viscous xylocaine can also be used.) Younger children are especially fearful of the pressurized atomizer or "squirt gun" and nasal speculum, so drops to the nose on one side are equally effective. The medication has a bitter taste and will, of course, provide some numbing to the oral cavity as well. Patients must be cautioned about eating or drinking immediately after the examination.

After a five-minute period, vasoconstriction and anesthesia are obtained and passage of the endoscope can take place. The use of the smaller 2.2 mm scope has markedly improved tolerance to the examination, which takes only minutes to perform. The posterior nose, nasopharynx, pharynx, tongue base, and larynx can be readily visualized and potential narrowing, masses, or obstructions identified.

Rigid endoscopy can be utilized as well, but this technical tool is less well tolerated than the small flexible scope.

Presumably, OSA is the result of some abnormality in patency of the upper airway during sleep. This can be due to structural abnormalities in muscle or bone surrounding those areas, or dynamic factors affecting nearby collapsible soft tissues. Examination of the nose, nasopharynx, oral cavity, oropharynx, and larynx should identify the potential site of obstruction. Fiberoptic examinations,

Table 2   Potential Sites of Obstruction

Nose
   Aperture-nasal aperture stenosis
   Valve collapse
   Septal deformities
   Polyps
   Encephaloceles
   Hemangiomas
   Gliomas
   Turbinate hypertrophy
Nasopharynx
   Adenoids
   Encephaloceles
   Retrusive maxilla
Oral cavity
   Palate abnormalities
   Tongue—anterior and posterior lesions
   Cysts—Internal thyroglossal, dermoids,
      lymphatic malformations
Hypopharynx
   Masses, extrinsic compression
Larynx
   Masses, cysts, tumors
   Neurogenic cause, vocal fold mobility

performed with the patient seated or supine, are almost a mandatory adjunct to the routine physical. In some cases, endoscopic examination can be coupled with a PSN if there remains doubt as to the location or site of obstruction. Often, there will be a multifactorial problem involving the tongue base, palate, and hypopharynx. In some cases, dynamic videography will help define the elements contributing to the obstruction and apneic events.

In any case, physical examination should lead to a likely site of the problem, leading to a potential surgical solution (Table 2).

Generally, the history will be sufficient to identify the site as being supraglottic. The need for tracheoscopy or bronchoscopy is unusual. However, in children where the history is confusing, or where there is a prior problem identified with the larynx or trachea, a complete airway endoscopy may need to be performed.

SPECIAL CIRCUMSTANCES (TABLE 3)

Down's syndrome presents a variety of factors that may contribute to the high rate of sleep apnea in children. There is a relative macroglossia, and the

Table 3 High-Risk Populations

Obesity
Down's syndrome
Mucopolysaccharidoses
Achondroplasia
Craniofacial disorders
  Craniosynostoses
  Apert's, Crouzon's, Pfeiffer's, and Saethre–Chotzen's syndromes
    Robin sequence
    Stickler syndrome
    CHARGE syndrome
    Choanal atresia
  Mandibulofacial dysostosis (Treacher Collins syndrome)
  Craniofacial microsomia (hemifacial microsomia,
    Goldenhar's syndrome, 1st and 2nd branchial arch syndrome)
Muscular dystrophy
  Cerebral palsy
  Klippel–Feil syndrome
  Beckwith–Weideman syndrome
  Prader–Willi syndrome
  Hallerman–Streiff syndrome
  Mucopolysaccharide storage diseases
  Post pharyngoplasty patients

combination of this with hypotonia may be the significant problem. In addition, obesity, maxillary hypoplasia, and other individual issues may provide incremental resistance to airflow, thus contributing to OSA, PS, or UARS (2).

Mucopolysaccharide (MPS) storage diseases such as Hunter's and Hurler's syndromes also create airway difficulties over time due to the increasing nonmetabolized storage products being deposited in tissues of the upper airway. Although they may initially respond to conservative surgery, progression of the disorder may lead to need for tracheostomy. Central apnea and hypoventilation are associated with MPS; in such high-risk patients a sleep study is almost always indicated.

Achondroplasia is another genetic disorder with a high proportion of sleep apnea in those affected (14). Midface hypoplasia and obesity may contribute to this condition. Adenotonsillectomy, weight reduction, continuous positive airway pressure (CPAP), and tracheostomy have all been used successfully to help mediate disturbed sleep.

Craniofacial disturbances such as the Robin sequence are commonly associated with airway issues requiring active management. Any craniofacial disturbance causing alterations in skull base development or maxillary or mandibular growth patterns can also contribute to nighttime-breathing problems. Individuals with these diagnoses should be screened for potential OSA and the general medical history taken. Other at-risk groups include children with cerebral palsy, muscular dystrophy, and hypothyroidism.

HOME VIDEO–AUDIO

Studies of audiotaping and videotaping have suggested some positive predictive ability, especially for video (83%). Although these studies may be helpful, they do not measure physiologic changes taking place during sleep. Oximetry during sleep and nap PSG have high rates of false negative results, although they can suggest a diagnosis if positive. Neither of these studies can determine the severity of the sleep disturbance, however—an important piece of information in determining management.

CONSERVATIVE MANAGEMENT

Infants and children under two represent a special population. They certainly fall outside of the two-to-eight-year-old range with the highest prevalence of SDB secondary to adenotonsillar hypertrophy. As a result, they require special vigilance and evaluation to diagnose the site and degree of sleep disturbance present.

Although surgery is a common option for management, antibiotics as well as oral and nasal steroids have all been used to try to relieve symptoms and restore normal sleep patterns.

CONCLUSION

Successful outcomes from surgical management are dependent on identification and localization of the etiology of obstruction. An appropriate, staged approach to intervention can only be planned with the performance of an accurate and thorough physical examination. Increasingly complex patients with multiple co-morbidities and of various ages require differing techniques and evaluation methodologies.

APPENDIX A: OBSTRUCTIVE SLEEP APNEA-18 SURVEY DOMAINS AND ITEMS

(S) Sleep disturbance
  S1 Loud snoring
  S2 Breath holding spells or pauses in breathing at night
  S3 Choking or gasping sounds while asleep
  S4 Restless sleep or frequent awakenings from sleep

(P) Physical suffering
  P1 Mouth breathing because of nasal obstruction
  P2 Frequent colds or upper respiratory tract infections
  P3 Nasal discharge or runny nose
  P4 Difficulty in swallowing foods

(E) Emotional distress
  E1 Mood swings or temper tantrums
  E2 Aggressive or hyperactive behavior
  E3 Discipline problems

(D) Daytime problems
  D1 Excessive daytime drowsiness or sleepiness
  D2 Poor attention span or concentration
  D3 Difficulty getting out of bed in the morning

(C) Caregiver concerns
  C1 Caused you to worry about your child's general health
  C2 Created concern that your child is not getting enough air
  C3 Interfered with your ability to perform daily activities
  C4 Made you frustrated

Notes: A point scale from 1 to 7 is to grade each item. (None of the time to all of the time.) The total score can be graded as mild <60, moderate 60–80, and severe >80. Each domain can also be assessed separately with the S domain having the highest likelihood of greatest change in mean score.

APPENDIX B: PEDIATRIC SLEEP QUESTIONNAIRE (CHERVIN)

A. While sleeping, does your child
  ...snore more than half the time?
  ...always snore?
  ...snore loudly?
  ...have "heavy" or loud breathing?
  ...have trouble breathing or struggle to breathe?

Have you ever...
  ...seen your child stop breathing during the night?

Does your child...
  ...tend to breathe through the mouth during the day?
  ...have a dry mouth on waking up in the morning?
  ...occasionally wet the bed?

B. Does your child...
  ...wake up feeling unrefreshed?
  ...have a problem with sleepiness during the day?
  Has a teacher or other supervisor commented that your child seems sleepy during the
    day?
  Is it hard to wake your child up in the morning?
  Does your child wake up with headaches in the morning?
  Did your child stop growing at a normal rate at any time since birth?
  Is your child overweight?

C. This child often...
  ...does not seem to listen when spoken to directly
  ...has difficulty organizing tasks and activities
  ...is easily distracted by extraneous stimuli
  ...fidgets with hands or feet or squirms in seat
  ...is "on the go" or often acts as if "driven by a motor"
  ...interrupts or intrudes on others (e.g., butts into conversations or games)

Notes: Each item is answered with either yes, no or don't know. Eight or more positive answers to the
22 questions are highly sensitive and specific for identifying SDB.

REFERENCES

1. Schechter M. Technical report: diagnosis and management of childhood obstructive schechter sleep apnea syndrome. Pediatr 2002; 109(4):e69.
2. Marcus C, Chapman D, Ward S, et al. Clinical practice guideline: diagnosis and management of childhood sleep apnea syndrome. Pediatr 2002; 109:704–712.
3. Lipton JL, Gozal D. Obstructive sleep apnea syndrome. eMedicine 2004; Section 1–11.
4. Carroll JL, Mc Colley SA, Marcus CL, et al. Inability of clinical history to distinguish primary snoring from obstructive sleep apnea in children. Chest 1995; 108:610–618.
5. Brouillette R, Hanson D, David A, et al. A diagnostic approach to suspected sleep apnea in children. J Pediatr 1984; 105:10–14.
6. Mitchell RB, Kelly J. Child behavior after adenotonsillectomy for obstructive sleep apnea syndrome. Laryngoscope 2005; 115:2051–2055.
7. Gozal D. Sleep disordered breathing and school performance in children. Pediatr 1998; 102:616–620.
8. Chan J, Edman JC, Koltai PJ. Obstructive sleep apnea in children. AmFamPhysician 2004; 69:1147–1154.
9. Redline S, Tishler PV, Schlucter M. Risk factors for sleep-disorderd breathing in children. Associations with obesity, race, and respiratory problems. Am J Respir Crit Care Med 1999; 159:1527–1532.
10. De Serres LM, Derkay C, Astley S, et al. Measuring quality of life in children with obstructive sleep disorders. Arch Otolaryngol Head Neck Surg 2000; 126:1423–1429.
11. Chervin RD, Hedger K, Dillon JE, et al. Pediatric sleep questionnaire (PSQ): Validity and reliability of scales for sleep-disordered breathing, snoring, sleepiness, and behavioral problems. Sleep Med 2000; 1(1):21–32.
12. Sohn H, Rosenfeld RM. Evaluation of sleep disordered breathing in children. Otolaryngol Head Neck Surg 2003; 128(3):344–352.
13. Friedman M, Ibrahim H, Bass L. Clinical staging of sleep disordered breathing. Otolaryngol Head Neck Surg 2002; 127:13–21.
14. Waters KA, Everett F, Sillence DO, et al. Treatment of obstructive sleep apnea in achondroplasia. Am J Med Genet 1995; 59(4):460–466.

6

Diagnostic Testing for Sleep-Disordered Breathing and Interpretation of the Polysomnogram

Norman R. Friedman

Department of Otolaryngology/Head and Neck Surgery, University of Colorado Health Sciences Center and The Children's Hospital, Denver, Colorado, U.S.A.

CHAPTER HIGHLIGHTS

- A recent meta-analysis revealed that only 55% of all children suspected to have obstructive sleep apnea (OSA) by clinical evaluation had OSA confirmed by polysomnography (PSG).
- An understanding of sleep terminology is essential to make appropriate clinical decisions.
- A normal oximetry study does not rule out the possibility of sleep-disordered breathing (SDB), and a formal PSG is necessary.
- A clinical role for ambulatory PSG in children has not been established.
- Pediatric sleep medicine may need to accept that adult electroencephalogram (EEG) arousal criteria are not sensitive enough to detect sleep fragmentation in children and should not be the gold standard to measure new diagnostic techniques.
- An obstructive apnea index of greater than one event may be statistically significant, but whether it is clinically relevant remains unclear.
- A child does not need to have severe SDB to experience clinically relevant symptoms.
- Recent investigations have suggested that habitual snoring may not be benign.

INTRODUCTION

One might expect a good patient history would predict the presence of SDB. Yet, multiple studies have shown that history alone fails to reliably predict the presence of SDB (1). A classic study from Johns Hopkins, which stratified patients' symptoms by severity of OSA, failed to demonstrate a high positive predictive value for clinical history. The study used overnight sleep studies (polysomnography) to determine whether a patient had primary snoring or OSA. The scoring criterion for an obstructive apnea (OA) was stringent. To diagnose an OA, the event must have an associated 4% oxygen desaturation (2).

Nowadays, one scores an OA when a child has a nearly complete absence of flow with a persistence of respiratory effort for at least two breaths (3,4). Of the 83 children, 48 were diagnosed with primary snoring, which was defined as an apnea hypopnea index (AHI) of less than one event per hour. The rest had OSA with an AHI of greater than one event per hour. As the study required a 4% oxygen desaturation, some of the primary snorers may actually have had OSA by applying current scoring criteria. Of note, the history did not predict OSA even when the index was raised, so that only the children with severe OSA (index >10 events per hour) were compared to the primary snorers. In a subanalysis of 26 patients who snored but had no scoreable respiratory events, the history did not distinguish the simple primary snorers from those who had obstruction (2). The parents could report loud snoring, mouth breathing, and pauses, but their history was not consistently confirmed by PSG. This implicates that the presence of snoring is not diagnostic of OSA. As the incidence of primary snoring is greater than OSA, most snoring children will not have OSA. The results from a recent systematic review of the medical literature confirmed the findings of Johns Hopkins' investigation. The meta-analysis, which combined the results from 10 studies, revealed that only 55% of all children suspected to have OSA by clinical evaluation had OSA confirmed by PSG (1).

The intention here is to introduce the reader to PSG and the other technology available to diagnose SDB. One will learn how to interpret the results of a sleep study. With technological advances, the clinical interpretation of sleep studies may become more complex. An understanding of the terminology and basic principles underlying PSG will facilitate clinicians' understanding of the results and enhance their ability to provide high-quality clinical care.

TERMINOLOGY

SDB is a relatively new medical specialty. The American Board of Sleep Medicine (ABSM) has recently been approved as a medical specialty by the Accreditation Council of Graduate Medical Education. Diplomates of the ABSM are board-certified physicians from a variety of medical specialties: internal medicine, especially pulmonary medicine, neurology, otolaryngology, pediatrics, and psychiatry. Some diplomates do not have medical degrees. As the field is in its infancy, terminology is only beginning to become standardized.

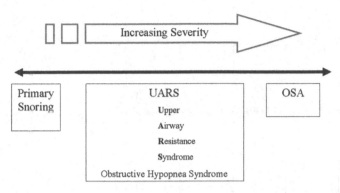

Figure 1   Sleep-disordered breathing is a spectrum of disease that ranges from primary snoring to upper airway resistance syndrome to obstructive sleep apnea. *Abbreviation*: OSA, obstructive sleep apnea.

The review of the literature is confusing because a variety of terms have been used to describe similar events. For example, OSA is now a specific diagnosis rather than a broad term. SDB is a newer term which describes a disrupted breathing pattern. SDB is a spectrum of disease that ranges from primary snoring to upper airway resistance syndrome (UARS) to OSA (Fig. 1) (4).

UARS describes an abnormal breathing pattern without discrete OAs or hypopneas but rather snoring, labored breathing, and paradoxical breathing. To detect UARS may require special equipment that many sleep labs do not use regularly, such as an esophageal manometer probe. OSA occurs when there are either partial or near-complete pauses in the breathing in the presence of persistent respiratory efforts. Some experts consider primary snoring to be the least severe manifestation of SDB and others say it is benign (5). With primary snoring, there is no associated apnea, hypoventilation, or cardiovascular effects on the individual. Recent research in children, however, has suggested that primary snoring may not be benign (6).

Since the first sleep studies in the 1950s, the scoring and quantification of respiratory events have evolved. Two major categories of respiratory events exist: central and obstructive. A central event occurs when airflow ceases secondary to a lack of respiratory effort (Fig. 2). Once again, obstructive respiration has

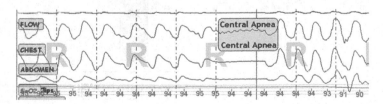

Figure 2   Polysomnogram recording of a central apnea.

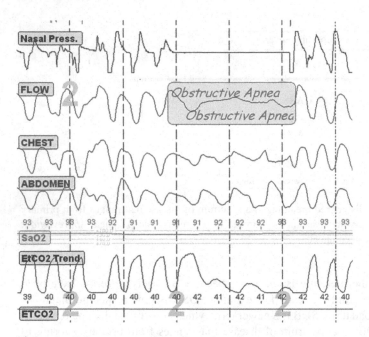

Figure 3   Polysomnogram recording of an obstructive apnea.

persistent respiratory effort but either near-complete cessation of airflow—OA—
or partial cessation of airflow—obstructive hypopnea (OH) (Figs. 3 and 4). The
AASM standard definition of an OA in adults is the near-complete absence of
airflow, with a persistence of respiratory effort for at least 10 seconds. No desaturation is necessary. The most dramatic terminology change occurred when
Medicare guidelines required that a hypopnea be associated with at least a 4%
oxygen desaturation. Previously, a hypopnea needed to have either a 3% to 4%

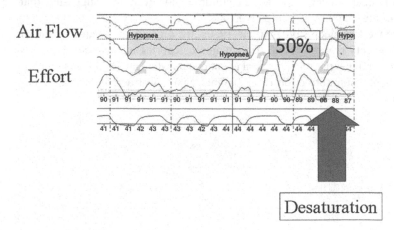

Figure 4   Polysomnogram recording of an obstructive hypopnea.

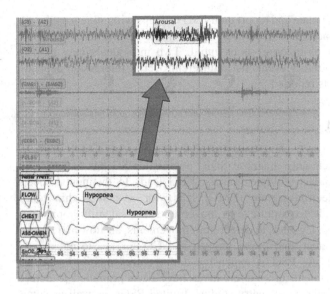

Figure 5 Polysomnogram recording of a respiratory event related arousal.

desaturation or an arousal. Currently, many laboratories score the old hypopnea with an associated arousal as a respiratory event related arousal (RERA) (Fig. 5) (7). Ten seconds was selected arbitrarily-but it does correspond to the amount of time an adult would be apneic if he is breathing at a normal rate of 12 times a minute and misses two breaths. As children have a faster respiratory rate that varies with age, the duration criterion in children is two missed breaths (3).

Besides the variability in scoring respiratory events, numerous indices exist to summarize the sleep study findings: AHI, central apnea index (CAI), respiratory disturbance index (RDI), obstructive apnea/hypopnea index (OAHI), and RERA index (Table 1). The AHI and RDI are the most commonly used terms to report sleep study findings.

Table 1 Indices to Report Polysomnogram Results

Index	Full name	Description
CAI	Central apnea index	Only central respiratory events
AHI	Apnea/hypopnea index	All respiratory events except for RERAs
RDI	Respiratory disturbance index	All respiratory events including RERAs
OAHI	Obstructive apnea/ hypopnea index	Includes OA, OH, and mixed apneas
RERA-I	Respiratory event related arousal index	Only includes RERAs

How clinicians tabulate and report their PSG findings will influence clinical decision-making. If one receives clinical reports from several sleep labs, an understanding of their terminology is essential. Two individuals may have a similar number of respiratory events but a different overall impression depending upon which index is reported.

POLYSOMNOGRAM

As history and examination alone have failed to demonstrate a high positive predictive value to accurately diagnose SDB, overnight PSG has become the gold standard. A PSG has multiple sensors: EEG leads to distinguish sleep from wakefulness, electromyogram (EMG) leads for assessing chin tone, electro-oculograph leads to capture eye movements and identify rapid eye movement (REM) sleep, leg leads to detect limb movements, air flow and respiratory effort belts to detect apnea, and oxygen and CO_2 probes to assess gas exchange (Fig. 6) (8). As PSG is expensive and requires monitoring away from the home environment, other alternatives have been promoted to detect SDB: audiotapes, videotapes, oximetry studies, limited PSGs, as well as some newer technologies. A limited PSG or cardiorespiratory study does not have the sensors which allow for sleep stage scoring: EEG, electro-oculograph, and chin leads. In simple terms, as one increases the number of sensors, the diagnostic accuracy improves. Redundancies are important, especially in children, who frequently either dislodge or intentionally remove the sensors during a sleep study. Importantly, the PSG is the only diagnostic test which has the capability to detect changes in the end tidal CO_2. Monitoring of the end tidal CO_2 is

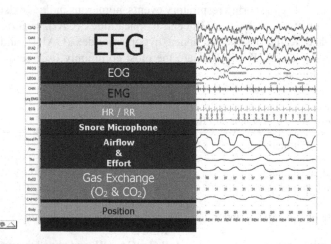

Figure 6 Multiple sensors utilized during polysomonography. *Abbreviations*: EEG, electroencephalogram; EMG, electromyogram; EOG, electro-oculogram; HR, Heart rate; RR, R to R interval.

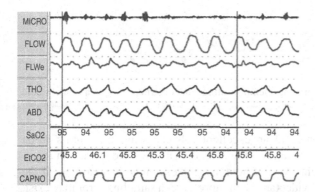

Figure 7 Polysomnogram tracing demonstrating partial obstructive hypoventilation. The end tidal CO_2 is persistently above 45 and the nasal pressure signal demonstrates flow limitation. *Abbreviations*: ABD, abdomen effort belt; CAPNO, capnogram; FLOW, thermistor flow signal; FLWe, nasal pressure flow signal; THO, thorax effort belt.

necessary to diagnose a common type of pediatric SDB, partial obstructive hypoventilation. Partial obstructive hypoventilation is present when the end-tidal CO_2 rises in association with prolonged periods of decreased airflow (Fig. 7) (3,8).

OTHER DIAGNOSTIC TOOLS

Audiotape

The simplest diagnostic tool for a parent is to place a tape recorder in the child's room and press "record." If the objective is to identify snoring, an audiotape is helpful. Cessation of snoring could be an apnea or resumption of breathing. Sounds of a struggle are more predictive for obstruction. A recent investigation which compared home audiotapes to PSG did not demonstrate a role for audiotapes. In this study, the audiotapes were independently rated for the presence of OSA. The PSG divided the subjects into two groups: primary snoring (AHI < 5) and OSA (AHI ≥ 5). The audiotapes' predictive value for either the presence or absence of OSA was not sufficient to promote the audiotape as a reliable test for OSA (9). The tape is a short window in time and does not provide a quantitative assessment. The method is also inefficient for the clinician because one cannot rapidly screen a 30-minute audiotape for OSA.

Videotape

Videotaping is occasionally utilized by parents "to capture" their concerns regarding their child's breathing pattern at night. Once again, the test is nonquantitative. Research has shown that the ability to detect OSA is quite good with a sensitivity of 94%; however, the low specificity (elevated number of false positives) indicated that the clinician review of videotapes actually overdiagnosed the

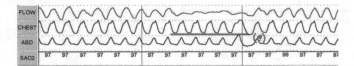

Figure 8   Polysomnogram tracing demonstrating an obstructive apnea with stable oxygenation.

condition (10). The parents did an excellent job capturing the child's worst periods of sleep in this investigation. However, the captured video was not representative of the entire night. Also of note, no gas exchange is measured. If the physician believes that the videotape is unimpressive, a sampling error may exist.

Oximetry

Oximetry would have a greater role in the diagnosis of OSA if all obstructive respiratory events were associated with oxygen desaturations. As previously mentioned, the AASM standard definition of an OA in adults is the near-complete absence of airflow, with a persistence of respiratory effort for at least 10 seconds (7). As an OA does not require an associated oxygen desaturation, one may have repetitive obstructive respiratory events without an oxygen desaturation (Fig. 8). Unless dips are present in the oxygen channel, an oximetry study may mistakenly classify a child with SDB as normal. Characteristically, an abnormal oximetry study has a sawtooth pattern (Fig. 9) (11). Despite the limitations of oximetry, a role for it does exist.

Dr. Broulitte has investigated the role of oximetry and OSA on several occasions. The initial study of 349 patients identified 210 subjects with PSG confirmed OSA. Of these 210 children, 93 also had a positive oximetry study. The positive predictive value was 97%; however, the oximetry study did not identify 56% of the children with PSG-proven OSA (12). A later study assigned grades to 230 oximetry studies, 178 of which were either normal or inconclusive; yet follow-up PSG studies identified OSA in 49% of these patients (13). These studies do not refute the value of oximetry. For a habitually snoring child without any underlying pulmonary conditions, an abnormal oximetry study may be diagnostic for OSA. So, if one has a high suspicion that OSA exists but desires some objective evidence, an abnormal oximetry study is valuable in this setting.

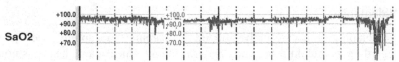

Figure 9   Oximetry tracing with a sawtooth pattern of intermittent oxygen desaturation, which is suggestive of sleep-disordered breathing in a child with snoring and no pulmonary disease.

Oximetry should not be used as a screening test for SDB because it has poor sensitivity. To rule out a clinical disorder, a diagnostic study should have high sensitivity (not many false negative results), otherwise the clinician would falsely assume that the patient is healthy (14). Subsequently, oximetry studies may produce negative results when there actually is a problem. In my experience, clinicians are falsely reassured when a child has a normal oximetry study. If an oximetry study is normal, a formal PSG is necessary. Personally, I feel that oximetry does have utility as a triage tool either to reassure parents who have heightened concern about their child's breathing pattern and access to a sleep study is limited, or to identify patients who have significant hypoxemia and require more urgent attention.

Nap Polysomnogram

If simple tests are unable to reliably diagnose OSA, is an abbreviated PSG or nap PSG sufficient? The nap PSG uses all of the same monitoring sensors as an overnight test, but the test occurs during the day and has a short sampling time (the child may only sleep for one hour). Recognize that while a nap test does not require overnight observation in the sleep unit, the sensor placement can take up to one hour prior to initiating the study. Unfortunately, similar to an oximetry study, a nap PSG has poor sensitivity. Thus, a negative nap PSG would require a confirmatory overnight PSG to conclusively rule out the possibility of OSA (15). The poor sensitivity for a nap PSG is multi-factorial: children over four years rarely nap, supine sleep may not occur, REM sleep is unlikely unless the child is asleep for over 1.5 hours, and all REM periods may not be equivalent.

Ambulatory Polysomnography

An ambulatory or unattended portable PSG, which is performed in a child's own bedroom, would be the ideal setting to evaluate sleep problems. Unfortunately, clinical investigations so far have not established a clinical role for ambulatory PSG in children. However, these studies did not use EEG sensors to accurately determine sleep versus wake states (16,17). The Tucson Children's Assessment of Sleep Apnea (TuCASA) study, which did utilize EEG sensors, advocates the use of a home PSG at least for research purposes. While they did report that 91% of the subjects had a technically acceptable study on the first attempt, limitations existed during the data acquisition that are worth noting. The flow sensors were that most problematic with the thermister and nasal cannula having a signal for at least six hours for only 59% and 52%, respectively. Their definition of "good quality study acquisition" was to have a readable signal from the oximetry, one EEG, and at least two respiratory channels (airflow, thoracic or abdominal) for over five hours. Of note, signal quality was poorer for younger children. Another limitation of this portable device was the inability to measure end tidal P_{CO_2} (18). This is significant because some children, rather than having discrete obstructive respiratory events, instead have prolonged periods of partial obstructive hypoventilation which is manifested by elevated end tidal P_{CO_2} levels (Fig. 7) (3,8). A systematic review of unattended ambulatory PSG studies in adults has found limited data to support a role for its use in detecting sleep apnea (19) and the Centers for Medicare and Medicaid Services have determined that unattended ambulatory PSGs will not be reimbursed, ambulatory PSG will have a minor role in the diagnosis of pediatric SDB.

The major advantage of an *attended* PSG is the constant monitoring provided by the technician overseeing the study. Technicians can note unusual events, correctly label events that are artifact, and replace dislodged data sensors, to name only a few of the many tasks they perform through the course of a night's work. As a technician is available for the entire study, one may add extra sensors to look for other sleep disorders: (*i*) end tidal P_{CO_2} signal for hypoventilation, (*ii*) limb leads for periodic limb movement disorder, and (*iii*) video taping of any unusual sleep disruptions which may be seizure activity or parasomnias. The technician is also able to intervene when necessary. Some patients may be hypoxemic and require oxygen. The addition of oxygen in a controlled environment minimizes the rare risk of unknowingly eliminating a child's respiratory drive.

NEW TECHNOLOGY TO DETECT SLEEP DISRUPTION

A major issue in pediatric sleep medicine is whether our current sleep systems can reliably detect physiological changes in children secondary to the obstructive respiratory events. For adults, obstructive respiratory events are typically associated with an EEG arousal. Arousals disrupt the sleep architecture and are associated with daytime symptoms (20–22). For children with OSA, the sleep architecture is reportedly preserved, making this less useful than for adults (23,24).

Peripheral Arterial Tonometry

Peripheral arterial tonometry (PAT) is a new tool to detect the disruption of the sleep architecture. As EEG (cortical) arousals occur less frequently in children with SDB, recent research is being directed at autonomic (subcortical) arousals. Typically, in response to obstructive respiration, the body has an increase in sympathetic nervous activity. PAT indirectly measures sympathetic activity by noninvasively assessing vasoconstriction in the finger. With an increase in sympathetic discharge, peripheral vasoconstriction occurs and peripheral arterial tone signal at the distal finger attenuates (Fig. 10). A recent investigation demonstrated a good correlation between arousals and PAT-signal attenuations. However, PAT could not distinguish between spontaneous and respiratory-related arousals (25). PAT is not ready to replace PSG, but one should be aware of its existence because it may play a larger clinical role in the future.

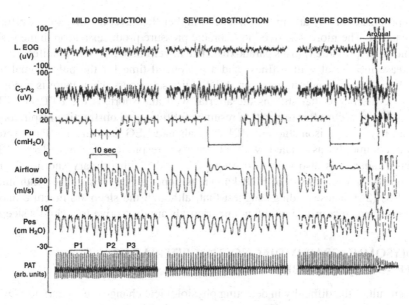

Figure 10 A representative tracing from one subject showing the changes in peripheral arterial tonometry during periods of mild inspiratory flow limitation without a detectable electroencephalogram (EEG) arousal (*left panel*), severe inspiratory flow limitation without a detectable EEG arousal (*middle panel*), and severe inspiratory flow limitation with arousal (*right panel*). L. EOG, left electro-oculogram; C_3-A_2, EEG placement; P_n, nasal pressure; P_{es}, esophageal pressure; $P1$, $P2$, and $P3$ represent periods of 10 cardiac cycles preceding the decrease in P_n ($P1$), at the end of the period of decreased P_n ($P2$), and immediately after P_n is restored to holding pressure ($P3$). *Abbreviation*: PAT, peripheral arterial tonometry. *Source*: Adapted from Ref. 45.

As many PAT events that were detected did not have an associated EEG arousal, PAT may be a more sensitive tool to assess sleep pattern disruption. Alternatively, recognize that PAT will be altered by any event which increases sympathetic tone, such as hypoxemia. Potentially, pediatric sleep medicine will need to accept that adult EEG arousal criteria are not sensitive enough to detect sleep fragmentation in children and should not be the gold standard to measure new diagnostic techniques.

Pulse Transit Time

Another novel diagnostic tool to detect autonomic arousals associated with respiratory events is the pulse transit time (PTT). PTT is an indirect measure of arterial wall stiffness. It measures the time for an arterial pulse pressure wave to travel from the heart to a peripheral site. PTT is inversely proportional to arterial stiffness. The premise underlying PTT is that when an individual with a compromised airway attempts to inhale, a higher than average inspiratory effort is required. The more negative intrathoracic pressure produces a drop in the systemic blood pressure (pulsus paradoxus). The lower blood pressure manifests as a decrease in arterial wall stiffness and a prolonged time for the pulse signal to reach the finger monitoring sensor. A PTT arousal occurs when there is a sympathetic discharge that stiffens the arterial wall and shortens the PTT. A PTT arousal may occur after respiration resumes following an obstructive respiratory event. In a comparison study of PTT arousals and EEG arousals, the PTT were more commonly associated with obstructive respiratory events. The PTT arousal index was also able to distinguish a child with primary snoring from the one with a mild form of SDB known as upper airway resistance syndrome (UARS) (26). These findings suggest that, although the sleep architecture may be preserved, subcortical or autonomic arousals are disruptive to a child's sleep.

POLYSOMNOGRAPHY DIAGNOSTIC CRITERIA FOR SLEEP-DISORDERED BREATHING

As a result of the difficulty in detecting physiological changes secondary to SDB, strict diagnostic criteria for PSG diagnosis of pediatric SDB have not been established. For adults, a distinction is made between OSA and OSA syndrome. To have the syndrome, one must have daytime symptoms, specifically excessive daytime sleepiness, and an index of greater than five obstructive respiratory events per hour is abnormal (27,28). The Wisconsin Sleep Cohort Study demonstrated that one is more likely to have an abnormal sleep study and be asymptomatic than actually have the syndrome of OSA (abnormal index with excessive daytime sleepiness). The prevalence of OSA (AHI >5 events per hour) for adults between 30 and 60 years of age was 24% in men and 9% in women. The prevalence of OSA syndrome was 4% and 2%, respectively (29). For research purposes, The Sleep Institute at Kosair Children's hospital has proposed a composite score for SDB severity (Table 2). In their investigation, children were divided into three groups by their OAHI as well as other PSG measures: (*i*) normal, OAHI <1; (*ii*) mild SDB, OAHI 1 to 5; (*iii*) OSA, OAHI >5 events per hour (30).

A consensus statement from the American Thoracic Society (ATS) states that a child with an OA of any duration with an index that exceeds one event per hour is abnormal (8). The major reference for this recommendation was an investigation that evaluated 50 normal children aged 1 to 18. These children were not suspected to have OSA secondary to their negative score on a standard OSA questionnaire developed by Brouillette. The study did not determine the number of hypopneas, i.e., partial pauses in the breathing (31). The broad age range and lack of hypopnea data force one to question this data as truly reflecting normative values. Recently, Dr. Marcus reviewed the raw data from her initial study and reported that the mean AHI was 0.2 ± 0.6. The statistically significant AHI (i.e., mean ± 2 SD) was 1.5 events per hour (32). Another study from her

Table 2 Composite Score for Polysomnography Severity Scale

	0	1	2	3
OAHI	0–0.9	1.0–4.9	5.0–9.9	≥10.0
RERA	0–0.9	1.0–4.9	5.0–9.9	≥10.0
Total arousal index	0–9.9	10.0–14.9	5.0–9.9	≥20.0
Sat Nadir (%)	≥90	85–89	80–84	≤79

0, normal; 1, mild; 2, moderate; 3, severe; hypopneas = 50% decrease with either 4% desat or arousal; RERA = arousal just after apnea, hypopnea, or snore; total arousal = RERA + technician + spontaneous.
Abbreviations: OAHI, obstructive apnea/hypopnea index; RERA, respiratory event related arousal.
Source: From Ref. 30.

group that evaluated healthy children without any symptoms of SDB determined that the mean OAHI was 0.2 ± 0.3 events per hour. As previously mentioned, a major issue is which technology is being used to identify the respiratory events. This study utilized an oro-nasal thermistor but not a nasal pressure cannula to detect respiratory events (33). As the nasal pressure cannula is recognized as a more sensitive tool for detecting airflow, the actual normative values may be higher. The second edition of the International Classification of Sleep Disorders states that, for children, more than one apnea or hypopnea per hour with a duration of at least two respiratory cycles is abnormal. However, the committee qualified its recommendation, stating that the criteria may be modified once more comprehensive data become available (3). In summary, an OAHI index of greater than one event may be statistically significant, but whether it is clinically relevant remains unclear.

CLINICAL RELEVANCE

The current research is aimed at identifying above what AHI threshold determines clinical relevance. The Sleep Institute at Kosair Children's hospital has developed a sleep pressure score (SPS) to provide an index of sleep disruption in children. Contrary to the other published reports, the sleep architecture was disrupted if the arousals were separated into different groups: spontaneous and respiratory. Despite the total number of arousals being preserved, a child with SDB experienced more RERA and less spontaneous arousals. The sleep pressure score is a mathematical calculation based on these findings (34). To assess the clinical relevance of the SPS, a group of children underwent neurobehavioral testing the day following an overnight PSG. They found that children with a high SPS were more likely to have abnormal testing (35). A high SPS score was associated with an AHI of seven events per hour. These findings have the potential to provide clinical relevance to an AHI threshold (34). The TuCASA also examined the relationship between SDB and daytime functioning, focussing on children between ages 6 and 12. Parents completed a questionnaire and all children underwent ambulatory PSG studies. However, instead of calculating an AHI, the group reported their results as an RDI. Both the Kosair Children's group and the TuCASA group included central apneas in their indices, allowing for comparison of each group's findings. The TuCASA group demonstrated that those children with an RDI greater than five were more likely to have parent-reported snoring, excessive daytime sleepiness, and learning problems. A suba-nalysis of the data, which evaluated gas exchange problems, revealed that the clinical relevance threshold dropped from five to one event per hour if the respir-atory events were associated with a 3% oxygen desaturation (36).

These findings suggest that gas exchange abnormalities contribute to the mor-bidity of SDB. A follow-up prospective study, using formal cognitive testing, sup-ports TuCASA group's initial findings (37). In summary, any child with an AHI of greater than five events per hour appears to have a clinically significant SDB. However, a lower AHI may be clinically relevant if the events are associated with oxygen desaturations. One should be aware that an index of greater than five events per hour is the lower threshold to diagnose OSA in adults (27).

In summary, any child with an AHI of greater than five events per hour appears to have a clinically significant SDB. However, a lower AHI may be clinically relevant if the events are associated with oxygen desaturations. Remember that an index of greater than five events per hour in adults is the lower threshold to diagnose OSA.

IMPLICATIONS OF HABITUAL SNORING

Habitual snoring is perceived as a benign process reflecting vibratory noise of the upper airway during inhalation while asleep. However, a recent study by O'Brien et al. on the neurobehavioral implications of habitual snoring raises concerns that snoring alone may have deleterious consequences. This study excluded any child with parent-reported ADHD or hyperactivity. However, their inclusion criteria allowed for the possibility that a child with occasional obstruction—an AHI of <5, as long as the child was not having obstructive apneic events of more than one per hour—could be included in the primary snoring group (6). The normative data published by the Marcus group contradicts this investigation's definition of primary snoring because an AHI of greater than 1.5 events per hour is statistically significant (32). The TuCASA group also reported that in chil-dren, an AHI less than five events was clinically relevant if the obstructive res-piratory events were associated with 3% oxygen desaturations (36).

In the O'Brien investigation, after identifying children with primary snoring, a comprehensive battery of neurobehavioral tests were administered: differential ability scale (DAS), the developmental neuropsychological assessment (NEPSY), Connor's parent rating scale, and child behavior checklist (CBCL). Significant effects on cognitive testing for reasoning and conceptual ability were demonstrated in all three domains of the DAS. General conceptual ability and verbal and nonverbal clusters are the three domains tested by the DAS. Furthermore, statistically significant differences were detected on language and visuospatial measures by the NEPSY—a cognitive test designed to assess neurobiological development. Subtle differences for hyperactivity and social problems were identified by the Connor scale. Several subscales of the CBCL were also abnormal: social problems, anxiety/depression, attention, delinquency, and internalizing behavior (6).

Recognizing a lack of consensus on the respiratory event threshold to diagnose SDB exists. Some sleep experts would assert that at least a few of these habitually snoring children actually have OSA. Regardless, a child does not need to have severe SDB to experience clinically relevant symptoms.

CLINICAL DIAGNOSIS OF SLEEP-DISORDERED BREATHING

While the gold standard to diagnose SDB remains the overnight PSG study, not every child requires a diagnostic test prior to intervention. One may defer a PSG study if clinically significant obstruction—apnea, retractions, and paradoxical respirations—is either observed by medical personnel or documented by audio–video recording. The expert panel included this exception so that a patient may have therapy expeditiously when the diagnosis is highly probable. If the diagnosis is uncertain or the child would require intensive postoperative monitoring (i.e., a high surgical risk), a preoperative PSG study is recommended (8). For children with nightly snoring, Figure 11 outlines a management algorithm. The pathway relies upon clinical symptoms and tonsil size to make critical decisions. The pharyngeal muscle tone also contributes to one's propensity to experience SDB. However, the measurement of muscle tone is not straightforward. Although the pathway states that an asymptomatic child with markedly enlarged tonsils (4+) should undergo an overnight PSG study, it is reasonable to consider an observation period where the child returns for re-evaluation. One's clinical suspicion of SDB should be heightened in the presence of enlarged tonsils, especially if the parents cannot provide a reliable history. If the child has no clinical symptoms and the tonsils are only moderately enlarged (3+), observation is appropriate. However, educating the parents of the risks of SDB and what to look for is paramount. A PSG study is recommended for a child who has no obvious source of anatomical obstruction (no adenotonsillar hypertrophy with a patent nose), but significant daytime symptoms of SDB. Other conditions, especially a periodic limb movement disorder, may mimic SDB. If the PSG does detect SDB in a child with no adenotonsillar hypertrophy, a complete evaluation of the upper airway by flexible laryngoscopy should be performed to look for other possible sites of obstruction: base of the tongue, lingual tonsils, or

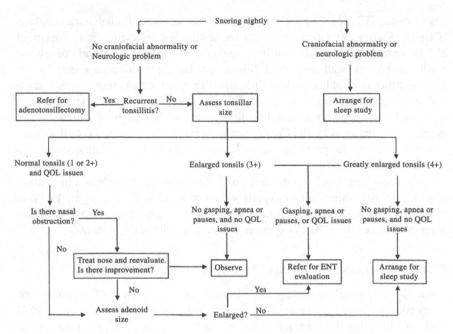

Figure 11 Management algorithm for children with nightly snoring. *Abbreviations*: QOL, quality of life; ENT, ear, nose, and throat. *Source*: Adapted from Ref. 46, Figures 17–19.

hypopharynx or larynx. Imaging studies are also available to help identify where the obstruction is (38–40). Recent investigations have suggested that habitual snoring may not be benign (6,41). If this observation is replicated, clinicians will need to lower their threshold for recommending intervention.

Sleep disorders detected by polysomnogram that are not obstructive:
    Central sleep apnea
    Central hypoventilation
    Parasomnia
    Periodic limb movement disorder
    Periodic breathing
    Obesity hypoventilation
    Seizure

TECHNOLOGY TO DETECT APNEA

SDB in children shows a spectrum of obstruction (4). The measurement techniques utilized in an overnight PSG study can help determine where on the spectrum a child may fall and help quantify the severity of SDB. It is important for a clinician to be aware of which airflow and respiratory effort sensors a sleep laboratory uses, as some airflow sensors are more sensitive in detecting airflow limitation (42). If one refers children to several sleep laboratories, awareness of the collection technique is even more important. Different measurement techniques can produce different results, which could ultimately affect patient care.

Airflow

Although the best method to quantify airflow is a pneumotachograph, most sleep laboratories utilize a nasal thermistor and nasal pressure cannula. The thermistor is a *qualitative* measurement that detects temperature fluctuations with respiration. It does not have a linear relationship to true airflow. A nasal pressure cannula is *quantitative* and does provide a linear approximation of airflow (19). Figure 12 clearly demonstrates that without the nasal pressure transducer, the OA events would go undetected. It is important to note that the nasal pressure is not accurate while the child is mouth breathing. Therefore, to score using the nasal pressure cannula, the monitoring technicians need to note when mouth breathing is present.

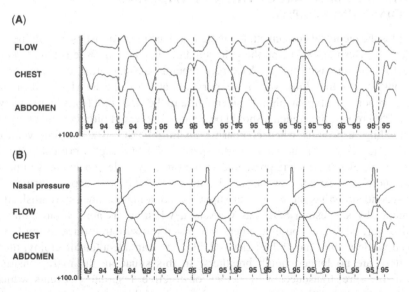

Figure 12 Demonstration of how the nasal pressure is a more sensitive tool to detect airflow limitation. Notice that (A) has only one flow sensor, which is a thermistor that detects fluctuation in temperature and (B) has repetitive obstructive respiratory events identified by a quantitative sensor, the nasal pressure sensor.

Respiratory Effort

Historically, to make a diagnosis of the UARS, an esophageal pressure transducer was considered necessary. Few laboratories, however, consistently use esophageal pressure monitoring. A more widely used airflow sensor is the nasal pressure transducer. A pediatric study that utilized both the nasal and esophageal pressure signals demonstrated good correlation between the two sensors. An increase in esophageal pressure was associated with flow limitation in the nasal pressure channel. Flow limitation suggests that the airway is compromised and SDB is present (43). However, one cannot state that the nasal pressure signal is equivalent to esophageal pressure because the investigators did not independently score respiratory events using the esophageal pressure channel. A study in adults did demonstrate that the nasal pressure signal is comparable to esophageal manometry (44). Addition of a nasal pressure signal to the PSG study will detect more obstructive respiratory events; subsequently, more children will be diagnosed with SDB. One would expect that some children who had previously been diagnosed with primary snoring or UARS by nasal thermister would actually have OSA if the PSG was repeated with a nasal cannula.

PITFALLS TO BE AWARE OF WHEN INTERPRETING A POLYSOMNOGRAPHY

Besides the technical equipment, the patient's sleep characteristics may influence outcomes. Despite PSG being the gold standard, it is not 100% sensitive, largely due to sampling issues. The ATS recommends consideration of repeating a normal PSG if the child does not experience at least one REM period or the parent reports an atypical night of sleep while in the sleep unit (8). When reviewing a PSG report, the clinician should be aware of potential pitfalls which may be misleading, especially when comparing an initial PSG to a post-intervention PSG. The percent of the entire night spent in REM sleep is critical because obstructive events are more prevalent during this stage. Sleep position is important to note, as obstructive events are also more common in the supine position. If the second study has more REM or supine sleep, a higher index may mislead a clinician by suggesting SDB has worsened, when it has not. Often, children with severe SDB are mouth breathers. The nasal pressure transducer is nonfunctional while a child mouth breathes (42,43). After an adenotonsillectomy, most children are no longer mouth breathers. In this situation, the more sensitive nasal pressure transducer will detect obstructive respiratory events which went undetected in the preoperative study, when children were prone to mouth breathe. When assessing gas exchange with the end tidal CO_2, both the numerical value and waveform pattern is important. If the waveform is poor (i.e., has a

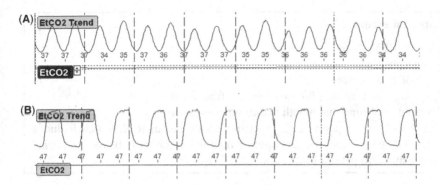

Figure 13 Demonstration of (**A**) "peaked" end tidal CO_2 waveform and (**B**) good or square end tidal CO_2 waveform.

peaked pattern), one will underestimate the actual end tidal CO_2 and may miss the diagnosis of partial obstructive hypoventilation (Fig. 13).

If a child undergoes PSG studies at different laboratories, the method of reporting results may produce further confusion. RDI, AHI, or OAHI are similar terms to quantitate the severity of the study. An RDI will include any respiratory event: OA, hypopnea, central apnea, and an RERA. The AHI includes both central and obstructive respiratory events. The OAHI only includes obstructive respiratory events. Needless to say, these terms are similar but not identical. For a general overview of PSG results, the hypnogram is an excellent resource. On a single page, one can view all the important information which was collected during the 10-hour study. One can review the oxygen status, assess the amount of REM sleep, identify the stage and sleep position when the respiratory events occur, and much more (Fig. 14).

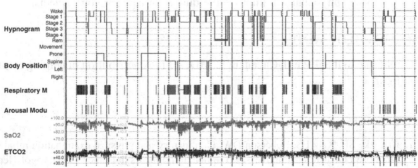

Figure 14 An example of hypnogram in a child with severe sleep-disordered breathing.

Potential errors

Lack of REM sleep
Supine position
Type of flow sensor
Percentage of time that flow sensors are functional
Percentage of time that mouth breathing is present
How results are reported e.g., reporting results as an RDI, which includes
    central apneas, does not accurately reflect the number of obstructive events
Poor waveform pattern for the end tidal CO_2

POSTOPERATIVE SLEEP STUDIES

After the diagnosis of SDB has been established and the child has been treated, what is the role of a postoperative PSG study? The ATS states that children with mild or moderate SDB do not require a follow-up PSG study if they have complete resolution of symptoms after intervention. A postoperative PSG is suggested in the following conditions:

1. persistent symptoms: snoring, disrupted sleep pattern
2. child <1 year of age
3. severe OSA, especially if they have associated hypoxemia and hypercarbia. However, neither the ATS guidelines from 1996 nor the American Academy of Pediatric guidelines from 2002 elaborate on what constitutes severe sleep apnea (8).

CONCLUSION

For the clinician who interprets PSG study results and treats children with SDB, a familiarity with the sleep laboratory that performs the testing is important. An understanding of the terminology is critical. Developing a close relationship between you and your sleep physician will improve the quality of care for your patients.

ACKNOWLEDGMENT

I would like to thank Keith Cavanaugh, MD, for his contribution in helping create the figures.

REFERENCES

1. Brietzke SE, Katz ES, Roberson DW. Can history and physical examination reliably diagnose pediatric obstructive sleep apnea/hypopnea syndrome? Otolaryngol Head Neck Surg 2004; 131(6):827–832.

2. Carroll JL, McColley SA, Marcus CL, Curtis S, Loughlin GM. Inability of clinical history to distinguish primary snoring from obstructive sleep Apnea Syndrome in Children. Chest 1995; 108:610–618.

3. American Academy of Sleep Medicine. International Classification of Sleep Disorders, Diagnostic and Coding Manual. 2nd ed. Westchester, IL: American Academy of Sleep Medicine, 2005:56–59.

4. Cardiorespiratory sleep studies in children. Establishment of normative data and polysomnographic predictors of morbidity. American Thoracic Society. Am J Respir Crit Care Med 1999; 160(4):1381–1387.

5. Clinical practice guideline: diagnosis and management of childhood obstructive sleep apnea syndrome. Pediatrics 2002; 109(4):704–712.

6. O'Brien LM, Mervis CB, Holbrook CR, et al. Neurobehavioral implications of habitual snoring in children. Pediatrics 2004; 114(1):44–49.

7. Kushida CA; Littner MR; Morgenthaler T, et al. Practice parameters for the indications for polysomnography and related procedures: an update for 2005. Sleep 2005; 28(4):499–521.

8. Standards and indications for cardiopulmonary sleep studies in children. American Thoracic Society. Am J Respir Crit Care Med 1996; 153(2):866–878.

9. Lamm C, Mandeli J, Kattan M. Evaluation of home audiotapes as an abbreviated test for obstructive sleep apnea syndrome (OSAS) in children. Pediatr Pulmonol 1999; 27(4):267–272.

10. Sivan Y, Kornecki A, Schonfeld T. Screening obstructive sleep apnoea syndrome by home videotape recording in children. Eur Respir J 1996; 9(10):2127–2131.

11. Shepart JW, Staats BA. Trend oximetry. In: Shepard JW Jr, ed. Shepard Atlas of Sleep Medicine. New York: Futura Publishing Company, 1991:159–169.

12. Brouillette RT, Morielli A, Leimanis A, Waters KA, Luciano R, Ducharme FM. Nocturnal pulse oximetry as an abbreviated testing modality for pediatric obstructive sleep apnea. Pediatrics 2000; 105(2):405–412.

13. Nixon GM, Kermack AS, Davis GM, Manoukian JJ, Brown KA, Brouillette RT. Planning adenotonsillectomy in children with obstructive sleep apnea: the role of overnight oximetry. Pediatrics 2004; 113(1 Pt 1):e19–e25.

14. Ransohoff DF, Feinstein AR. Problems of spectrum and bias in evaluating the efficacy of diagnostic tests. N Engl J Med 1978; 299(17):926–930.

15. Saeed MM, Keens TG, Stabile MW, Bolokowicz J, Davidson Ward SL. Should children with suspected obstructive sleep apnea syndrome and normal nap sleep studies have overnight PSG studies? Chest 2000; 118(2):360–365.

16. Zucconi M, Calori G, Castronovo V, Ferini-Strambi L. Respiratory monitoring by means of an unattended device in children with suspected uncomplicated obstructive sleep apnea: a validation study. Chest 2003; 124(2):602–607.

17. Poels PJ, Schilder AG, van den Berg S, Hoes AW, Joosten KF. Evaluation of a new device for home cardiorespiratory recording in children. Arch Otolaryngol Head Neck Surg 2003; 129(12):1281–1284.

18. Goodwin JL, Enright PL, Kaemingk KL, et al. Feasibility of using unattended polysomnography in children for research—report of the Tucson Children's Assessment of Sleep Apnea study (TuCASA). Sleep 2001; 24(8):937–944.

19. Flemons WW, Littner MR, Rowley JA, et al. Home diagnosis of sleep apnea: a systematic review of the literature. An evidence review cosponsored by the American

Academy of Sleep Medicine, the American College of Chest Physicians, and the American Thoracic Society. Chest 2003; 124(4):1543–1579.

20. Stepanski E, Lamphere J, Badia P, Zorick F, Roth T. Sleep fragmentation and daytime sleepiness. Sleep 1984; 7(1):18–26.

21. Stepanski E, Lamphere J, Roehrs T, Zorick F, Roth T. Experimental sleep fragmentation in normal subjects. Int J Neurosci 1987; 33(3–4):207–214.

22. Chugh DK, Weaver TE, Dinges DF. Neurobehavioral consequences of arousals. Sleep 1996; 19(suppl 10):S198–S201.

23. McNamara F, Issa FG, Sullivan CE. Arousal pattern following central and obstructive breathing abnormalities in infants and children. J Appl Physiol 1996; 81(6): 2651–2657.

24. Wong TK, Galster P, Lau TS, Lutz JM, Marcus CL. Reliability of scoring arousals in normal children and children with obstructive sleep apnea syndrome. Sleep 2004; 27(6):1139–1145.

25. Tauman R, O'Brien LM, Mast BT, Holbrook CR, Gozal D. Peripheral arterial tonometry events and electroencephalographic arousals in children. Sleep 2004; 27(3):502–506.

26. Katz ES, Lutz J, Black C, Marcus CL. Pulse transit time as a measure of arousal and respiratory effort in children with sleep-disordered breathing. Pediatr Res 2003; 53(4):580–588. Epub 2003 Feb 05.

27. Sleep-related breathing disorders in adults: recommendations for syndrome definition and measurement techniques in clinical research. Sleep 1999; 22:667–689.

28. American Academy of Sleep Medicine. International Classification of Sleep Disorders, Diagnostic and Coding Manual. 2nd ed. Westchester, IL: American Academy of Sleep Medicine, 2005:51–55.

29. Young T, Palta M, Dempsey J, Skatrud J, Weber S, Badr S. The occurrence of sleep-disordered breathing among middle-aged adults. N Engl J Med 1993; 328(17): 1230–1235.

30. Montgomery-Downs HE, O'Brien LM, Holbrook CR, Gozal D. Snoring and sleep-disordered breathing in young children: subjective and objective correlates. Sleep 2004; 27(1):87–94.

31. Marcus CL, Omlin KJ, Basinki DJ, et al. Normal polysomnographic values for children and adolescents. Am Rev Respir Dis 1992; 146(5 Pt 1):1235–1239.

32. Witmans MB, Keens TG, Davidson Ward SL, Marcus CL. Obstructive hypopneas in children and adolescents: normal values. Am J Respir Crit Care Med 2003; 168:1540.

33. Traeger N, Schultz B, Pollock AN, Mason T, Marcus CL, Arens R. Polysomnographic values in children 2–9 years old: additional data and review of the literature. Pediatr Pulmonol 2005; 40(1):22–30.

34. Tauman R, O'Brien LM, Holbrook CR, Gozal D. Sleep pressure score: a new index of sleep disruption in snoring children. Sleep 2004; 27(2):274–278.

35. O'Brien LM, Tauman R, Gozal D. Sleep pressure correlates of cognitive and behavioral morbidity in snoring children. Sleep 2004; 27(2):279–282.

36. Goodwin JL, Kaemingk KL, Fregosi RF, et al. Clinical outcomes associated with sleep-disordered breathing in Caucasian and Hispanic children—the Tucson Children's Assessment of Sleep Apnea study (TuCASA). Sleep 2003; 26(5):587–591.

37. Kaemingk KL, Pasvogel AE, Goodwin JL, et al. Learning in children and sleep disordered breathing: findings of the Tucson Children's Assessment of Sleep Apnea (TuCASA) prospective cohort study. J Int Neuropsychol Soc 2003; 9(7):1016–1026.
38. Donnelly LF, Shott SR, LaRose CR, Chini BA, Amin RS. Causes of persistent obstructive sleep apnea despite previous tonsillectomy and adenoidectomy in children with down syndrome as depicted on static and dynamic cine MRI. AJR Am J Roentgenol 2004; 183(1):175–181.
39. Rama AN, Tekwani SH, Kushida CA. Sites of obstruction in obstructive sleep apnea. Chest 2002; 122(4):1139–1147.
40. Shepard J, Gefter W, Guilleminault C, et al. Evaluation of the upper airway in patients with obstructive sleep apnea. Sleep 1991; 14:361–371.
41. Goldstein NA, Pugazhendhi V, Rao SM, et al. Clinical assessment of pediatric obstructive sleep apnea. Pediatrics 2004; 114(1):33–43.
42. Serebrisky D, Cordero R, Mandeli J, Kattan M, Lamm C. Assessment of inspiratory flow limitation in children with sleep-disordered breathing by a nasal cannula pressure transducer system. Pediatr Pulmonol 2002; 33(5):380–387.
43. Trang H, Leske V, Gaultier C. Use of nasal cannula for detecting sleep apneas and hypopneas in infants and children. Am J Respir Crit Care Med 2002; 166:464–468.
44. Ayappa I, Norman RG, Krieger AC, Rosen A, O'malley RL, Rapoport DM. Noninvasive detection of respiratory effort-related arousals (REras) by a nasal cannula/pressure transducer system. Sleep 2000; 23(6):763–771.
45. O'Donnell CP, Allan L, Atkinson P, Schwartz AR. The effect of upper airway obstruction and arousal on peripheral arterial tonometry in obstructive sleep apnea. Am J Respir Crit Care Med 2002; 166(7):965–971.
46. Johnson CE, Kelley PE, Friedman NR, Chan KH, Berman S. Ear, nose and throat. In: Hay W, Hayward A, Levin M, Sondheimer JM, eds. Current Pediatric Diagnosis and Treatment. 16th ed. New York: The McGraw Hill Companies, 2003:487.

7

Sleep-Disordered Breathing in High-Risk Children

Ron B. Mitchell

Department of Otolaryngology and Pediatrics, Saint Louis University School of Medicine, Cardinal Glennon Children's Medical Center, St. Louis, Missouri

James Kelly

Department of Surgery, University of New Mexico, Albuquerque, New Mexico, U.S.A.

CHAPTER HIGHLIGHTS

- High-risk children are those affected by obesity, neuromuscular or craniofacial disorders, Down syndrome, and mucopolysaccharidoses as well as a number of other disorders such as cerebral palsy (CP), Prader-Willi syndrome (PWS), achondroplasia, Arnold-Chiari malformations, and sickle cell disease.
- The prevalence of sleep-disordered breathing (SDB) in these children is higher than in the general population of children. There is a temptation to downplay the significance of sleep disturbances in these children, given the other grave problems that affect them, and the problem is frequently underestimated.
- High-risk children are more likely to have upper airway obstruction that is multifactorial in etiology, they more commonly have perioperative complications, and adenotonsillectomy may lead to only partial resolution of SDB.
- Surgical therapy should be viewed as beneficial rather than uniformly curative.

INTRODUCTION

Adenotonsillar hypertrophy is the most common cause of SDB in children, and adenotonsillectomy has been shown to be an effective treatment in the majority of these children (1). However, the surgical management of SDB is more complex in children considered to be at high risk. Such children are more likely to have upper airway obstruction that is multifactorial in etiology, they more commonly have perioperative complications, and adenotonsillectomy may lead to only partial resolution of SDB. Surgical management in these cases requires a multidisciplinary approach including general pediatrics, pediatric pulmonology, anesthesiology, and otolaryngology. Furthermore, in recent years, there has been increasing recognition of the association between SDB and both nighttime and daytime behavioral problems in children. These problems are often exacerbated in high-risk children, and resolution of behavioral problems after surgery is more difficult to evaluate.

In this chapter the prevalence, surgical management, and outcome of adenotonsillectomy for SDB in specific populations of high-risk children will be discussed. High-risk children are those affected by obesity, neuromuscular or craniofacial disorders, Down syndrome, and mucopolysaccharidoses as well as a number of other disorders such as CP, PWS, achondroplasia, Arnold-Chiari malformations, and sickle cell disease. Emphasis will be placed on the prevalence of SDB in the populations of high-risk children encountered most frequently. The specific precautions that may be necessary when adenotonsillectomy is undertaken as therapy for SDB in these children is discussed, as well as recent studies of the outcome of surgical therapy for SDB in high-risk children.

OBESITY

- The prevalence of childhood obesity in the United States has doubled over the last quarter century.
- The prevalence of SDB in children with obesity is 25% to 40%.
- Adenotonsillectomy leads to improvement but not resolution of the underlying sleep disorder in the majority of obese children.

The prevalence of childhood obesity in the United States has risen from 6% to 14% over the last quarter century (2,3). There is also increasing evidence that childhood obesity is a worldwide problem (4). The prevalence of SDB in children with obesity is 25% to 40% (5). SDB in obese children is associated with a decrease in the cross-sectional area of the upper airway caused by adipose tissue immediately adjacent to the pharynx (6). In addition, there may be external compression of the upper airway by fat in the subcutaneous tissues of the neck (7). Enlarged tonsils and adenoids in obese children further decrease the cross-sectional area of the pharynx.

There are relatively few studies that have examined the outcome of adenotonsillectomy for SDB in obese children. Kudoh and Sanai (8) studied 25 obese children prospectively for a period of five to six days after adenotonsillectomy for SDB. They showed that during this brief follow-up period surgery was effective in decreasing irregular breathing and oxygen desaturation during sleep, as measured by pulse oximetry. Marcus et al. (9) studied eight obese children with SDB diagnosed by polysomnography (PSG). After adenotonsillectomy caregivers reported an improvement in sleep disturbances. Postoperative PSG was performed in two of these children and this showed resolution of SDB in both. Soultan et al. (10) reported a retrospective study of 17 obese children with SDB after adenotonsillectomy. The caregivers of eight of these children reported resolution of the symptoms of SDB after surgery. One child continued to have persistent snoring and in another child no improvement was reported. The remaining children were lost to follow-up. These studies were limited by the absence of data from PSG before and after adenotonsillectomy and by the small populations of children studied.

Mitchell and Kelly (11) studied 30 children who underwent adenotonsillectomy for SDB (Fig. 1). PSG was used preoperatively to diagnose the severity of SDB in each child and postoperatively to evaluate the outcome of surgery. The study showed that obese children with SDB have a clear improvement in physiological parameters of sleep and in quality of life after adenotonsillectomy. The respiratory distress index decreased from a mean of 30.0 before surgery to

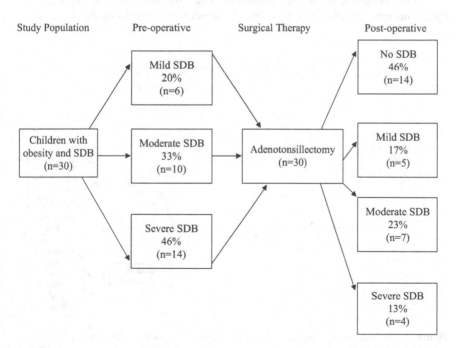

Figure 1 Adenotonsillectomy for sleep-disordered breathing in obese children. *Abbreviation*: SDB, sleep-disordered breathing.

11.6 after surgery. However, 16 of the 30 children (54%) continued to have significant SDB after surgery. The improvements in sleep disturbances occurred without any significant change in age- and gender-corrected body mass index (BMI) for the study population. This suggests that adenotonsillectomy for SDB leads to improvement but not resolution of the underlying sleep disorder in the majority of obese children.

Obese children with SDB have been shown to have neurocognitive abnormalities including reduced learning, memory, and language skills (12). It has been postulated that decreased activity and hypersomnolence, both known to be consequences of SDB in children, may lead to obesity (13,14). Therefore, it is logical to propose that treating SDB by adenotonsillectomy would lead to increased activity, weight loss, and improved learning. Surprisingly, Soultan et al. (10) showed that surgical treatment of SDB is associated with increased weight in obese children. Kudoh and Sanai (8) reported no decrease in weight after adenotonsillectomy for obstructive sleep apnea in obese children, despite the fact that dietary treatment was given before surgery. These reports suggest that adenotonsillectomy may improve SDB but does not lead to weight reduction. Clearly, the treatment of obese children with SDB is complex (Fig. 2) and involves dietary, behavioral, and surgical therapies as well as a greater understanding of the causes of obesity in children (15).

In conclusion, obesity in children is increasing and consequently more of these children are likely to be referred for adenotonsillectomy to treat SDB.

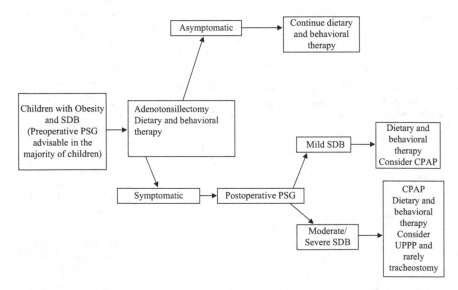

Figure 2 Treatment of sleep-disordered breathing in children with obesity. *Abbreviations*: CPAP, continuous positive airway pressure; PSG, polysomnography; SDB, sleep-disordered breathing; UPPP, uvulopalatopharyngoplasty.

Surgical therapy improves but does not always resolve SDB. Obese children with SDB who remain symptomatic should be studied postoperatively with PSG. Those with persistent SDB may benefit from treatment with continuous positive airway pressure (CPAP) (16).

DOWN SYNDROME

- Anatomical abnormalities along with generalized hypotonia and a tendency to obesity make the prevalence of SDB in children with Down syndrome very high.
- A delay in diagnosis of SDB in children with Down syndrome is the rule.
- Even though adenotonsillectomy may be successful initially, recurrence of symptoms of SDB is high. It is important to inform caregivers that multiple interventions are often required.

Children with Down syndrome have multiple anatomic and physiologic factors that predispose them to SDB. These include midfacial and mandibular hypoplasia, macroglossia, a narrow nasopharynx, and a shortened palate (17,18). These anatomical abnormalities along with generalized hypotonia and a tendency to obesity make the prevalence of SDB in children with Down syndrome much higher than in the general population of children. Furthermore, gastroesophageal reflux disease (GERD) (19) and chronic lung disease (20) are also common in children with Down syndrome and may worsen airway problems.

The prevalence of SDB in children with Down syndrome is reported to be between 50% and 100% (21–23). Marcus et al. (22) reported SDB documented by PSG in all 53 children with Down syndrome enrolled in their study. Levanon et al. (24) found that all children with Down syndrome whose parents reported a sleep disturbance had SDB when they were studied using PSG. However, several other studies reported a lower prevalence of SDB in children with Down syndrome. Dyken et al. (21) studied 19 children with Down syndrome using PSG. They found that SDB was present in 79% of these children and the severity of the sleep disturbance was directly related to BMI and inversely related to age. Miguel-Diez et al. (23) showed a 55% prevalence of SDB in children with Down syndrome and this was higher in younger male children but was not increased by a higher BMI. Mitchell et al. (11) studied 23 children with Down syndrome and upper airway obstruction who presented to an otolaryngology clinic and found that laryngomalacia was the most common cause of the obstruction in children under two, but SDB was more common in children older than two.

As noted earlier, SDB may have several different clinical presentations including daytime somnolence, behavioral problems, poor school performance and, in younger children, developmental delay and enuresis (25). Since many of these factors are also associated with Down syndrome, a delay in diagnosis of SDB in children with Down syndrome is usually the rule. Nevertheless, it is evident that the prevalence of SDB in children with Down syndrome is high.

The difference in reported prevalence rates between studies is likely to be a result of selection bias. Children with Down syndrome who present to a sleep or otolaryngology clinic are more likely to have SDB than children with Down syndrome in the general population. However, the prevalence of SDB in children with Down syndrome appears to be underestimated by both caregivers and healthcare providers. In addition, assessing improvements in behavior following surgery for SDB in children with Down syndrome may be extremely complex (26).

Adenotonsillectomy remains the treatment of choice for children with Down syndrome and SDB (20). Additional procedures such as uvulopalatopharyngoplasty (UPPP) and tracheostomy may be necessary in selected children (Fig. 3). Strome et al. (27) recommended UPPP for all children with Down syndrome since the results were better than tonsillectomy alone. However, when UPPP is performed, the alteration in the oropharyngeal anatomy may convert a child with SDB into a "silent obstructor." Nonetheless, significant SDB demonstrated by postoperative PSG has been reported in up to 60% of children with Down syndrome (20,28). Donnelly et al. (29) studied 27 children with Down syndrome and persistent SDB after adenotonsillectomy using cine magnetic resonance imaging (MRI). The most common causes of obstruction in these children included macroglossia, glossoptosis, recurrent enlargement of the adenoids, and enlarged

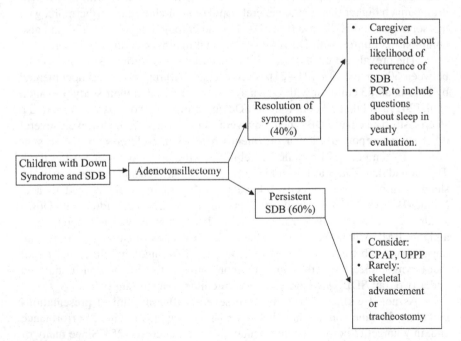

Figure 3 Treatment of sleep-disordered breathing in children with Down syndrome. *Abbreviations*: CPAP, continuous positive airway pressure; PCP, primary care physician; SDB, sleep-disordered breathing; UPPP, uvulopalatopharyngoplasty.

lingual tonsils. The outcome of other therapies for children with Down syndrome and SDB such as CPAP and skeletal advancement remains unknown (30).

Thus children with Down syndrome have a high prevalence of SDB that is multifactorial and responds partially to adenotonsillectomy (Fig. 3). Even though surgery may be successful initially, recurrence of symptoms of SDB is high. It is important to inform caregivers that multiple interventions are often required and that the success rate is lower than what is expected in the general population of children.

NEUROMUSCULAR DISEASE

- The symptoms of SDB in children with neuromuscular disease is probably underestimated and often difficult to distinguish from the underlying disease.
- Outcome studies of the benefits of surgical therapy for SDB in these children are limited by difficulties in obtaining study populations of children with comparable disorders.
- The possible treatment options include adenotonsillectomy with or without UPPP, tracheostomy, or bi-level positive airway pressure (BiPAP).

Neuropathies, congenital myopathies, muscular dystrophies, myotonias, and myasthenia gravis usually lead to both central and obstructive apneas (31). Children with neuromuscular disease have loss of respiratory muscle function and a drop in central respiratory drive. However, it is likely that some central apneas are in effect obstructive but appear central because of weak respiratory effort (32). This is worsened by diaphragmatic dysfunction that limits the ability to compensate for the sleep-related drop in alveolar ventilation. SDB commonly presents as hypopneas and desaturations during rapid eye movement (REM) sleep that progresses to include nonREM sleep.

SDB in children with neuromuscular disease often manifests as daytime sleepiness, fatigue, drowsiness, morning headaches, and failure to thrive. It can be difficult to distinguish clinically between the underlying neuromuscular disease and SDB. Equally, this limits attempts to determine the prevalence of SDB in these children, which is probably underestimated (33,34).

The possible treatment options in children with neuromuscular disease and SDB include adenotonsillectomy with or without UPPP (35), tracheostomy, or BiPAP. The latter can be used by mask or through a tracheostomy with good results (36,37). Children with neuromuscular disease are at risk of malignant hyperthermia and this should be discussed with the anesthesiologist prior to surgery (38). Therapeutic options should be individualized with careful follow-up including clinical assessment and PSG.

Children with neuromuscular diseases form a heterogeneous group based on the etiology of individual disorders. As a consequence, outcome studies of

the benefits of adenotonsillectomy for SDB in these children are limited by difficulties in obtaining study populations of children with comparable disorders. It is
quite possible that children with different neuromuscular diseases respond selec-
tively to surgical therapy for SDB, but this remains to be determined in future
outcome studies.

MUCOPOLYSACCHARIDOSES

- SDB is common in children with mucopolysaccharidosis because of
  upper airway narrowing caused by hypertrophy of the tongue, tonsils,
  adenoids, and mucous membranes.
- More than 50% of children with mucopolysaccharidosis have symptoms of SDB.
- Children with mucopolysaccharidosis can be difficult to intubate
  because of soft tissue deposits in the hypopharynx and larynx as well
  as reduced extension of the neck.
- It is essential to realize that SDB is a severe and progressive consequence of mucopolysaccharidosis and not infrequently the cause of
  death in these children.

Mucopolysaccharidoses are a group of genetic disorders characterized by
enzyme deficiencies that lead to defective catabolism of lysosomal glycosamino-
glycans and accumulation of mucopolysaccharides in the soft tissues of the body.
The specific enzyme deficiency determines the type of mucopolysaccharidosis
and includes Hurler and Scheie syndrome (α-L-iduronidase deficiency), Hunter
syndrome (iduronate sulfatase deficiency), and Sly syndrome (β-glucuronidase
deficiency) (39).

SDB is common in children with mucopolysaccharidosis because of upper
airway narrowing caused by hypertrophy of the tongue, tonsils, adenoids, and
mucous membranes. This narrowing is worsened by a physiological decrease
in tone of the supporting muscles of the pharynx and increased airway resistance.
The lower airway is narrowed by glycosaminoglycan deposits in the tracheo-
bronchial mucosa, scoliosis, and thoracic hyperkyphosis. Abdominal dimensions
are reduced due to spinal problems and hepatosplenomegaly. It is, therefore,
not surprising that SDB is often severe in these children and may be a cause of
death.

The prevalence of SDB in children with mucopolysaccharidosis is high.
Semenza et al. (40) reported that more than 50% of children with mucopolysaccharidosis had symptoms of SDB and 89% of those tested had moderate to severe
SDB confirmed by PSG. Leighton et al. (39) studied 26 children with mucopolysaccharidosis using PSG and reported a high prevalence of SDB in these children
(88%). The sleep disturbance was often severe and was related to the type of
mucopolysaccharidosis. For example, all children with Hurler or Hunter
syndromes had significant SDB, while the two children with Maroteaux-Lamy

syndrome had normal PSG examinations. Clearly, any further conclusions were limited by the small size of the study population.

The therapeutic options in children with mucopolysaccharidosis and SDB include adenotonsillectomy (41), nasal CPAP (42), and tracheostomy (40). Children with mucopolysaccharidosis can be difficult to intubate because of reduced extension of the neck and this should be anticipated preoperatively. Pre- and postoperative PSG is essential to assess the outcome of surgery since caregivers' reports of the severity of SDB tend to be inaccurate. Caregivers often underestimate the severity of SDB in moderate or severe cases and overestimate the severity in mild cases (39). When considering surgery as a therapeutic option, it is essential to realize that SDB is a severe and progressive consequence of mucopolysaccharidosis and not infrequently the cause of death in these children (43).

CRANIOFACIAL SYNDROMES

- These include craniofacial anomalies such as Apert, Crouzon, and Pfeiffer syndromes.
- The prevalence of SDB in these children is estimated at 40% to 50%.
- Causes of SDB in these children result in a complex clinical picture that may vary over time.
- Surgical therapy is rarely curative.

Craniofacial deformities result from abnormal development of the brain, cranium, and facial skeleton. Premature fusion of cranial growth plates as well as abnormal facial bone development lead to craniofacial anomalies such as Apert, Crouzon, and Pfeiffer syndromes. Children with such craniofacial syndromes are at a high risk for SDB. The structural abnormalities of the upper airway include a hypoplastic maxilla and a high-arched palate that lead to crowding of the nasopharynx, a hypoplastic mandible that leads to reduced dimensions of the oropharynx, and a number of congenital laryngeal abnormalities including subglottic stenosis (44). Upper airway obstruction due to these structural abnormalities is worsened by frequent upper respiratory infections and GERD.

The prevalence of SDB in children with craniofacial syndromes is estimated at 40% to 50% (45). The variety of causes of SDB in these children results in a complex clinical picture that may vary over time. In young children, the causes of SDB may be primarily nasal, while as the child gets older, oropharyngeal obstruction secondary to tonsillar hypertrophy may become increasingly important. In a retrospective study, Hoeve et al. (45) reported that symptoms of SDB were recorded in 26% of children with craniofacial syndromes, and that only a small number of these children underwent PSG. In another retrospective study, Pijpers et al. (46) showed that 26% of children with Apert, Crouzon, or Pfeiffer syndromes had clinical symptoms of SDB, while a questionnaire sent to caregivers indicated a prevalence of SDB in 53% of the same children. Both studies concluded that there was a tendency for healthcare providers to under-estimate SDB in children with craniofacial syndromes and recommended more awareness of the importance of diagnosing sleep problems in these children.

PSG is the investigation of choice both for diagnosis of SDB and for the evaluation of treatment outcomes in children with craniofacial deformities. Endoscopy and cephalometry may also be helpful in preoperative planning (45). Therapeutic options include adenotonsillectomy, UPPP, CPAP, maxillary and mandibular advancement, and tracheostomy. Nishikawa et al. (44) reported a successful outcome after adenotonsillectomy in six out of nine children with SDB and craniofacial deformities. They also reported good results in two patients on long-term CPAP. Pijpers et al. (46) reported on 24 children with craniofacial syndromes who underwent adenotonsillectomy. Four of these children required oxygen the first night postoperatively. A further 11 children underwent maxillary and mandibular advancement and four of these required a postoperative tra-cheostomy. Two children were treated with CPAP. Unfortunately, pre- and post-operative PSG were not reported on these children. The relative effectiveness of different modalities for the treatment of SDB in children with craniofacial syn-dromes remains unknown because most reports are limited to retrospective case series with very small study populations.

OTHER HIGH-RISK POPULATIONS

Cerebral Palsy

- Poor neuromuscular control, seizure disorders, GERD, and increased oropharyngeal secretions lead to a high prevalence of SDB in children with CP.
- A tracheostomy is often considered a first-line treatment for SDB but may not always be the best option.
- Good results have also been reported with adenotonsillectomy, UPPP, tongue hyoid advancement, mandibular advancement, and tongue reduction.

Children with CP are at a high risk for SDB because of poor neuromuscular control, seizure disorders, GERD, and increased oropharyngeal secretions. Adenotonsillar hypertrophy together with decreased tone of the pharyngeal mus-culature during sleep contribute to upper airway collapse. Children with CP and spastic quadriplegia are also less able to compensate for upper airway obstruction by repositioning their bodies (47). The prevalence of SDB in children with CP is unknown but is likely to be high. Kotagal et al. (47) reported SDB in five of nine children with CP [22] studied using PSG. These children also had a high number of respiratory disturbances per hour of sleep.

A tracheostomy is often considered a first-line treatment for SDB in children with CP. However, a tracheostomy may not always be the best option.

A tracheostomy can limit the child's daycare options and may lead to a significant increase in the caregiver's responsibilities. Good results have also been reported with adenotonsillectomy, UPPP, tongue hyoid advancement, mandibular advancement, and tongue reduction (48,49). Occasionally, an ethics consult can help direct care.

Prader-Willi Syndrome

- Children with PWS have severe infantile hypotonia, craniofacial abnormalities, and obesity that all contribute to SDB.
- Early detection and treatment of SDB in children with PWS may delay the development of cor pulmonale, the most common cause of death in these children.

PWS is a genetic disorder caused by loss of paternal genes located on chromosome 15. Children with PWS have severe infantile hypotonia, feeding difficulties, developmental delay, craniofacial abnormalities, and obesity. They often have sleep abnormalities including SDB. The causes of SDB in children with PWS include facial dysmorphism, hypotonia, and obesity. Adenotonsillar hypertrophy is a contributing factor (50).

The prevalence of SDB in children with PWS is difficult to establish and depends on the selection criteria used in different studies (50). However, SDB may not be universal in these children and the severity of the sleep disorder, when it occurs, does not appear to be directly related to the degree of obesity (51). Early detection and treatment of SDB in children with PWS may delay the development of cor pulmonale, the most common cause of death in these children (50). Adenotonsillectomy is the first-line treatment. Pre- and postoperative PSG should be performed routinely in children with PWS. Other operative procedures such as UPPP or tracheostomy need to be considered on a case-by-case basis as does the use of CPAP (52).

Achondroplasia

- Children with achondroplasia are predisposed to SDB because of midfacial hypoplasia, dysplasia of the basi-occiput, foramen magnum stenosis with compression of the cervical spinal cord, and thoracic cage restriction.
- Surgical management of SDB in these children includes adenotonsillectomy, ventriculoperitoneal shunt, and foramen magnum decompression.

Achondroplasia, the most common form of dwarfism, is an autosomal dominant syndrome that is most commonly caused by a mutation in fibroblast growth factor receptor-3 (53). Children with achondroplasia are predisposed to SDB because of midfacial hypoplasia, dysplasia of the basi-occiput, foramen magnum stenosis with compression of the cervical spinal cord, and thoracic cage restriction. The prevalence of SDB in children with achondroplasia is about 40% (54). Tasker et al. (55) identified three distinct groups of children with achondroplasia and SDB. Group 1 (35%) were the least symptomatic and had only SDB. Group 2 (35%) had SDB as well as hydrocephalus and a small foramen magnum. Group 3 (30%), the most severely affected group, also had cor pulmonale and cardiorespiratory failure. PSG (56) as well as neurological and respiratory physiological assessments should be used preoperatively in children with achondroplasia and SDB (55). Preoperatively, an MRI scan of the cervical spine can demonstrate spinal cord compression. Surgical management of SDB in these children includes adenotonsillectomy, ventriculoperitoneal shunt, and foramen magnum decompression. In the study by Tasker et al., adenotonsillectomy was most successful in Group 1. Over 80% of these children showed improvement or resolution of SDB after surgery (54,55).

Arnold-Chiari Malformations

- Apnea occurs as a consequence of brainstem compression.
- Both central and obstructive apneic episodes are usually seen in these children.
- Surgical management involves decompression of the Chiari malformation.

These intracranial malformations are caused by elongation of the hindbrain and lead to apnea as a consequence of brainstem compression. The diagnosis is by MRI. Type I, which usually presents in young adulthood, is caused by elongation of the cerebellar tonsils that are displaced into the upper cervical canal. Type II is associated with myelodysplasia and meningomyelocele. It is the most common form of the disorder and presents in childhood. Type III also includes cervical spina bifida and herniation of the cerebellum (57). Both central and obstructive apneic episodes are usually seen in these children, and preoperative PSG is essential. There is evidence that SDB is underestimated in these children (57,58). Surgical management involves decompression of the Chiari malformation.

Sickle Cell Anemia

- Adenotonsillectomy is advisable as early as possible since SDB could be an important predisposing factor in the etiology of cerebrovascular accidents in these children.
- Children should be admitted to the hospital one night before surgery for hydration, transfused with red blood cells to reduce the concentration of sickle cell hemoglobin to less than 30%, and discharged only after adequate oral intake is achieved.

Sickle cell anemia is an autosomal recessive disorder of hemoglobin that alters the properties of red blood cells and is associated with varying degrees of anemia (59). Strokes, transient ischemic attacks, and seizures are common in sickle cell disease. Hypoxia promotes polymerization of sickle hemoglobin and the adhesion of red cells to endothelium. Both episodic and continuous nocturnal hypoxemia are common in sickle cell disease, possibly because of upper-airway obstruction secondary to adenotonsillar hypertrophy (60). Children with sickle cell anemia and a clinical history of SDB should have routine preoperative PSG. If hypoxemia is present, adenotonsillectomy is advisable as early as possible since SDB could be an important predisposing factor in the etiology of cerebrovascular accidents in these children. Preoperative management includes admission to the hospital one night before surgery for hydration, transfusion of red blood cells to reduce the concentration of sickle cell hemoglobin to less than 30% (61), and discharge only after adequate oral intake. A good outcome with resolution of symptoms and improvement in alveolar hypoventilation has been shown in a number of studies of adenotonsillectomy in children with sickle cell anemia (61–63).

CONCLUSIONS

Early recognition of the symptoms and consequences of SDB is important for practitioners involved in the care of high-risk children. These are children with obesity, neuromuscular or craniofacial disorders, Down syndrome, mucopolysaccharidoses, and a number of other disorders including CP, PWS, achondroplasia, Arnold-Chiari malformations, and sickle cell disease. There is a temptation to downplay the significance of sleep disturbances in these children, given the other grave problems that affect them. However, it should be recognized that SDB, when left untreated in high-risk children, may lead to complications such as right heart failure, cor pulmonale, or even sudden death.

A multidisciplinary approach is essential in the surgical management of SDB in high-risk children. In addition to general pediatrics, the team for management of these children should include pulmonology, anesthesiology, and otolaryngology. With respect to surgical therapy for SDB in high-risk children, adenotonsillectomy should be viewed as beneficial rather than uniformly curative. However, adenotonsillectomy not only improves the symptoms of SDB but also preserves the integrity of the airway so that more aggressive surgical treatment can be avoided. Evaluation of the outcome of adenotonsillectomy for SDB in high-risk children is complex, since this surgery does not address the other comorbidities that affect them. It is the goal of future research to establish adjunct therapies to maximize the benefits of adenotonsillectomy for SDB in high-risk children.

REFERENCES

1. Suen JS, Arnold JE, Brooks, LJ. Adenotonsillectomy for treatment of obstructive sleep apnea in children. Arch Otolaryngol Head Neck Surg 1995; 121:525–530.
2. National Center for Health Statistics. Health, United States. Washington, DC, 2001.

3. National Center for Health Statistics. Prevalence of overweight among children and adolescents: United States. Washington, DC, 1999. http://www.cdc.gov/nchs/products/pubs/pubd/hestats/overwght99.htm.
4. Reilly JJ. Physical activity and obesity in childhood and adolescence. Lancet 2005; 366:268–269.
5. Wing YK, Hui SH, Pak WM, et al. A controlled study of sleep related disordered breathing in obese children. Arch Dis Child 2003; 88:1043–1047.
6. Shelton KE, Woodson H, Gay S, et al. Pharyngeal fat in obstructive sleep apnea. Am Rev Respir Dis 1993; 148:462–466.
7. Koenig JS, Thach BT. Effects of mass loading on the upper airway. J Appl Physiol 1988; 64:2294–2299.
8. Kudoh F, Sanai A. Effect of tonsillectomy and adenoidectomy on obese children with sleep-associated breathing disorders. Acta Otolaryngol Suppl 1996; 523:216–218.
9. Marcus CL, Curtis S, Koerner CB, et al. Evaluation of pulmonary function and polysomnography in obese children and adolescents. Pediatr Pulmonol 1996; 21: 176–183.
10. Soultan Z, Wadowski S, Rao M, et al. Effect of treating obstructive sleep apnea by tonsillectomy and/or adenoidectomy on obesity in children. Arch Pediatr Adolesc Med 1999; 153:33–37.
11. Mitchell RB, Kelly J. Adenotonsillectomy for obstructive sleep apnea in obese children. Otolaryngol Head Neck Surg 2004; 131:104–108.
12. Rhodes SK, Shimoda KC, Waid LR, et al. Neurocognitive deficits in morbidly obese children with obstructive sleep apnea. J Pediatr 1995; 127:741–744.
13. Gupta NK, Mueller WH, Chan W, et al. Is obesity associated with poor sleep quality in adolescents? Am J Hum Biol 2002; 14:762–768.
14. von Kries R, Toschke AM, Wurmser H, et al. Reduced risk for overweight and obesity in 5- and 6-y-old children by duration of sleep—a cross-sectional study. Int J Obes Relat Metab Disord 2002; 26:710–716.
15. Slyper AH. Childhood obesity, adipose tissue distribution, and the pediatric practitioner. Pediatrics 1998; 102:e4.
16. Marcus CL, Ward SL, Mallory GB, et al. Use of nasal continuous positive airway pressure as treatment of childhood obstructive sleep apnea. J Pediatr 1995; 127:88–94.
17. Miller JD, Capusten BM, Lampard R. Changes at the base of skull and cervical spine in Down syndrome. Can Assoc Radiol J 1986; 37:85–89.
18. Shapiro BL, Gorlin RJ, Redman RS, et al. The palate and Down's syndrome. N Engl J Med 1967; 276:1460–1463.
19. Thompson LD, McElhinney DB, Jue KL, et al. Gastroesophageal reflux after repair of atrioventricular septal defect in infants with trisomy 21: a comparison of medical and surgical therapy. J Pediatr Surg 1999; 34:1359–1363.
20. Jacobs IN, Teague WG, Bland JW Jr. Pulmonary vascular complications of chronic airway obstruction in children. Arch Otolaryngol Head Neck Surg 1997; 123:700–704.
21. Dyken ME, Lin-Dyken DC, Poulton S, et al. Prospective polysomnographic analysis of obstructive sleep apnea in Down syndrome. Arch Pediatr Adolesc Med 2003; 157:655–660.
22. Marcus CL, Keens TG, Bautista DB, et al. Obstructive sleep apnea in children with Down syndrome. Pediatrics 1991; 88:132–139.
23. Miguel-Diez J, Villa-Asensi JR, Alvarez-Sala JL. Prevalence of sleep-disordered breathing in children with Down syndrome: polygraphic findings in 108 children. Sleep 2003; 26:1006–1009.

24. Levanon A, Tarasiuk A, Tal A. Sleep characteristics in children with Down syndrome. J Pediatr 1999; 134:755–760.
25. Gozal D. Sleep-disordered breathing and school performance in children. Pediatrics 1998; 102:616–620.
26. Lefaivre JF, Cohen SR, Burstein FD, et al. Down syndrome: identification and surgical management of obstructive sleep apnea. Plast Reconstr Surg 1997; 99: 629–637.
27. Strome SE, Chang AE, Shu S, et al. Secretion of both IL-2 and IL-4 by tumor cells results in rejection and immunity. J Immunother Emphasis Tumor Immunol 1996; 19:21–32.
28. Wiet GJ, Bower C, Seibert R, et al. Surgical correction of obstructive sleep apnea in the complicated pediatric patient documented by polysomnography. Int J Pediatr Otorhinolaryngol 1997; 41:133–143.
29. Donnelly LF, Shott SR, LaRose CR, et al. Causes of persistent obstructive sleep apnea despite previous tonsillectomy and adenoidectomy in children with Down syndrome as depicted on static and dynamic cine MRI. AJR Am J Roentgenol 2004; 183:175–181.
30. Bell RB, Turvey TA. Skeletal advancement for the treatment of obstructive sleep apnea in children. Cleft Palate Craniofac J 2001; 38:147–154.
31. Gordon N. Sleep apnoea in infancy and childhood. Considering two possible causes: obstruction and neuromuscular disorders. Brain Dev 2002; 24:145–149.
32. McNicholas WT. Clinical diagnosis and assessment of obstructive sleep apnoea syndrome. Monaldi Arch Chest Dis 1997; 52:37–42.
33. Labanowski M, Schmidt-Nowara W, Guilleminault C. Sleep and neuromuscular disease: frequency of sleep-disordered breathing in a neuromuscular disease clinic population. Neurology 1996; 47:1173–1180.
34. Mellies U, Ragette R, Schwake C, et al. Daytime predictors of sleep disordered breathing in children and adolescents with neuromuscular disorders. Neuromuscul Disord 2003; 13:123–128.
35. Sudo A, Fukumizu M, Sugai K, et al. Improvement of obstructive sleep apnea by uvulopalatopharyngoplasty and tonsillectomy in a case of Duchenne muscular dystrophy. No To Hattatsu 2000; 32:352–357.
36. Guilleminault C, Philip P, Robinson A. Sleep and neuromuscular disease: bilevel positive airway pressure by nasal mask as a treatment for sleep disordered breathing in patients with neuromuscular disease. J Neurol Neurosurg Psychiatry 1998; 65:225–232.
37. Padman R, Hyde C, Foster P, et al. The pediatric use of bilevel positive airway pressure therapy for obstructive sleep apnea syndrome: a retrospective review with analysis of respiratory parameters. Clin Pediatr (Phila) 2002; 41:163–169.
38. Litman RS, Rosenberg H. Malignant hyperthermia: update on susceptibility testing. JAMA 2005; 293:2918–2924.
39. Leighton SE, Papsin B, Vellodi A, et al. Disordered breathing during sleep in patients with mucopolysaccharidoses. Int J Pediatr Otorhinolaryngol 2001; 58:127–138.
40. Semenza GL, Pyeritz RE. Respiratory complications of mucopolysaccharide storage disorders. Medicine (Baltimore) 1988; 67:209–219.
41. Ruckenstein MJ, Macdonald RE, Clarke JT, et al. The management of otolaryngological problems in the mucopolysaccharidoses: a retrospective review. J Otolaryngol 1991; 20:177–183.

42. Ginzburg AS, Onal E, Aronson RM, et al. Successful use of nasal-CPAP for obstructive sleep apnea in Hunter syndrome with diffuse airway involvement. Chest 1990; 97:1496–1498.

43. Shapiro J, Strome M, Crocker AC. Airway obstruction and sleep apnea in Hurler and Hunter syndromes. Ann Otol Rhinol Laryngol 1985; 94:458–461.

44. Nishikawa H, Pearman K, Dover S. Multidisciplinary management of children with craniofacial syndromes with particular reference to the airway. Int J Pediatr Otorhinolaryngol 2003; 67(suppl 1):S91–S93.

45. Hoeve LJ, Pijpers M, Joosten KF. OSAS in craniofacial syndromes: an unsolved problem. Int J Pediatr Otorhinolaryngol 2003; 67(suppl 1):S111–S113.

46. Pijpers M, Poels PJ, Vaandrager JM, et al. Undiagnosed obstructive sleep apnea syndrome in children with syndromal craniofacial synostosis. J Craniofac Surg 2004; 15:670–674.

47. Kotagal S, Gibbons VP, Stith JA. Sleep abnormalities in patients with severe cerebral palsy. Dev Med Child Neurol 1994; 36:304–311.

48. Cohen SR, Lefaivre JF, Burstein FD, et al. Surgical treatment of obstructive sleep apnea in neurologically compromised patients. Plast Reconstr Surg 1997; 99:638–646.

49. Magardino TM, Tom LW. Surgical management of obstructive sleep apnea in children with cerebral palsy. Laryngoscope 1999; 109:1611–1615.

50. Nixon GM, Brouillette RT. Sleep and breathing in Prader-Willi syndrome. Pediatr Pulmonol 2002; 34:209–217.

51. Butler JV, Whittington JE, Holland AJ, et al. Prevalence of, and risk factors for, physical ill-health in people with Prader-Willi syndrome: a population-based study. Dev Med Child Neurol 2002; 44:248–255.

52. Hiroe Y, Inoue Y, Higami S, et al. Relationship between hypersomnia and respiratory disorder during sleep in Prader-Willi syndrome. Psychiatry Clin Neurosci 2000; 54:323–325.

53. Rousseau F, Bonaventure J, Legeai-Mallet L, et al. Mutations in the gene encoding fibroblast growth factor receptor-3 in achondroplasia. Nature 1994; 371: 252–254.

54. Sisk EA, Heatley DG, Borowski BJ, et al. Obstructive sleep apnea in children with achondroplasia: surgical and anesthetic considerations. Otolaryngol Head Neck Surg 1999; 120:248–254.

55. Tasker RC, Dundas I, Laverty A, et al. Distinct patterns of respiratory difficulty in young children with achondroplasia: a clinical, sleep, and lung function study. Arch Dis Child 1998; 79:99–108.

56. Zucconi M, Weber G, Castronovo V, et al. Sleep and upper airway obstruction in children with achondroplasia. J Pediatr 1996; 129:743–749.

57. Hershberger ML, Chidekel A. Arnold-Chiari malformation type I and sleep-disordered breathing: an uncommon manifestation of an important pediatric problem. J Pediatr Health Care 2003; 17:190–197.

58. Kirk VG, Morielli A, Brouillette RT. Sleep-disordered breathing in patients with myelomeningocele: the missed diagnosis. Dev Med Child Neurol 1999; 41: 40–43.

59. Kirkham FJ, Hewes DK, Prengler M, et al. Nocturnal hypoxaemia and central-nervous-system events in sickle-cell disease. Lancet 2001; 357:1656–1659.

60. Wali YA, Al Lamki Z, Soliman H, et al. Adenotonsillar hypertrophy: a precipitating factor of cerebrovascular accident in a child with sickle cell anemia. J Trop Pediatr 2000; 46:246–248.

61. Derkay CS, Bray G, Milmoe GJ, et al. Adenotonsillectomy in children with sickle cell disease. South Med J 1991; 84:205–208.
62. Maddern BR, Reed HT, Ohene-Frempong K, et al. Obstructive sleep apnea syndrome in sickle cell disease. Ann Otol Rhinol Laryngol 1989; 98:174–178.
63. Samuels MP, Stebbens VA, Davies SC, et al. Sleep related upper airway obstruction and hypoxaemia in sickle cell disease. Arch Dis Child 1992; 67:925–929.

8

Adenotonsillectomy

Sara I. Pai and David E. Tunkel

*Department of Otolaryngology/Head and Neck Surgery,
Johns Hopkins University School of Medicine, Baltimore, Maryland, U.S.A.*

CHAPTER HIGHLIGHTS

- Adenotonsillar hypertrophy is the leading cause of childhood obstructive sleep apnea syndrome (OSAS) and adenotonsillectomy is the mainstay of treatment.
- New surgical techniques for removal of the tonsils and adenoids continue to evolve in order to reduce the risk of postoperative complications, such as pain and hemorrhage.
- Children younger than three years of age, those with severe OSAS, and those with neuromotor or craniofacial anomalies are at increased risk for perioperative complications such as respiratory compromise.
- Appropriate preoperative risk assessment and postoperative monitoring are necessary for high-risk patients.
- In children with complex medical conditions that affect upper airway anatomy and tone, OSAS may persist after adenotonsillectomy and they may require additional evaluation and treatment.

INTRODUCTION AND HISTORICAL PERSPECTIVE

Tonsillectomy has been practiced for at least 3000 years. Writings from the Hindu literature, dating from approximately 1000 B.C., describe a condition wherein (1):

> ... the phlegm and blood are deranged in the soft palate or tonsils, [and] they become large ... accompanied with thirst, cough, and difficult

breathing. When troublesome, they are to be seized between the blades
of a forceps and drawn forward, and with a semicircular knife the third
of the swelled part is to be removed... ·

In the first century A.D., Cornelius Celsus described the removal of
inflamed tonsils using finger dissection. After the tonsils were removed, the
oropharynx was rinsed with vinegar and medication was applied to provide
hemostasis (2). Subsequent reports of tonsillectomy focused on technical
advances in the surgical tools used to remove the tonsils. The precursors of the
modern instruments used for tonsillectomy were devices aimed at shortening the
uvula. Forceps, snares, and guillotine-type instruments were developed, some of
which were prototypes for instruments used in modern tonsil surgery (3,4).

Tonsillectomy was initially a popular method for treating a variety of respiratory and/or systemic diseases (5,6). In the early twentieth century, the
primary indication for adenotonsillectomy was recurrent tonsillar infection (7).
The popularity of the procedure peaked in the 1930s, and by the 1960s and
1970s approximately two million individuals a year underwent tonsillectomy,
adenoidectomy, or adenotonsillectomy in the United States (6,8–10). The development of antibiotics and improved medical management of pharyngeal infections, as well as the development of a better understanding of the appropriate
surgical indications for the treatment of such infections, led to a progressive
decrease in the number of adenotonsillectomies performed (11). An increasing
awareness of the prevalence and significance of adenotonsillar hypertrophy as
a cause of upper-airway obstruction and obstructive sleep apnea (OSA) in children has led to a recent upward trend in the number of adenotonsillectomies performed in the United States (12–14). In fact, adenotonsillar hypertrophy with
obstructive symptoms has now replaced infection as the most common indication
for such surgery (15).

PATHOPHYSIOLOGY OF OBSTRUCTIVE SLEEP APNEA
SYNDROME/ADENOTONSILLAR ENLARGEMENT

Nocturnal upper-airway obstruction occurs from a variety of factors that are
discussed elsewhere in this textbook. In otherwise healthy children, adenotonsillar hypertrophy is a significant risk factor in the development of OSAS
(16). However, a number of studies have shown that there is no absolute
correlation between the size of the tonsils and adenoids and the severity of
OSAS (17,18). The etiology of OSAS is multi-factorial, involving a combination of the structural characteristics of the upper airway, including adenotonsillar size as related to the overall pharyngeal dimensions and geometry, as well
as dynamic changes in neuromotor control of upper-airway tone during sleep.
Genetic and hormonal factors also seem to play a role. Ovchinsky et al. (19)
have found that 20% of first-degree relatives of 115 index cases with pediatric
OSAS have symptoms highly suggestive of OSA. With the incidence of this

syndrome in the general population at about 2% to 4%, these findings support the idea that genetic factors may predispose children to nocturnal upper-airway obstruction (19).

Although adenotonsillar hypertrophy is the leading cause of childhood OSAS, OSAS is also associated with a number of other pediatric medical conditions that affect neural control of the upper airway, reduce airway caliber, or increase its collapsibility. These conditions include systemic disorders that affect both neuromotor tone and craniofacial anatomy (i.e., trisomy 21, achondroplasia, mucopolysaccharidoses, obesity), neuromotor diseases that create abnormal airway tone during sleep (i.e., cerebral palsy, muscular dystrophy), and craniofacial anomalies that narrow the upper airway (i.e., mandibular hypoplasia from the Pierre Robin triad) (20–29). Although the underlying cause of OSAS in these children may not be adenotonsillar enlargement, removal of the tonsils and/or adenoids is often the first and perhaps the most effective treatment of OSAS in these cases.

PREOPERATIVE ASSESSMENT

Diagnosis and Clinical Evaluation

Early diagnosis and treatment of OSAS in children result in decreased morbidity, and may be cost-effective as well. A recent study has found that children with OSAS have a 226% increase in healthcare utilization as compared with controls during the one year prior to their appropriate evaluation and treatment (30). The mean period between the onset of symptoms and treatment of OSAS has been reported to be 3.3 years (31). Once children with OSAS are treated with an adenotonsillectomy, total annual healthcare costs are reduced by one-third (32). Adenotonsillectomy is associated with a 60% reduction in the number of new admissions, 39% reduction in emergency department visits, 47% reduction in the number of consultations, and 22% reduction in costs for prescribed drugs for these children. The clinical practice guideline on the diagnosis and management of OSAS in children released by the American Academy of Pediatrics in 2002 recommends screening of all children for snoring (33). If snoring is reported and the patient has symptoms or a physical examination that is suggestive of OSAS, additional diagnostic testing with subsequent consideration for adenotonsillectomy, when appropriate, is recommended.

The diagnosis of childhood OSAS is suggested by the history and physical examination, and can be confirmed by polysomnography (PSG). PSG is particularly useful for assessing the severity of OSAS, and to help predict both the likelihood of postoperative respiratory complications and the likelihood of cure after adenotonsillectomy.

Tonsil and adenoid size should be assessed in children with symptoms of nocturnal upper-airway obstruction. Signs of adenoidal hypertrophy include decreased nasal airflow despite an adequate nasal airway on rhinoscopy, a hyponasal speech pattern, and an open-mouth breathing posture. Nasal examination should be focused to exclude obstructive septal deviation, intranasal masses, or mucosal or turbinate swelling within the nose. The oral examination should focus on tonsil size and symmetry, pharyngeal dimensions, palate shape and size, tongue size and motion, and signs of decreased pharyngeal tone such as drooling or stertor. When sleep-disordered breathing (SDB) is accompanied by awake symptoms such as stridor or hoarseness, laryngotracheal examination with flexible or rigid endoscopy should be performed.

Routine oral and nasal examinations can be supplemented with fiberoptic nasal endoscopy to assess nasal patency, adenoid size, and the effect of tonsil size and anatomy on awake respiration (34). Fiberoptic endoscopy can be used to identify the sites of obstruction in children with OSAS. Croft et al. (18) have identified distinct adenoidal, adenotonsillar, tongue base, and laryngeal sites of obstruction based on fiberoptic endoscopy, and have based successful surgical plans on these findings (18).

Most healthy children undergo adenotonsillectomy for the treatment of nocturnal upper-airway obstruction without preoperative PSG (35). This reflects a number of issues, including a lack of general availability of pediatric sleep laboratories, a lack of consensus about normal and abnormal polysomnographic values in children, and the notion that the need for tonsillectomy and/or adenoidectomy may be best decided on clinical grounds [quality of life (QOL) changes, behavioral and learning issues, etc.]. The quantitative data obtained from PSG can be used to help predict which children are at risk for perioperative complications, including postoperative respiratory compromise. We advocate that PSG be performed before adenotonsillectomy to treat OSAS in high-risk patients, including those with craniofacial anomalies, neuromotor disease, or associated medical conditions that may complicate surgery.

Other diagnostic tests that may be useful in the preoperative evaluation of a child with OSAS include a chest radiograph, an electrocardiogram, or an echocardiogram. These tests are usually reserved for those with symptoms or signs of cardiovascular complications of OSAS, such as left or right ventricular hypertrophy, pulmonary hypertension, congestive heart failure, or systemic hypertension. Children with multiple, lengthy, or extreme episodes of hypoxemia on PSG may require formal cardiopulmonary evaluation before surgery. Airway radiography, cephalometric studies, and imaging such as magnetic resonance or computed tomography have limited utility in the diagnosis of OSAS, but may assist in the treatment plan for high-risk children with OSAS caused by unusual anatomic abnormalities (Fig. 1).

Hemostatic Assessment

Postoperative bleeding is the most common serious complication of adenotonsillectomy, and strategies for minimizing the risk of posttonsillectomy hemorrhage continue to evolve. Preoperative laboratory studies of coagulation are not

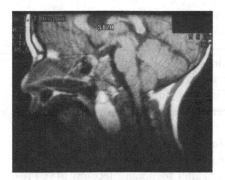

Figure 1 Magnetic resonance imaging T2-weighted sagittal image of a retropharyngeal lymphangioma. The child presented with new-onset obstructive sleep apnea.

performed routinely before adenotonsillectomy, as they have limited predictive value in the general pediatric population and are not cost-effective. In a retrospective review of 994 patients undergoing tonsillectomy, adenoidectomy, or adenotonsillectomy, the prothrombin time and partial thromboplastin time had positive predictive values too low to justify their use to exclude coagulation abnormalities such as von Willebrand (vWD) disease or hemophilia (36). A subsequent retrospective study of 4373 patients confirmed these findings (37). This study described other factors, including surgical technique, perioperative infection, or postoperative dehydration, which may predict postoperative bleeding better than coagulation studies. The American Academy of Otolaryngology-Head and Neck Surgery published guidelines in the 1999 Clinical Indicators Compendium, recommending preoperative coagulation studies and bleeding workup in select patients when an abnormality is suspected by history or if family history is unavailable (38).

A set of questions to reveal any history of abnormal bleeding should be included in the preoperative assessment, including queries about previous surgeries, dental extractions, or loss of primary teeth. Questions regarding easy bruising, frequent nosebleeds, or abnormal bleeding after cuts may lower the threshold for obtaining coagulation or bleeding studies. A family history of bleeding or coagulation disorders should also be assessed. If the family history is suggestive of coagulopathy, further preoperative laboratory studies or consultations are often warranted.

PREANESTHESIA ASSESSMENT AND PREOPERATIVE MEDICAL MANAGEMENT

The perioperative anesthesia management of children undergoing adenotonsillectomy for OSAS is focused on the potential for serious respiratory compromise in these children. Children younger than three years of age (39–43), children with severe OSAS documented by PSG (40,41,44), and those with craniofacial anomalies or neuromotor impairment are at greatest risk for perioperative respiratory compromise (42,45,46).

Children with active and recent history of upper respiratory infections have a greater incidence of perioperative adverse respiratory events such as major oxygen desaturations or more episodes of breath-holding (47). A history of reactive airway disease increases the risk of perioperative adverse respiratory events in children with active upper respiratory infections (47). Such children should have their medical regimen optimized before adenotonsillectomy.

Patients with sickle cell disease have a higher risk of postoperative complications, especially pulmonary complications, after adenotonsillectomy (48). Protocols for preparation of children with sickle cell disease for adenotonsillectomy include aggressive preoperative hydration as well as transfusion regimens to reduce the hemoglobin S percentage to less than 30% to 40% (49,50). Modern transfusion therapy consists of multiple small transfusions of Hb A erythrocytes administered over several weeks prior to the operation, with the goal of correcting the chronic anemia as well as suppressing erythropoiesis of HbS-containing cells in the patient's bone marrow (49,51).

Children with coagulopathies such as vWD disease and hemophilia are at increased risk for perioperative hemorrhage. Children with predominantly type I vWD have safely undergone adenotonsillectomy using perioperative intravenous desmopressin (1-deamino-8-D-arginine vasopressin, also referred to as DDAVP) and the use of an antifibrinolytic, ε-aminocaproic acid, without the need for plasma-derived products (52,53). Patients with an inadequate response to DDAVP, such as vWD type 2B, 2N, or 3, require the use of plasma-derived factor VIII concentrate (such as Humate P or Alphanate) that contains vWD factor (54).

Patients with hemophilia A are deficient in factor VIII coagulant, and those who suffer from mild to moderate hemophilia A will benefit from the use of intravenous or intranasal DDAVP, which can raise factor VIII levels two- to three-fold. Factor VIII replacement, in the form of lyophilized concentrates or recombinant factor, is the mainstay of therapy (55). Those with hemophilia B are deficient in factor IX clotting activity, and replacement of factor IX products prepared from plasma and recombinant factor IX (rFIX) (BeneFix, Genetics Institute, Cambridge, Massachusetts) have been shown to result in safe and effective surgical hemostasis (56).

PERIOPERATIVE ANESTHETIC CONCERNS

Sedation

Sedative drugs, anesthetic agents, and opioid analgesics can worsen upper-airway obstruction, particularly in children with OSAS, by decreasing pharyngeal muscle tone and inhibiting the arousal and ventilatory response to hypoxia, hypercapnia, and obstruction (57). One recent study suggests that preoperative sedation with midazolam may be safely administered to children with mild or moderate SDB, and possibly to children with severe OSA, if the children are closely observed for signs of airway obstruction, hypoventilation, and lethargy (58). However, further prospective studies are needed to confirm these results.

The use of anticholinergic drugs such as atropine or glycopyrrolate may reduce the risk of laryngospasm by reducing pharyngeal secretions. In addition, they may reduce the risk of bradycardia that can occur from some anesthetic agents as well as from hypoxemia that may occur if the airway becomes obstructed on induction (59).

Anesthetic Induction

Induction of general anesthesia is difficult in many children, and the challenges of the dynamic and static airway in the child with OSAS complicate induction several-fold. The anesthesia and surgical teams must anticipate the likelihood of upper-airway obstruction on induction, and should have several plans for airway management should such obstruction occur. There are advocates for induction using mask administration of inhaled anesthetics and those for induction using intravenous medications. While this discussion is complex and beyond the scope of this chapter, the method of anesthetic induction in children with OSAS should depend upon the experience of the anesthesia team, the severity of OSAS in the child, anatomic issues with regard to the upper airway, and the presence and type of medical comorbidities.

SURGERY

Adenotonsillectomy is the treatment of choice for OSAS and perhaps for sleep-related upper-airway obstruction of lesser severity in otherwise healthy children. Brodsky et al. (60) have found that children undergoing adenotonsillectomy for upper-airway obstruction have decreased lateral oropharyngeal dimensions compared with children undergoing adenotonsillectomy for chronic infection. They suggest that decreased oropharyngeal size, in addition to adenotonsillar hyperplasia, may contribute to OSAS in children (60). Removal of enlarged lymphoid tissue in Waldeyer's ring should be curative for most of these children (61–63).

Dr. S. J. Crowe, the first chairman of otolaryngology at Johns Hopkins Hospital, first described a technique for tonsillectomy (Fig. 2) that combined meticulous surgical dissection for complete tonsil removal, hemostasis to prevent postoperative hemorrhage, and anesthetic management to prevent lung abscess formation (1). Crowe introduced his technique in 1912, and in 1917 he reported a postoperative hemorrhage rate of only 1.2% (64). In 1930, Fowler described the modern tonsillectomy as removing the entire tonsil by dissecting between the tonsillar capsule and the superior constrictor muscle (65). When

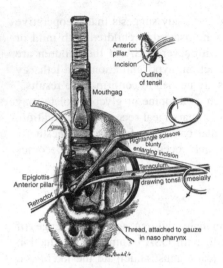

Figure 2   Dr. Crowe's surgical technique for tonsillectomy as depicted by Max Brödel. *Source*: Courtesy of Charles C. Thomas Publisher, Springfield, Illinois.

the goal of tonsillectomy was the treatment of chronic infection, the emphasis was on complete removal of the tonsil in order to avoid remnants that could allow persistent disease. As the indications for adenotonsillectomy have evolved more toward the treatment of upper-airway obstruction, subtotal tonsil resection has been reconsidered.

Surgical Techniques

The considerable postoperative discomfort after tonsillectomy as well as the small but finite rate of delayed hemorrhage after surgery has led to a number of different techniques. These include cold dissection, monopolar and bipolar electrocautery dissection, plasma-mediated excision, ultrasonic dissection, microdebrider intracapsular tonsillectomy, radiofrequency thermal ablation, and other methods. Adenoidectomy can be performed with curettes (66), electrocautery (67,68), microdebrider (69,70), and other devices, but the morbidity from adenoidectomy tends to be minimal and the differences among these techniques less appreciable.

The time honored "cold-dissection" technique of tonsillectomy involves grasping the tonsil, pulling it into the midline, incising the anterior tonsillar pillar sharply, performing blunt and sharp dissection in the plane between the pharyngeal constrictors and the tonsillar capsule, snaring the base of the tonsil, and removing it from the fossa with gentle manipulation. Electrocautery or ligatures are then used for hemostasis. Monopolar cautery has replaced the cold technique over the last two to three decades as the most popular technique used for tonsillectomies in the United States (71). In general, the monopolar cautery dissection techniques afford greater hemostasis during dissection with reduced blood loss, but may have longer healing times with worsened postoperative pain.

Nunez et al. (72) prospectively compared electrocautery tonsillectomy with cold dissection in a group of 54 children. Cold dissection resulted in double the intraoperative blood loss (33.7 mL vs. 15.1 mL). Recovery in the first 24 hours after surgery was similar in both groups. However, additional follow-up of the children revealed increased pain in the electrodissection group when compared with the cold dissection (72). Other studies have supported these findings (73–75). Electrocautery techniques may be useful in patients with coagulopathies or small children (with small blood volumes), whereas the cold dissection technique may be useful in adult populations who seem to have longer periods with postoperative pain.

Other Surgical Techniques

Bipolar Cautery

Bipolar cautery allows less electrical energy leak to surrounding tissues, providing precise coagulation with less tissue injury. The use of small bipolar bayonet forceps for tonsillectomy combined with magnification of the operative field with the operating microscope was popularized by Andrea (76). Variations of the bipolar cautery include bipolar electrosurgical scissors (PowerStar Ethicon, Inc., Somerville, New Jersey, U.S.A.) that cut and coagulate simultaneously. In a prospective, randomized trial of 200 patients undergoing tonsillectomy, Raut et al. (77) compared bipolar scissors with cold dissection. While the morbidity with regard to postoperative pain and hemorrhage was similar between the bipolar scissors and cold dissection groups, the median intraoperative blood loss was 5 mL with the bipolar scissors technique and 115 mL with cold dissection. The mean operating time was also much shorter with bipolar scissors (13 minutes with the bipolar scissors vs. 20 minutes with cold dissection) (77). This has been confirmed by other authors (78,79).

Plasma Excision (Coblation)

Plasma-mediated excision (ArthroCare Corporation, Sunnyvale, California, U.S.A.) uses electrical current that is conducted through a medium such as normal saline fluid or gel. The radiofrequency energy excites the saline solution and creates a field of active protons that are able to break molecular bonds between tissues. By operating at lower temperatures and frequencies, the method theoretically reduces the thermal injury from conventional electrocautery and may reduce postoperative pain. The studies comparing coblation to conventional cold dissection tonsillectomy or monopolar conventional electrosurgery have not consistently shown any statistical differences in postoperative pain or recovery (80–81). A double-blind, randomized, controlled study comparing coblation to bipolar cautery dissection did report less postoperative pain experienced by the coblation tonsillectomy group (82). Belloso et al. (83) demonstrated a reduced incidence of postoperative bleeding with coblation tonsillectomy, Divi et al. (84) reported no significant difference in postoperative bleeding rates, and other groups reported increased postoperative hemorrhage using coblation (85,86). It appears that coblation allows for an efficient tonsillectomy, perhaps with an associated learning curve prior to its proficient use by the surgeon; additional analyses are needed to confirm any clear advantages over other techniques.

Harmonic Scalpel

The ultrasonically activated scalpel (UltraCision® Harmonic Scalpel, Ethicon Endosurgery, Cincinnati, Ohio, U.S.A.) is a relatively new surgical tool that uses ultrasonic vibration to transfer mechanical energy sufficient to break hydrogen bonds. It is equipped with vibrating titanium blades that cut at a frequency of approximately 55.5 kHz. This device generates minimal heat and therefore results in minimal surrounding tissue damage. Several studies have compared the harmonic scalpel to electrocautery for tonsillectomy. A prospective, randomized study performed by Walker and Syed (87) used a questionnaire to compare the postoperative course after tonsillectomy with the harmonic scalpel (155 patients) with that after electrocautery (161 patients). While intraoperative blood loss and postoperative hemorrhage did not differ with technique, those undergoing harmonic scalpel tonsillectomy had a significantly earlier return to normal diet and activity (87). A study of 117 children undergoing tonsillectomy who were randomly assigned to surgery with the harmonic scalpel (61 patients) or electrocautery (59 patients) also showed equivalent blood loss in the two groups (88). Operative time was significantly longer in the harmonic scalpel group, and there was a trend toward lower pain scores on postoperative days 2, 3, and 4. However, this trend did not reach statistical significance (88).

Intracapsular Tonsillectomy/Tonsillotomy

In 1999, Linder et al. (89) reported the use of a CO_2 laser for tonsillotomy (partial tonsil resection). Tonsillotomy leaves the tonsillar capsule in situ but removes the obstructive portion of the tonsil. By maintaining the integrity of the capsule covering the pharyngeal constrictor muscles, deep pharyngeal injury and local inflammation can be minimized. Clinically, this leads to reduced postoperative pain and faster recovery time. This is significant, as postoperative pain is the principal morbidity after tonsillectomy.

A prospective randomized study compared the long-term effects of intracapsular tonsillotomy versus the traditional total blunt tonsillectomy using a questionnaire that addressed issues such as postoperative snoring, apnea events, difficulty in eating, infections, and general health, up to six years after surgery. There were no differences in the answers between the two groups and it was concluded that tonsillotomy with CO_2 laser provided the same long-term benefits for symptoms of obstruction as traditional total dissection of the tonsils, with less postoperative morbidity such as pain and risk of bleeding (90).

Subtotal tonsillectomy without use of the laser has been popularized in the last five to seven years as the use of powered dissectors has become routine throughout otolaryngology. The microdebrider has been used to both reduce tonsil volume and remove adenoids. Advocates of this "powered intracapsular tonsillectomy and adenoidectomy" note that preservation of the tonsillar capsule while removing the obstructive portion of the tonsils can reduce pain and perhaps postoperative hemorrhage (91,92). Remaining tonsillar tissue after such surgery has the potential to harbor infection or regrow. A retrospective review comparing 150 children after powered intracapsular tonsillectomy (combined with adenoidectomy) with 162 children after standard tonsillectomy during the same time period has demonstrated intracapsular tonsillectomy to be as effective as standard tonsillectomy for relief of obstructive SDB as judged by questionnaires and clinical assessment. The powered intracapsular tonsillectomy also affords less postoperative pain and a significantly more rapid recovery (91,92). Powered intracapsular tonsillectomy and adenoidectomy have been used in very young children for treatment of OSAS with clinical effectiveness and low morbidity (93). This technique is promising, but long-term follow-up is needed with regard to both effectiveness in treating OSA and recurrence of tonsillar disease.

Radiofrequency Volume Reduction

Radiofrequency tonsil reduction is a new technique that has been introduced to treat OSAS in children. With this method, the temperature-controlled radiofrequency probe (e.g., Somnoplasty, Somnus Medical Technologies, Inc., Mountain View, California, U.S.A.) is inserted directly into the tonsillar tissue. The current density around the electrode tip is high enough to create a region of tissue destruction that contracts over time, with consequent reduction in total tissue volume. A pilot study of this technique demonstrates less pain when compared with conventional tonsillectomy, as well as an improvement in several clinical and polysomnographic parameters of OSAS up to one year following surgery (94–96). Preliminary trials of radiofrequency procedures have yielded promising results, but larger studies evaluating costs and benefits are still needed. The principal benefit of this method when applied to adults is the ability to perform tonsil volume reduction in the office under local anesthesia; in children, general anesthesia would be required with this technique because of the issues with cooperation of young children, as well as the need for concomitant adenoidectomy.

Adjuvant Therapies

The benefits of perioperative antibiotics with adenotonsillectomy have not been studied extensively. Antibiotics have been found to reduce postoperative morbidities such as pain, fever, and mouth odor (97,98). In addition, one study demonstrates that tonsillectomy patients treated with antibiotics have an earlier return to normal activity and diet by one day as compared with those who do not receive postoperative antibiotics (99).

The impact of perioperative steroid administration on the recovery from tonsillectomy has been studied. A meta-analysis of several double-blind, randomized, placebo-controlled studies suggest that a single intravenous dose of dexamethasone is an effective, relatively safe and inexpensive treatment for reducing morbidity from pediatric tonsillectomy. Children receiving a single intraoperative dose of dexamethasone (dose range, 0.15–1.0 mg/kg; maximum dose range, 8–25 mg) are two times less likely to vomit in the first 24 hours than children receiving placebo (RR = 0.54, CI95 = 0.42, 0.69; $P < 0.00001$) (100). Additionally, children receiving dexamethasone are more likely to advance to a soft/solid diet on posttonsillectomy day 1 (RR = 1.69, CI95 = 1.02, 2.79; $P = 0.04$) than those receiving placebo (101–103).

POSTOPERATIVE MANAGEMENT

Recovery Setting

The majority of children who undergo adenotonsillectomy for mild OSAS have immediate improvement of their obstruction as demonstrated by sleep studies performed on the first postoperative night (104,105). However, children with severe OSAS as documented by PSG or children with comorbidities such as obesity, neuromuscular, or craniofacial disorders may experience a prolonged recovery or incomplete relief of their OSAS after an adenotonsillectomy. Consequently, these children are at risk for respiratory difficulties in the immediate postoperative period. These high-risk children require inpatient postoperative management in a monitored setting. This setting should allow for prompt recognition of the signs of upper-airway obstruction as well as intervention to prevent morbidity.

Airway Management

Extubation before the return of laryngeal and pharyngeal reflexes may result in upper-airway obstruction in children with obstructive apnea after pharyngeal surgery. Therefore, extubation should be performed in a setting where the patient has a return of laryngeal reflexes to protect the airway, while trying to avoid excessive coughing or agitation in the presence of the endotracheal tube. The insertion of an oral and/or nasopharyngeal airway can help maintain an airway if upper-airway obstruction on extubation is anticipated. Brown et al. (106) have reported the use of endotracheal intubation and mechanical ventilation for several days after an adenotonsillectomy in children with severe OSAS and cor pulmonale. Patients with risk factors such as obesity, neurological disorders, asthma, or those less than three years of age may be predisposed to persistent respiratory difficulties in the immediate postoperative period and may require the respiratory assistance of continuous positive airway pressure (CPAP) or bilevel positive airway pressure (BiPAP) after an adenotonsillectomy (41,107).

POSTOPERATIVE COURSE

While the recovery process after tonsillectomy with or without an adenoidectomy can vary depending on patient factors and operative technique, the postoperative course usually has the following features. Throat discomfort often worsens during the first week after surgery, with gradual improvement in pain starting one week after surgery. Otalgia that occurs several days after surgery is referred from the pharyngeal surgical site, and is not usually indicative of otitis media. Halitosis can occur during the first ten days after surgery, often from the eschar at the tonsillectomy and/or adenoidectomy site. The examination of the pharynx after surgery shows healing raw tonsil beds for several days after surgery, and the dark eschar is replaced by white to green healing tonsil beds over the first few days. This appearance in the posttonsillectomy patient is often erroneously interpreted as postoperative infection. Fortunately, pharyngeal infection is exceedingly rare in these well-vascularized open surgical beds. Full healing and remucosalization of the tonsillar fossa may take several weeks depending on the surgical technique used. Swelling of the uvula is not uncommon after adenotonsillectomy.

As postoperative hemorrhage is the most common serious complication of adenotonsillectomy, any report of red blood from the mouth warrants attention. The presence of clot in the tonsillar bed suggests a recent bleeding event as well. The most common time we see postoperative bleeding after tonsillectomy is on the sixth and seventh days after surgery.

Nausea and vomiting after adenotonsillectomy can occur from anesthetic issues, swallowed bloody secretions, and adverse reaction to narcotic analgesics. This is usually self-limited, but on rare occasions will lead to an admission for intravenous hydration and observation.

Our patients are instructed to maintain a liquid and soft diet for 10 to 14 days after surgery. They are told to report any episodes of bleeding from the mouth, and are encouraged to return urgently for evaluation should this occur. Antibiotics are used for the first postoperative week, and analgesics are used liberally within the guidelines addressed elsewhere in this chapter. We expect a gradual return to normal activity over this 10- to 14-day period, and we advise close supervision of children during this period.

When adenoidectomy is performed without tonsillectomy, postoperative discomfort is limited, as is the risk of bleeding. Halitosis is common. Some children experience neck discomfort, particularly on extension, which may develop over several days after surgery. We do not restrict the diet or activity of children recovering from adenoidectomy.

COMPLICATIONS

Respiratory Compromise

The most severe complication of adenotonsillectomy, when performed for childhood OSAS, is perioperative respiratory compromise. Upper-airway obstruction can occur on induction of general anesthesia, on emergence from anesthesia, and during the immediate perioperative period. Several large retrospective series (40,41,44) have helped to identify clinical risk factors that can predict respiratory difficulties after an adenotonsillectomy for OSAS in most high-risk children. Children with severe OSAS, children with complex issues of upper-airway tone or craniofacial anatomy, and children less than three years of age are at increased risk for respiratory compromise or prolonged recovery (40,41,45). The use of preoperative PSG can quantify the severity of OSAS in such high-risk children and can provide a baseline for the assessment of postoperative respiratory compromise during sleep.

High-risk children require careful monitoring of their cardiopulmonary status after surgery (39,40,108). Narcotic analgesics and other sedating medications should be used judiciously, and postoperative oxygen supplementation should be administered with attention to signs of depression of ventilatory drive. The postoperative setting should allow for the use of nasopharyngeal airways, CPAP or BiPAP, or even endotracheal intubation in the unusual high-risk child who has respiratory compromise after adenotonsillectomy for upper-airway obstruction (41,106,107). In general, we can use clinical and polysomnographic information to predict whether a child is at risk for respiratory compromise. Intraoperative management and postoperative care can be tailored to avoid or treat such respiratory difficulties.

Pain Management

The search for a "better tonsillectomy" is primarily driven by the significant postoperative discomfort experienced by many patients. The analgesic management of children undergoing adenotonsillectomy for OSAS is complicated by concerns about the effects of narcotics on respiration and the effects of nonsteroidal anti-inflammatory agents on postoperative hemorrhage risk. Brown et al. (109) have found that children with recurrent hypoxemia due to OSAS have a reduced morphine requirement for analgesia after adenotonsillectomy, perhaps due to a change in opiate receptor function. Narcotics should be used with discretion in these patients. Acetaminophen is a standard postoperative medication given to children after adenotonsillectomy. In a prospective, randomized, double-blind study of acetaminophen compared with acetaminophen with codeine, the children who receive acetaminophen alone consume a significantly higher percentage of a normal diet on the first six postoperative days, with no difference in pain scores, as compared with those who receive acetaminophen with codeine (110).

Dehydration/Hyponatremia

Postoperative pain can lead to poor oral intake of fluids and subsequent dehydration. Small children, those with developmental delays or pre-existing swallowing problems may be at greatest risk. Novel approaches have been used to prevent dehydration, including the use of intravenous fluids administered at home (111). Pain management, parental counseling, and patient selection can help prevent these problems.

Hyponatremia is a potentially lethal complication following tonsillectomy in children (112). It is caused by the inappropriate administration of hypotonic solutions in a patient who has intravascular volume depletion, which is the principal stimulus to increased antidiuretic hormone (ADH) release following surgery. Rehydration should be performed with isotonic solutions in volumes that are appropriate for the needs of the child, calculating maintenance, fluid needs, volume deficit, blood loss, and other fluid losses such as vomiting. Judd et al. (113,114) have found that the administration of a hypotonic solution maintains elevated ADH levels, whereas ADH is lowered by the administration of plasma, blood, or isotonic saline.

Severe hyponatremia has also been reported as a cause of death following tonsillectomy in children with vWD disease after administration of desmopressin (115). Desmopressin, a synthetic analog of naturally occurring ADH, stimulates the resorption of free water in the kidney. Predisposing factors for hyponatremia reported in the literature include young age, weight less than 10 kg, the administration of hypotonic intravenous fluids, liberal fluid replacement, emesis, multiple doses of desmopressin, and an increased release of endogenous ADH during stress (52). Hypotonic intravenous solutions should be avoided in such patients, with close monitoring of fluid status and electrolytes (116).

Hemorrhage

Postoperative hemorrhage is the most common severe complication after tonsillectomy. Posttonsillectomy hemorrhage can be classified into primary or delayed hemorrhage. Primary bleeding occurs within the first 24 hours of surgery and is considered to be related to surgical technique. It is considered more dangerous because of the possible risk of aspiration and laryngospasm (117). Therefore, these patients will often need to be admitted for further observation. In a survey of pediatric otolaryngologists, two-thirds of practitioners attempt to control active bleeding in the emergency room, whereas one-third proceed directly to the operating room (118).

Repeated bleeding episodes after tonsillectomy are unusual, and a diagnostic workup for coagulopathy should be considered. In a prospective study of 1516 patients, nearly one-half of the patients who experienced postoperative hemorrhage had undetected coagulation diseases (primarily vWD disease) that were diagnosed after surgery in a hematological study (118,119). Severe bleeding may indicate an injury to a large vessel, with resultant pseudoaneurysm formation. Angiography and selective embolization may be necessary to diagnose and treat these rare but serious complications of tonsillectomy (120). Delayed hemorrhage occurs within the first 10 postoperative days and is most likely attributed to infection, dehydration, or slough of eschar. However, there is little difference in the management of immediate or delayed hemorrhage.

The need for blood transfusions for postoperative hemorrhage in the pediatric population is unusual. In a retrospective study of 7743 children undergoing tonsillectomies and/or adenoidectomies, 18 patients (0.2%) required transfusions because of severe blood loss postoperatively (121). In another retrospective study of 1720 patients who underwent tonsillectomy for chronic tonsillitis, the average transfusion rate was 0.52%. A low hemoglobin and hematocrit before surgery are risk factors that predict the need for transfusion after postoperative bleeding (122).

Velopharyngeal Insufficiency/Nasopharyngeal Stenosis

Tonsillectomy and adenoidectomy can affect velar closure. Adenoidectomy can cause nasal air emission during speech, but this velopharyngeal insufficiency is usually temporary. Tonsillectomy alone can cause problems with velar closure in some instances as well, although tonsillectomy in fact has been used to treat such voice problems in children where tonsil anatomy is impeding velar closure (123,124). Nasopharyngeal stenosis has been described after adenotonsillectomy, presumably from cicatricial scarring of the nasopharyngeal inlet. A variety of repairs have been described for this difficult problem, including the use of pharyngeal flaps, incision of scar with steroid injection, and dilatations (125).

EXPECTED OUTCOMES

Cure Rates

Several authors have documented the clinical effectiveness of adenotonsillectomy for nocturnal upper-airway obstruction in children (61,126). Helfaer et al. (105) performed PSG on otherwise healthy children with mild OSAS on the first night after adenotonsillectomy. The number of apnea events decreased and the oxygen saturation during sleep improved immediately after surgery in these children. Such rapid relief of obstructive symptoms after adenotonsillectomy in children with mild or moderate OSAS can be expected, but OSAS may persist in severe cases [respiratory disturbance index (RDI) > 19.1 on preoperative PSG] or in patients with asthma, cerebral palsy, morbid obesity, Down syndrome, or other syndromes (127,128).

A prospective study of 30 obese children (BMI greater than the 95th percentile) who were followed postoperatively for a mean period of 5.6 months revealed a marked improvement in RDI after an adenotonsillectomy, with a mean preoperative RDI of 30.0 and a mean postoperative RDI of 11.6

($P < 0.001$). While QOL as measured by OSA-18 improved significantly for these obese children after surgery, the OSA was not cured in the majority of children (129).

Similarly, 29 children with severe OSA identified by an RDI ≥ 30 were studied prospectively after adenotonsillectomy. The most common co-morbidities were obesity, asthma, and allergic disease. The mean preoperative RDI was 63.9 and the mean postoperative RDI was 14.2 ($P < 0.0001$). These children with severe OSA showed a significant improvement in RDI and in QOL over a period of several months after surgery, but were by no means reliably cured. Postoperative PSG is recommended in such cases to identify those who may require additional therapy (130).

Quality of Life

Recently, several authors have examined the effects of adenotonsillectomy on patient's QOL. Validated instruments for measuring QOL changes for children after adenotonsillectomy for sleep apnea include the OSD-6 developed by de Serres et al. (131), and the OSA-18 developed by Franco et al. (132). Both instruments survey caregivers on their child's sleep disturbance, physical and emotional symptoms, daytime activity, and caregiver concerns. A pre- and post-adenotonsillectomy study using the OSD-6 instrument detected large improvements in at least short-term QOL in most children. Specifically, large, moderate, and small improvements in QOL were seen in 74.5%, 6.1%, and 7.1% of children, respectively. The most improved areas were sleep disturbance, caregiver concern, and physical suffering (131).

The OSA-18 was used with the child behavior checklist by Goldstein et al. (133) to evaluate the changes in behavior and QOL after adenotonsillectomy in 64 children with SDB. They found improvements in the QOL with concomitant improvement in behavior after adenotonsillectomy (133). Another prospective study of 60 children (mean age, 7.1, range 3–12 years) supported the benefits of adenotonsillectomy on QOL. Mitchell et al. (134) using the OSA-18 survey, compared survey results obtained prior to surgery with those obtained within six months after surgery and found that children with OSA diagnosed by PSG demonstrated a statistically significant improvement in sleep disturbance, physical suffering, emotional distress, and daytime problems after adenotonsillectomy for OSA. Caregiver concerns were also reduced. The mean total OSA-18 score was 71.4 before surgery and 35.8 after adenotonsillectomy, with the greatest change in mean score observed in the area of sleep disturbance ($P < 0.002$) (134).

Another study surveyed caregivers on changes in QOL in children 9–24 months after adenotonsillectomy, and there appeared to be a mild recurrence of symptoms of sleep disturbance and physical suffering such as snoring, mouth breathing, nasal discharge, and breath-holding spells in some children. However, caregivers perceived a long-term improvement in QOL after adenotonsillectomy despite the recurrence of these symptoms (135). This study was limited by a large number of children lost to follow-up (43%).

Growth Effects

Failure to thrive often can be associated with childhood OSA and the pathophysiology is not clearly understood. Marcus et al. (136) measured energy expenditure during sleep in children before and after adenotonsillectomy. Children with OSA had an energy expenditure during sleep of $51 \pm 6 \, kcal/kg/day$ and this energy expenditure decreased to $46 \pm 7 \, kcal/kg/day$ ($P < 0.005$) after an adenotonsillectomy. While these children gained weight after surgery, the caloric intake of the children did not change. This group concluded that the poor growth seen in some children with OSAS is secondary to increased caloric expenditure caused by increased work of breathing during sleep (136). Other theories for growth impairment in these children include reduced growth hormone secretion (137) and altered insulin-like growth factor-I secretion (138), both of which can be reversed after an adenotonsillectomy.

Cognitive/Behavioral Effects

Daytime behavioral and learning disturbances have been causally associated with OSAS. In 1982, Brouillette et al. (139) reported that 5 of 22 children with OSAS presented with behavioral disturbances and developmental delay, both of which improved following treatment for upper-airway obstruction. Gozal, in a prospective study of 297 children who were in the lowest 10th percentile in their first-grade class, found that 54 children (18.1%) had sleep-associated gas-exchange abnormalities. Children who underwent adenotonsillectomy had improved school performance when compared with those children with sleep-related gas-exchange abnormalities who did not have surgery (140). In another prospective study of 39 children diagnosed with OSAS, impaired neurocognitive function appeared to have improved when studied six to ten months after adenotonsillectomy (141). These studies emphasize the importance of the early diagnosis and treatment of childhood OSAS in order to reduce the potential for impaired neurocognitive function.

CONCLUSIONS

Adenotonsillectomy is the mainstay for treatment of children with OSA. A variety of methods have been developed in attempts to reduce the two principal postoperative problems, pain and bleeding. Children with OSAS are at increased risk for respiratory compromise in the period surrounding the adenotonsillectomy. Preoperative risk assessment, anesthetic and surgical care tailored to reduce such risks, and postoperative monitoring are necessary for these children. While most children will be cured of OSAS after adenotonsillectomy, persistent disease will be seen in some children with complex medical problems. These children may need additional evaluation and treatment.

Signs and symptoms of adenoid hypertrophy include decreased nasal airflow, hyponasal speech, and open-mouth breathing posture.

Preoperative bleeding studies are indicated only if a child has a history of easy bleeding/bruising or there is a family history of bleeding disorders.

Preoperative PSG is indicated in patients who are high-risk for perioperative complications, including those with craniofacial anomalies, neuromotor diseases, or associated medical conditions that may complicate surgical management of OSAS.

REFERENCES

1. Proctor DF. History of the development of surgical techniques and concepts. In: Proctor DF, ed. The Tonsils and Adenoids in Childhood. Illinois: Charles C. Thomas Publisher, 1960:3.
2. Thornval A. Wilhelm Meyer and the adenoids. Arch Otolaryngol 1969; 90(3):383–386.
3. Physick PS. Description of a forceps, employed to facilitate the extirpation of the tonsil. Am J Med Sci 1828; 2:116–117.
4. Younis RT, Lazar RH. History and current practice of tonsillectomy. Laryngoscope 2002; 112(8 Pt 2 suppl 100):3–5.
5. Macbeth RG. The tonsil problem. Proc R Soc Med 1950; 43(5):324–328.
6. Kornblut AD. A traditional approach to surgery of the tonsils and adenoids. Otolaryngol Clin North Am 1987; 20(2):349–363.
7. Rosenfeld RM, Green RP. Tonsillectomy and adenoidectomy: changing trends. Ann Otol Rhino Laryngol 1990; 99(3 Pt 1):187–191.
8. Faigel H. Tonsillectomy: a bloody mess. Clin Pediatr (Phila) 1966; 5(11):652–653.
9. Gibb AG. Unusual complications of tonsil and adenoid removal. J Laryngol Otol 1969; 83(12):1159–1174.
10. Shaikh W, Vayda E, Feldman W. A systematic review of the literature on evaluative studies of tonsillectomy and adenoidectomy. Pediatrics 1976; 57(3):401–407.
11. Derkay CS. Pediatric otolaryngology procedures in the United States: 1977–1987. Int J Pediatr Otorhinolaryngol 1993; 25(1–3):1–12.
12. Kozak, LJ, Hall MJ, Pokras R, et al. Ambulatory Surgery in the United States, 1994, Advance Data 283. Washington, DC: U.S. Department of Health and Human Services, National Center for Health Statistics, Centers for Disease Control and Prevention, 1997:1–16.
13. Hall MJ, Lawrence L. Ambulatory Surgery in the United States, 1995, Advance Data 296. Washington, DC: U.S. Department of Health and Human Services, National Center for Health Statistics, Centers for Disease Control and Prevention, 1997:1–16.

14. Hall MJ, Lawrence L. Ambulatory Surgery in the United States, 1996, Advance Data 300. Washington DC: U.S. Department of Health and Human Services, National Center for Health Statistics, Centers for Disease Control and Prevention, 1998:1–16.
15. Darrow DH, Siemens C. Indications for tonsillectomy and adenoidectomy. Laryngoscope 2002; 112(8 Pt 2 suppl 100):6–10.
16. Leach J, Olson J, Hermann J, et al. Polysomnographic and clinical findings in children with obstructive sleep apnea. Arch Otolaryngol Head Neck Surg 1992; 118(7):741–744.
17. Ahlqvist-Rastad J, Hultcrantz E, Svanholm H. Children with tonsillar obstruction: indications for and efficacy of tonsillectomy. Acta Paediatr Scand 1988; 77(6):831–835.
18. Croft CB, Thomson HG, Samuels MP, et al. Endoscopic evaluation and treatment of sleep-associated upper airway obstruction in infants and young children. Clin Otolaryngol Allied Sci 1990; 15(3):209–216.
19. Ovchinsky A, Rao M, Lotwin I, et al. The familial aggregation of pediatric obstructive sleep apnea syndrome. Arch Otolaryngol Head Neck Surg 2002; 128(7):815–818.
20. Bredenkamp JK, Smith ME, Dudley JP, et al. Otolaryngologic manifestations of the mucopolysaccharidoses. Ann Otol Rhinol Laryngol 1992; 101(6):472–478.
21. Shapiro J, Strome M, Crocker AC. Airway obstruction and sleep apnea in Hurler and Hunter syndromes. Ann Otol Rhinol Laryngol 1985; 94(5 Pt 1):458–461.
22. Reid CS, Pyeritz RE, Kopits SE, et al. Cervicomedullary compression in young patients with achondroplasia: value of comprehensive neurologic and respiratory evaluation. J Pediatr 1987; 110(4):522–530.
23. Nelson FW, Hecht JT, Horton WA, et al. Neurological basis of respiratory complications in achondroplasia. Ann Neurol 1988; 24(1):89–93.
24. Marcus CL, Keens TG, Bautista DB, et al. Obstructive sleep apnea in children with Down syndrome. Pediatrics 1991; 88(1):132–139.
25. Marcus CL, Carroll JL. Obstructive sleep apnea syndrome. In: Loughlin GM, Eigen H, eds. Respiratory Disease in Children: Diagnosis and Management. Baltimore: Williams and Wilkins, 1994:475–499.
26. Khan Y, Heckmatt JZ. Obstructive apnoeas in Duchenne muscular dystrophy. Thorax 1994; 49(2):157–161.
27. Waters KA, Everett F, Silence DO, et al. Treatment of obstructive sleep apnea in achondroplasia: evaluation of sleep, breathing, and somatosensory-evoked potentials. Am J Med Genet 1995; 59(4):460–466.
28. Bower CM, Gungor A. Pediatric obstructive sleep apnea syndrome. Otolaryngol Clin North Am 2000; 33(1):49–75.
29. Monasterio FO, Drucker M, Molina F, et al. Distraction osteogenesis in Pierre Robin sequence and related respiratory problems in children. J Craniofac Surg 2002; 13(1):79–83.
30. Reuveni H, Simon T, Tal A, et al. Health care services utilization in children with obstructive sleep apnea syndrome. Pediatrics 2002; 110(1 Pt 1):68–72.
31. Richards W, Ferdman RM. Prolonged morbidity due to delays in the diagnosis and treatment of obstructive sleep apnea in children. Clin Pediatr (Phila) 2000; 39(2):103–108.

32. Tarasiuk A, Simon T, Tal A, et al. Adenotonsillectomy in children with obstructive sleep apnea syndrome reduces health care utilization. Pediatrics 2004; 113(2): 351–356.

33. Section on Pediatric Pulmonology, Subcommittee on Obstructive Sleep Apnea Syndrome, American Academy of Pediatrics. Clinical practice guideline: diagnosis and management of childhood obstructive sleep apnea syndrome. Pediatrics 2002; 109(4):704–712.

34. Wang D, Clement P, Kaufman L, et al. Fiberoptic evaluation of the nasal and nasopharyngeal anatomy in children with snoring. J Otolaryngol 1994; 23(1):57–60.

35. Weatherly RA, Ruzicka DL, Marriott DJ, et al. Polysomnography in children scheduled for adenotonsillectomy. Otolaryngol Head Neck Surg 2004; 131(5):727–731.

36. Manning SC, Beste D, McBride T, et al. An assessment of preoperative coagulation screening for tonsillectomy and adenoidectomy. Int J Pediatr Otorhinolaryngol 1987; 13(3):237–244.

37. Zwack GC, Derkay CS. The utility of preoperative hemostatic assessment in adenotonsillectomy. Int J Pediatr Otorhinolaryngol 1997; 39(1):67–76.

38. American Academy of Otolaryngology-Head Neck Surgery. Clinical Indicators Compendium. Alexandria, VA, 1999.

39. Wiatrak BJ, Myer CM 3rd, Andrews TM. Complications of adenotonsillectomy in children under 3 years of age. Am J Otolaryngol 1991; 12(3):170–172.

40. McColley SA, April MM, Carroll JL, et al. Respiratory compromise after adenotonsillectomy in children with obstructive sleep apnea. Arch Otolaryngol Head Neck Surg 1992; 118(9):940–943.

41. Rosen GM, Muckel RP, Mahowald MW, et al. Postoperative respiratory compromise in children with obstructive sleep apnea syndrome: can it be anticipated? Pediatrics 1994; 93(5):784–788.

42. Gerber ME, O'Connor DM, Adler E, et al. Selected risk factors in pediatric adenotonsillectomy. Arch Otolaryngol Head Neck Surg 1996; 122(8):811–814.

43. Biavati MJ, Manning SC, Phillips DL. Predictive factors for respiratory complications after tonsillectomy and adenoidectomy in children. Arch Otolaryngol Head Neck Surg 1997; 123(5):517–521.

44. Wilson K, Lakheeram I, Morielli A, et al. Can assessment for obstructive sleep apnea help predict postadenotonsillectomy respiratory complications? Anesthesiology 2002; 96(2):313–322.

45. Grundfast K, Berkowitz R, Fox L. Outcome and complications following surgery for obstructive adenotonsillar hypertrophy in children with neuromuscular disorders. Ear Nose Throat J 1990; 69(11):756–760.

46. Seid AB, Martin PJ, Pransky SM, et al. Surgical therapy of obstructive sleep apnea in children with severe mental insufficiency. Laryngoscope 1990; 100(5): 507–510.

47. Tait AR, Malviya S, Voepel-Lewis T, et al. Risk factors for perioperative adverse respiratory events in children with upper respiratory tract infections. Anesthesiology 2001; 95(2):299–306.

48. Griffin TC, Buchanan GR. Elective surgery in children with sickle cell disease without preoperative blood transfusion. J Pediatr Surg 1993; 28(5):681–685.

49. Derkay CS, Bray G, Milmoe GJ, et al. Adenotonsillectomy in children with sickle cell disease. South Med J 1991; 84(2):205–208.

50. Halvorson DJ, McKie V, McKie K, et al. Sickle cell disease and tonsillectomy. Preoperative management and postoperative complications. Arch Otolaryngol Head Neck Surg 1997; 123(7):689–692.

51. Ware RE, Filston HC. Surgical management of children with hemoglobinopathies. Surg Clin North Am 1992; 72(6):1223–1236.

52. Allen GC, Armfield DR, Bontempo FA, et al. Adenotonsillectomy in children with von Willebrand disease. Arch Otolaryngol Head Neck Surg 1999; 125(5):547–551.

53. Jimenez-Yuste V, Prim MP, De Diego JI, et al. Otolaryngologic surgery in children with von Willebrand disease. Arch Otolaryngol Head Neck Surg 2002; 128(12): 1365–1368.

54. Mannucci PM. Treatment of von Willebrand's disease. N Engl J Med 2004; 351(7):683–694.

55. Dunn AL, Abshire TC. Recent advances in the management of the child who has hemophilia. Hematol Oncol Clin North Am 2004; 18(6):1249–1276.

56. Raqni MV, Pasi KJ, White GC, et al. Use of recombinant factor IX in subjects with haemophilia B undergoing surgery. Haemophilia 2002; 8(2):91–97.

57. Biro P, Kaplan V, Bloch KE. Anesthetic management of a patient with obstructive sleep apnea syndrome and difficult airway access. J Clin Anesth 1995; 7(5):417–421.

58. Cultrara A, Bennett GH, Lazar C, et al. Preoperative sedation in pediatric patients with sleep-disordered breathing. Int J Pediatr Otorhinolaryngol 2002; 66(3):243–246.

59. Roffe C, Smith MJ, Basran GS. Anticholinergic premedication for fibreoptic bronchoscopy. Monaldi Arch Chest Dis 1994; 49(2):101–106.

60. Brodsky L, Moore L, Stanievich JF. A comparison of tonsillar size and oropharyngeal dimensions in children with obstructive adenotonsillar hypertrophy. Int J Pediatr Otorhinolaryngol 1987; 13(2):149–152.

61. Potsic WP, Pasquariello PS, Baranak CC, et al. Relief of upper airway obstruction by adenotonsillectomy. Otolaryngol Head Neck Surg 1986; 94(4):476-480.

62. Strandling JR, Thomas G, Warley AR, et al. Effect of adenotonsillectomy on nocturnal hypoxaemia, sleep disturbance, and symptoms in snoring children. Lancet 1990; 335(8684):249–253.

63. Brooks LJ. Treatment of otherwise normal children with obstructive sleep apnea. Ear Nose Throat J 1993; 72(1):77–79.

64. Crowe SJ, Watkins SS, Rothholz AS. Relation of tonsillar and nasopharyngeal infections to general systemic disorders. Bull Johns Hopkins Hosp 1917; 28:1–63.

65. Fowler RH. Tonsil Surgery. Philadelphia: FA Davis, 1930.

66. Shaalan HF. What is the right size of the adenoid curette? J Laryngol Otol 2003; 117(10):796–800.

67. Clemens J, McMurray JS, Willging JP. Electrocautery versus curette adenoidectomy: comparison of postoperative results. Int J Pediatr Otorhinolaryngol 1998; 43(2):115–122.

68. Elluru RG, Johnson L, Myer CM 3rd. Electrocautery adenoidectomy compared with curettage and power-assisted methods. Laryngoscope 2002; 112(8 Pt 2 suppl 100): 23–25.

69. Murray N, Fitzpatrick P, Guarisco JL. Powered partial adenoidectomy. Arch Otolaryngol Head Neck Surg 2002; 128(7):792–796.

70. Rodriguez K, Murray N, Guarisco JL. Power-assisted partial adenoidectomy. Laryngoscope 2002; 112(8 Pt 2 suppl 100):26–28.

71. Kay DJ, Mehta V, Goldsmith AJ. Perioperative adenotonsillectomy management in children: current practices. Laryngoscope 2003; 113(4):592–597.
72. Nunez DA, Provan J, Crawford M. Postoperative tonsillectomy pain in pediatric patients: electrocautery (hot) vs cold dissection and snare tonsillectomy—a randomized trial. Arch Otolaryngol Head Neck Surg 2000; 126(7):837–841.
73. Weimert TA, Babyak JW, Richter HJ. Electrodissection tonsillectomy. Arch Otolaryngol Head Neck Surg 1990; 116(2):186–188.
74. Leinbach RF, Markwell SJ, Colliver JA, et al. Hot versus cold tonsillectomy: a systematic review of the literature. Otolaryngol Head Neck Surg 2003; 129(4): 360–364.
75. Silveira H, Soares JS, Lima HA. Tonsillectomy: cold dissection versus bipolar electrodissection. Int J Pediatr Otorhinolaryngol 2003; 67(4):345–351.
76. Andrea M. Microsurgical bipolar cautery tonsillectomy. Laryngoscope 1993; 103(10):1177–1178.
77. Raut V, Bhat N, Kinsella J, et al. Bipolar scissors versus cold dissection tonsillectomy: a prospective, randomized, multi-unit study. Laryngoscope 2001; 111(12): 2178–2182.
78. Isaacson G, Szeremeta W. Pediatric tonsillectomy with bipolar electrosurgical scissors. Am J Otolaryngol 1998; 19(5):291–295.
79. Saleh HA, Cain AJ, Mountain RE. Bipolar scissor tonsillectomy. Clin Otolaryngol Allied Sci 1999; 24(1):9–12.
80. Philpott CM, Wild DC, Mehta D, et al. A double-blinded randomized controlled trial of coblation versus conventional dissection tonsillectomy on post-operative symptoms. Clin Otolaryngol 2005; 30(2):143–148.
81. Stoker KE, Don DM, Kang DR, et al. Pediatric total tonsillectomy using coblation compared to conventional electrosurgery: a prospective, controlled single-blind study. Otolaryngol Head Neck Surg 2004; 130(6):666–675.
82. Timms MS, Temple RH. Coblation tonsillectomy: a double blind randomized controlled study. J Laryngol Otol 2002; 116(6):450–452.
83. Belloso A, Chidambaram A, Morar P, et al. Coblation tonsillectomy versus dissection tonsillectomy: postoperative hemorrhage. Laryngoscope 2003; 113(11):2010–2013.
84. Divi V, Benninger M. Postoperative tonsillectomy bleed: coblation versus non-coblation. Laryngoscope 2005; 115(1):31–33.
85. Noon AP, Hargreaves S. Increased post-operative haemorrhage seen in adult coblation tonsillectomy. J Laryngol Otol 2003; 117(9):704–706.
86. Lowe D, van der Meulen J. National Prospective Tonsillectomy Audit: tonsillectomy technique as a risk factor for postoperative haemorrhage. Lancet 2004; 364(9435):697–702.
87. Walker RA, Syed ZA. Harmonic scalpel tonsillectomy versus electrocautery tonsillectomy: a comparative pilot study. Otolaryngol Head Neck Surg 2001; 125(5):449–455.
88. Willging JP, Wiatrak BJ. Harmonic scalpel tonsillectomy in children: a randomized prospective study. Otolaryngol Head Neck Surg 2003; 128(3):318–325.
89. Linder A, Markstrom A, Hultcrantz E. Using the carbon dioxide laser for tonsillotomy in children. Int J Pediatr Otorhinolaryngol 1999; 50(1):31–36.
90. Hultcrantz E, Linder A, Markstrom A. Long-term effects of intracapsular partial tonsillectomy (tonsillotomy) compared with full tonsillectomy. Int J Pediatr Otorhinolaryngol 2005; 69(4):463–469.

91. Koltai PJ, Solares CA, Mascha EJ, et al. Intracapsular partial tonsillectomy for tonsillar hypertrophy in children. Laryngoscope 2002; 112(8 Pt 2 suppl 100):17–19.

92. Koltai PJ, Solares CA, Koempel JA, et al. Intracapsular tonsillar reduction (partial tonsillectomy): reviving a historical procedure for obstructive sleep disordered breathing in children. Otolaryngol Head Neck Surg 2003; 129(5):532–538.

93. Bent JP, April MM, Ward RF, et al. Ambulatory powered intracapsular tonsillectomy and adenoidectomy in children younger than 3 years. Arch Otolaryngol Head Neck Surg 2004; 130(10):1197–1200.

94. Nelson LM. Radiofrequency treatment for obstructive tonsillar hypertrophy. Arch Otolaryngol Head Neck Surg 2000; 126(6):736–740.

95. Nelson LM. Temperature-controlled radiofrequency tonsil reduction: extended follow-up. Otolaryngol Head Neck Surg 2001; 125(5):456–461.

96. Nelson LM. Temperature-controlled radiofrequency tonsil reduction in children. Arch Otolaryngol Head Neck Surg 2003; 129(5):533–537.

97. Telian SA, Handler SD, Fleisher GR, et al. The effect of antibiotic therapy on recovery after tonsillectomy in children: a controlled study. Arch Otolaryngol Head Neck Surg 1986; 112(6):610–615.

98. Colreavy MP, Nanan D, Benamer M, et al. Antibiotic prophylaxis post-tonsillectomy: is it of benefit? Int J Pediatr Otorhinolaryngol 1999; 50(1):15–22.

99. Burkart CM, Steward DL. Antibiotics for reduction of posttonsillectomy morbidity: a meta-analysis. Laryngoscope 2005; 115(6):997–1002.

100. Steward DL, Welge JA, Myer CM. Do steroids reduce morbidity of tonsillectomy? Meta-analysis of randomized trials. Laryngoscope 2001; 111(10):1712–1718.

101. April MM, Callan ND, Nowak DM, et al. The effect of intravenous dexamethasone in pediatric adenotonsillectomy. Arch Otolaryngol Head Neck Surg 1996; 122(2):117–120.

102. Goldman AC, Govindaraj S, Rosenfeld RM. A meta-analysis of dexamethasone use with tonsillectomy. Otolaryngol Head Neck Surg 2000; 123(6):682–686.

103. Steward DL, Welge JA, Myer CM. Steroids for improving recovery following tonsillectomy in children. Cochrane Database Syst Rev 2003; (1):CD003997.

104. Nixon GM, Kermack AS, McGregor CD, et al. Sleep and breathing on the first night after adenotonsillectomy for obstructive sleep apnea. Pediatr Pulmonol 2005; 39(4):332–338.

105. Helfaer MA, McColley SA, Pyzik PL, et al. Polysomnography after adenotonsillectomy in mild pediatric obstructive sleep apnea. Crit Care Med 1996; 24(8):1323–1327.

106. Brown OE, Manning SC, Ridenour B. Cor pulmonale secondary to tonsillar and adenoidal hypertrophy: management considerations. Int J Pediatr Otorhinolaryngol 1988; 16(2):131–139.

107. Friedman O, Chidekel A, Lawless ST, et al. Postoperative bilevel positive airway pressure ventilation after tonsillectomy and adenoidectomy in children—a preliminary report. Int J Pediatr Otorhinolaryngol 1999; 51(3):177–180.

108. Price SC, Hawkins DB, Kahlstrom EJ. Tonsil and adenoid surgery for airway obstruction: perioperative respiratory morbidity. Ear Nose Throat J 1993; 72(8):526–531.

109. Brown KA, Laferriere A, Moss IR. Recurrent hypoxemia in young children with obstructive sleep apnea is associated with reduced opioid requirement for analgesia. Anesthesiology 2004; 100(4):806–810.

110. Moirs MS, Bair E, Shinnick P, et al. Acetaminophen versus acetaminophen with codeine after pediatric tonsillectomy. Laryngoscope 2000; 110(11):1824–1827.

111. Park AH, Kim H. Intravenous home hydration in pediatric patients following adenotonsillectomy. Int J Pediatr Otorhinolaryngol 2002; 66(1):17–21.

112. McRae RG, Weissburg AJ, Chang KW. Iatrogenic hyponatremia: a cause of death following pediatric tonsillectomy. Int J Pediatr Otorhinolaryngol 1994; 30(3): 227–232.

113. Judd BA, Haycock GB, Dalton RN, et al. Hyponatraemia in premature babies and following surgery in older children. Acta Paediatr Scand 1987; 76(3):385–393.

114. Judd BA, Haycock GB, Dalton RN, et al. Antidiuretic hormone following surgery in children. Acta Paediatr Scand 1990; 79(4):461–466.

115. Peeters A, Claes J, Saldien V. Lethal complications after tonsillectomy. Acta Otorhinolaryngol Belg 2001; 55(3):207–213.

116. Weinstein RE, Bona RD, Altman AJ, et al. Severe hyponatremia after repeated intravenous administration of desmopressin. Am J Hematol 1989; 32(4):258–261.

117. Windfuhr JP, Chen YS, Remmert S. Hemorrhage following tonsillectomy and adenoidectomy in 15,218 patients. Otolaryngol Head Neck Surg 2005; 132(2):281–286.

118. Cressman WR, Myer CM 3rd. Management of tonsillectomy hemorrhage: results of a survey of pediatric otolaryngology fellowship programs. Am J Otolaryngol 1995; 16(1):29–32.

119. Prim MP, De Diego JI, Jimenez-Yuste V, et al. Analysis of the causes of immediate unanticipated bleeding after pediatric adenotonsillectomy. Int J Pediatr Otorhinolaryngol 2003; 67(4):341–344.

120. Simoni P, Belloe JA, Kent B. Pseudoaneurysm of the lingual artery secondary to tonsillectomy treated with selective embolization. Int J Ped Otorhinolaryngol 2001; 59(2):125–128.

121. Mutz I, Simon H. Hemorrhagic complications after tonsillectomy and adenoidectomy: experiences with 7,743 operations in 14 years. Wien Klin Wochenschr 1993; 105(18):520–522.

122. Meyer JE, Jeckstrom W, Ross DA, et al. Incidence and clinical background of posttonsillectomy bleeding related blood transfusion over 12 years. Otolaryngol Pol 2004; 58(6):1065–1069.

123. Haapanen ML, Ignatius J, Rihkanen H, et al. Velopharyngeal insufficiency following palatine tonsillectomy. Eur Arch Otorhinolaryngol 1994; 251(3):186–189.

124. D'Antonio LL, Snyder LS, Samadani S. Tonsillectomy in children with or at risk for velopharyngeal insufficiency: effects on speech. Otolaryngol Head Neck Surg 1996; 115(4):319–323.

125. McLaughlin, KE, Jacobs IN, Todd NW, et al. Management of nasopharyngeal and oropharyngeal stenosis in children. Laryngoscope 1997; 107(10):1322–1331.

126. Zucconi M, Strambi LF, Pestalozza G, et al. Habitual snoring and obstructive sleep apnea syndrome in children: effects of early tonsil surgery. Int J Pediatr Otorhinolaryngol 1993; 26(3):235–243.

127. Suen JS, Arnold JE, Brooks LJ. Adenotonsillectomy for treatment of obstructive sleep apnea in children. Arch Otolaryngol Head Neck Surg 1995; 121(5):525–530.

128. Wiet GJ, Bower C, Seibert R, et al. Surgical correction of obstructive sleep apnea in the complicated pediatric patient documented by polysomnography. Int J Pediatr Otorhinolaryngol 1997; 41(2):133–143.

129. Mitchell RB, Kelly J. Adenotonsillectomy for obstructive sleep apnea in obese children. Otolaryngol Head Neck Surg 2004; 131(1):104–108.

130. Mitchell RB, Kelly J. Outcome of adenotonsillectomy for severe obstructive sleep apnea in children. Int J Pediatr Otorhinolaryngol 2004; 68(11):1375–1379.

131. de Serres LM, Derkay C, Sie K, et al. Impact of adenotonsillectomy on quality of life in children with obstructive sleep disorders. Arch Otolaryngol Head Neck Surg 2002; 128(5):489–496.

132. Franco RA Jr, Rosenfeld RM, Rao M. First place—resident clinical science award 1999: quality of life for children with obstructive sleep apnea. Otolaryngol Head Neck Surg 2000; 123(1 Pt 1):9–16.

133. Goldstein NA, Fatima M, Campbell TF, et al. Child behavior and quality of life before and after tonsillectomy and adenoidectomy. Arch Otolaryngol Head Neck Surg 2002; 128(7):770–775.

134. Mitchell RM, Kelly J, Call E, et al. Quality of life after adenotonsillectomy for obstructive sleep apnea in children. Arch Otolaryngol Head Neck Surg 2004; 130(2):190–194.

135. Mitchell RM, Kelly J, Call E, et al. Long-term changes in quality of life after surgery for pediatric obstructive sleep apnea. Arch Otolaryngol Head Neck Surg 2004; 130(4):409–412.

136. Marcus CL, Carroll JL, Koerner CB, et al. Determinants of growth in children with obstructive sleep apnea syndrome. J Pediatr 1994; 125(4):556–562.

137. Nieminen P, Lopponen T, Tolonen U, et al. Growth and biochemical markers of growth in children with snoring and obstructive sleep apnea. Pediatrics 2002; 109(4):55.

138. Bar A, Tarasiuk A, Segev Y, et al. The effect of adenotonsillectomy on serum insulin-like growth factor-I and growth in children with obstructive sleep apnea syndrome. J Pediatr 1999; 135(1):76–80.

139. Brouillette RT, Fernbach SK, Hunt CE. Obstructive sleep apnea in infants and children. J Pediatr 1982; 100(1):31–40.

140. Gozal D. Sleep-disordered breathing and school performance in children. Pediatrics 1998; 102(3 Pt 1):616–620.

141. Friedman BC, Hendeles-Amitai A, Kozminsky E, et al. Adenotonsillectomy improves neurocognitive function in children with obstructive sleep apnea syndrome. Sleep 2003; 26(8):999–1005.

9

Advanced Surgical Treatment of Obstructive Sleep Apnea Syndrome in the Pediatric Patient

Jerome E. Hester, Nelson B. Powell, and Robert R. Riley
Lucille Packard Children's Hospital, Stanford University Hospital, Palo Alto, California, U.S.A.

CHAPTER HIGHLIGHTS

- Great care must be taken when managing the airway of any patient with sleep apnea.
- One should manage pediatric sleep-disordered breathing (SDB) using a "stepwise protocol for therapy."
- Bypassing a stepwise approach in favor of more aggressive treatment exposes the patient to the increased morbidity of advanced procedures, which may not be necessary.
- Skeletal surgery (genioglossus advancement, maxillary-mandibular advancement) may be appropriate in an adolescent with a mature facial skeleton and dentition.
- In an adolescent without significant adenotonsillar hypertrophy and significant craniofacial abnormalities, skeletal surgery may be considered as a first step.
- A careful and stepwise technique to identify the levels of obstruction and treat them with minimal morbidity should be the goal of the physician.

INTRODUCTION

Acknowledgment of obstructive sleep apnea syndrome (OSAS) as a significant cause of morbidity in the pediatric community has met with slow acceptance. Recent studies outlining its effects on cognitive development, memory, behavior, and growth certainly should accelerate its acceptance, and these factors, as well as others, have led the pediatric community to recommend evaluation of all children with signs and/or symptoms of OSAS (1–4). However, it is imperative that, as more children are diagnosed, our treatment options expand and improve.

Certainly, the standard surgical approach has been tonsillectomy and adenoidectomy. Perhaps the first documentation of the surgical relief of airway obstruction having a causal relationship with a child's behavior dates back to 1889, when Dr. Hill published "On some causes of backwardness and stupidity in children and the relief of the symptoms in some instances by nasopharyngeal scarifications" (5). Subsequent studies have shown "cure" rates of 60% to 90% depending on the criteria and follow-up used (6). Marked improvement in cognitive functioning, bite deformities, growth, and quality of life measurements have all been shown after adenotonsillectomy (7,8). However, even the most optimistic results still demonstrate a failure rate, that is, those patients who show persistent SDB after surgery (9). For the majority of these children, no further treatment is recommended or even offered. This is likely due to the lack of systematic studies of more advanced surgical treatments and may be prejudiced in some situations by a lack of understanding of the seriousness of untreated disease. Additionally, there are concerns regarding the effect on the development and growth of the facial skeleton when altered by surgery in the pre-adolescent.

It is necessary to follow a systematic protocol for evaluating and treating the pediatric airway. A similar approach has been followed at Stanford University in the adult population with documented success (10). In this manner, surgical treatment can be guided by the physical findings of the individual patient, all the time understanding that no evaluation method has been shown to be perfect. Recommendations can then be made that will accomplish a high success rate without performing more aggressive surgery than is necessary.

PREOPERATIVE EVALUATION

There has been great discussion in the literature regarding the indications and accuracy of sleep studies for children (11). This debate is beyond the scope of this chapter. However, if one is considering any of the advanced surgical procedures, polysomnogram is mandatory. This allows the surgeon not only to confirm the diagnosis, but also to document the severity of the disease. This information indicates what is actually happening to the airway during sleep and helps identify what type of monitoring will be needed postoperatively.

A full medical history is taken. Although overt cardiac issues are very rare, studies have shown right side heart enlargement in children with sleep apnea (12). Identification of such medical issues will allow full evaluation prior to surgery. A head and neck examination is performed in these patients; fiberoptic laryngoscopy is done to visualize and assess the hypopharyngeal airway and rule out other uncommon findings such as neoplasms.

A cephalometric X-ray will also help define the hypopharyngeal airway and diagrams the facial skeleton. Laboratory data including a complete blood count and general metabolic survey are obtained.

PERIOPERATIVE MANAGEMENT

Great care must be taken when managing the airway of any patient with sleep apnea. Except where noted, all of the procedures we will describe are performed in the operating room with an anesthesiologist well trained in the specific airway concerns in these patients. Most procedures are under general anesthesia. Any procedures done using sedation must be performed with great caution, as it may be difficult to maintain an airway in the heavily sedated and relaxed sleep apneic patients.

Generally, these patients are admitted overnight for observation. The patients who undergo multilevel surgery will be observed in the intensive care unit. Pulse oximetry is continuously monitored. Intravenous narcotics are only prescribed for those patients in the intensive care unit. Patient-controlled anesthesia devices are never used. It has been demonstrated that the sleep apnea patient is more sensitive to narcotics, and the window of safety is much narrower, specifically in the postoperative patient who will have some airway edema (13). In those patients undergoing hypopharyngeal reconstruction, fiberoptic laryngoscopy is repeated prior to discharge. We have shown that significant airway findings can be present in these patients, even if they are asymptomatic (14). The patients are discharged home generally after 48 hours of observation if their exam is satisfactory and they are able to take in adequate oral intake.

STEPWISE PROTOCOL FOR THERAPY

The thought process that led to the development of our surgical protocol for adults certainly is valid for the pediatric population. This reasoning is again based on the imperfection of assessment of the airway preoperatively. Bypassing a stepwise approach in favor of more aggressive treatment exposes the patient to the increased morbidity of these procedures.

Concern for the airway postoperatively should be similar to that in the adult. Consideration should be given to starting the patients on continuous positive airway pressure (CPAP) at least two weeks prior to their surgery if their disease is severe [respiratory disturbance index (RDI) > 40 and oxygen desaturation <80%]. These patients are uncommon in the pediatric population. Patients with an RDI > 60 and oxygen desaturation <70% should be considered for a tracheostomy if they are intolerant of CPAP (15).

SURGICAL PROCEDURES

Temperature-Controlled Radiofrequency Reduction of the Turbinates

Certainly, adenoidal hypertrophy can play a large role in nasal obstruction, especially in the young child. Persistent nasal obstruction can lead to abnormal maxillomandibular development, worsening airway obstruction, and perhaps establishing the framework to develop sleep apnea as an adult (16).

Concerns regarding the alteration of midface growth have limited the use of septoplasty in the pre-adolescent. However, turbinate hypertrophy can also play a major role in nasal resistance. Surgical reduction of the inferior turbinate is associated with crusting, bleeding, and the need for postoperative packing. However, the advent of temperature-controlled radiofrequency reduction of the turbinates markedly reduces these potential morbidities (17).

The procedure is most commonly performed at the same time as other airway procedures, although in older children with isolated turbinate hypertrophy, it may be done under local anesthesia in the office. In these patients, topical anesthetic (1% lidocaine) is applied by cottonoids prior to injection. Approximately 1 to 2 mL of the same local anesthetic is injected into the turbinate. The radiofrequency probe is then inserted into the soft tissue of the turbinate. The amount of energy given is usually dependent on the size of the turbinate, but we have used between 250 and 450 J in this patient group. The patient typically describes the recovery as painless, although nasal congestion will persist for five to seven days.

Complications, which may include bleeding, crusting, and ulceration, are uncommon. Our recent review of 60 consecutive procedures did not yield any complications. Efficacy appears to be very high, although there are no published reports regarding the success rate of reduction of the turbinates using radiofrequency in children. Reported success in the adult population has been reported as 91% (18).

Surgery for Retropalatal Obstruction

Uvulopalatopharyngoplasty and Uvulopalatal Flap

Uvulopalatopharyngoplasty (UPPP) was initially described by Ikematsu in 1964 as a treatment for snoring and was then adopted by Fujita for sleep apnea (19,20). It is perhaps the most widely recommended surgery for sleep apnea in adults. UPPP, when performed correctly, is a successful technique for solving retropalatal obstruction. Published reports have noted only a 40% cure rate when performed alone (21). However, this incomplete response is most commonly due to persistent obstruction at the other regions of the airway. Not understanding this issue may occasionally lead the surgeon to overly aggressive resection, thinking that this will increase success. Unfortunately, this may also lead to an increase of complications without actually improving surgical cure.

This perceived limited rate of success, along with likely 7 to 10 days of significant postoperative pain, has led many in the medical community to shun it as a viable option. This assumption may also have slowed its use in the pediatric age group.

Currently, we do not have any absolute indications for considering palatal surgery in children. In the pre-adolescent who still has tonsils in place, a standard adenotonsillectomy would likely still be recommended (Table 1). However, in a child who has had previous tonsillectomy and has persistent disease, or in the adolescent who has evidence of palatal obstruction, consideration will be given to performing a palatal procedure.

The surgical technique of UPPP has been well documented in the literature with numerous variations described. The procedure is performed in the operating

Table 1 Indications for Advanced Surgical Treatment

In pre-adolescent:
  Persistent disease after adenotonsillectomy: may consider palatal surgery, turbinate reduction, or radiofrequency of tongue base as dictated by exam.

In adolescent:
  Persistent disease after adenotonsillectomy: may consider palatal surgery, turbinate reduction, or radiofrequency of tongue base.
  Skeletal surgery (genioglossus advancement, maxillary-mandibular advancement) may be appropriate if facial skeleton and dentition mature.
  In adolescent without significant adenotonsillar hypertrophy and significant craniofacial abnormalities, skeletal surgery may be considered as a first step.

room under general anesthesia. The technique is outlined in Figure 1. The uvulopalatal flap was originally described as a modification of the UPPP by our group in 1996 (22). Its goal was to reduce the risk of velopharyngeal incompetence and nasal stenosis. It has subsequently been shown to also result in less postoperative pain than the standard UPPP.

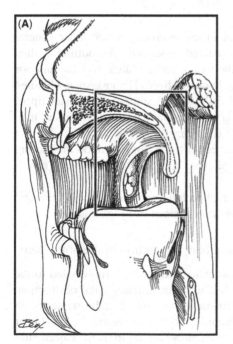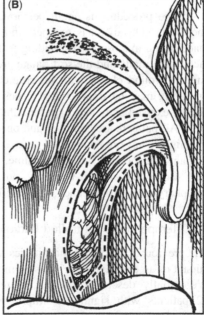

Figure 1 (**A**) Sagittal view of operative site. (**B**) Outline of surgical incision. Care must be taken to preserve mucosa at the anterior and post pillars. (**C**) Site after surgical excision. (**D**) Closure of uvulopalatopharyngoplasty and tonsillectomy (*continued on following page*).

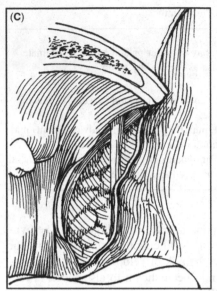 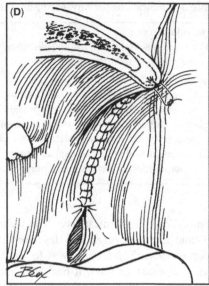

Figure 1 (*Continued*).

The procedure is again performed in the operating room under general anesthesia. The uvula is grasped and reflected superiorly. An outline is then made in the mucosa corresponding to the uvula, and the area over the anterior face of the uvula and the soft palate are demucosalized. Hemostasis is obtained and the wound closed with interrupted 3-0 Vicryl® sutures. The distal tip of the uvula may be transected if necessary. Redundant lateral wall tissue may also be excised and closed appropriately (Fig. 2).

All patients are admitted and observed with oxygen saturation monitoring overnight. They are maintained on a soft diet for 10 days and may require narcotic pain management during that time.

Complications are very low, but may include postoperative hemorrhage, velopharyngeal insufficiency, and various descriptions of dysphagia.

Temperature-Controlled Radiofrequency Reduction of the Soft Palate

The previously described morbidities associated with palatal surgery led to the pursuit of an effective, less invasive method to improve retropalatal obstruction. We initially described the use of temperature-controlled radiofrequency in 22 patients with significant improvement in RDI and snoring (23). Other reports have confirmed its success and safety. However, no trials have been published in the pediatric age group. This technique may have a role in treating persistent retropalatal obstruction. Its limitations may be tolerance of the pediatric patient to the procedure itself, as it is usually performed under local anesthesia

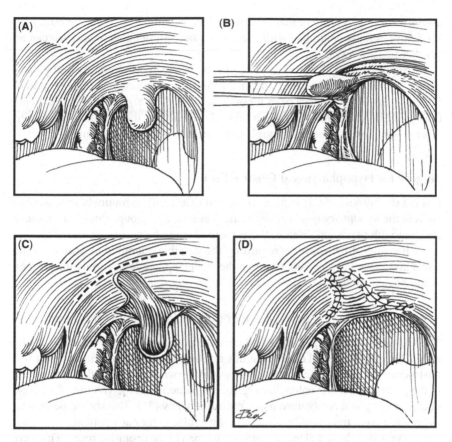

Figure 2 (A) Preoperative view. (B) The uvula is elevated superiorly and its outline marked on the palate. (C) Operative site after excision of the mucosa. (D) Closure of the wound. *Note*: Tonsillectomy can be incorporated when indicated.

and requires significant patient cooperation. In addition, two to four treatments are generally required for success, and even a cooperative child may not wish to return for subsequent treatments, due to the somewhat uncomfortable nature of the injection of local anesthetic.

The procedure is performed with the patient seated upright. Topical anesthetic (20% benzocaine) is sprayed onto the soft palate and posterior tongue. Local anesthetic (0.5% bupivacaine) is then injected into the paramedian areas of the soft palate. The probe of the radiofrequency delivery system is then placed vertically into the palate. It is very important that the surgeon verifies that the probe is within the tissue of the palate. If the lesion is created too superficially, an ulceration will occur. There have also been reports of the probe penetrating into the posterior pharyngeal wall (24). We will typically deliver a dose of 400 to 600 J to each spot in the adult population. Adolescents would receive dosages at the lower end of that spectrum. The patient will likely have mild pain for 5 days, usually controlled with acetaminophen. Subsequent treatments can be given 4 to 12 weeks later.

Reported complications have been low, but include ulceration and palatal fistula, therefore emphasizing the need for proper placement of the probe. Success rates in adults have been reported to be 65% to 80% in selected patients (25). It is likely that this will have a limited use only for those patients with mild disease who are also mature enough to cooperate with the treatment.

Surgery for Hypopharyngeal Obstruction

It is not the purpose of this section to suggest that it will be routinely necessary to address the hypopharyngeal region in the pediatric age group. However, in those children with persistent disease, these methods may be necessary.

Because of the concerns regarding the possible alteration of growth of the upper and lower jaws, consideration of the skeletal procedures is only undertaken in the postpubertal child.

Temperature-Controlled Radiofrequency Reduction of the Tongue

The relaxation of the hypopharyngeal musculature may lead to obstruction during apnea. Surgical treatment directed at this region generally attempts to correct this obstruction by moving the skeletal framework forward. Initial studies performed in the porcine model revealed that significant reduction in the volume of the base of the tongue could be obtained using radiofrequency (26). This should be viewed as an alternative treatment, evaluating its usefulness for each patient.

Typically, the initial treatment is performed in the operating room. This may be performed in conjunction with palatal surgery, or even as an adjunct to the genioglossus advancement. The patient is admitted overnight for oxygen saturation monitoring. Subsequent treatments may be done in the office under local anesthetic, although once again patient compliance in the pediatric age group may limit this, thus necessitating use of intravenous sedation in the operating room.

The procedure is performed by first applying topical anesthetic (20% benzocaine) to the base of the tongue. After grasping the anterior tongue, approximately 2 to 5 mL of 0.25% bupivacaine is injected into the desired location, generally, in the paramedian or median of the tongue posterior to the circumvallate papillae. The probe is then inserted into the tongue musculature. Settings of 85°C and delivery of between 400 to 800 J are given to each lesion. We are generally conservative with each lesion to prevent confluence of the sites. This can lead to a large area of necrotic tissue and increase the chance for infection. Treatments are spaced 4 to 12 weeks apart. Usually, improvement is documented by a polysomnogram after four treatments, although this may vary because of clinician judgment.

Certainly a major appeal of this treatment is the low morbidity. Localized infections and even abscesses have been reported, but serious complications are very rare (27). Studies in adults have shown a reduction in the RDI from 39.6 pretreatment to 17.8 posttreatment (28).

Mandibular Osteotomy with Genioglossus Advancement

The genioglossus muscle is a major dilator of the pharynx. Numerous studies have documented its role in airway obstruction in sleep apnea. The genioglossus advancement procedure was first described by Riley et al. (29) in 1984 and relies on the firm attachment of this muscle to the genial tubercle. Several modifications have been made over the past two decades trying to reduce potential morbidity.

Cephalometric and panorex radiographs are taken preoperatively to assess the position of the genial tubercle and of the tooth root tips. Typically, the procedure is performed under general anesthesia. The tubercle is palpated prior to the incision. The incision is transmucosal in the anterior gingival buccal sulcus. Dissection is then carried out subperiostally to the inferior border of the mandible. The mental nerves are generally not visualized, as the lateral aspect of the dissection is the canine. A rectangular osteotomy is then outlined through the outer cortex using a sagittal saw. This outline is typically 9 × 18 mm and centered 5 mm inferior to the root apices and 10 mm above the inferior border of the mandible, making sure to incorporate the tubercle. A 10 × 2-mm titanium screw is placed in the center of the fragment to facilitate its advancement. The cuts are then completed through the inner cortex. Hemostasis is obtained, and the fragment is then advanced and rotated to overlap the mandible. The outer cortex and marrow are removed and a 10 × 2-mm titanium screw is used to fixate the fragment inferiorly. The wound is then closed using absorbable suture (Fig. 3).

The patient is then admitted and observed under the precautions outlined earlier. Ecchymosis and edema may occur in the floor of mouth, which is generally self-limited, but must be closely monitored. Hypesthesia or paresthesia of the anterior chin or lower teeth will typically be present, but will resolve over a few months. Injury to the tooth roots and mandibular fracture have been reported but generally are avoided by careful placement of the osteotomy.

Hyoid Myotomy-Suspension

Anterior advancement of the hyoid bone has been shown to widen the posterior airway space. Hyoid myotomy with advancement has been performed for over 15 years with significant improvement in the patients' airway. However, in many patients, the genioglossus advancement alone or in concert with radiofrequency of the tongue base provides adequate treatment. The hyoid advancement is also the only one of these procedures that results in an external scar, which may be of particular concern in the adolescent patient.

A horizontal incision is made in a pre-existing neck crease at a level to allow easy access to the hyoid and the superior aspect of the thyroid cartilage. Dissection is continued to identify the hyoid itself. The hyoid is mobilized by transecting the infrahyoid musculature. The upper segment of the thyroid cartilage is identified. The hyoid is then advanced and secured to the cartilage

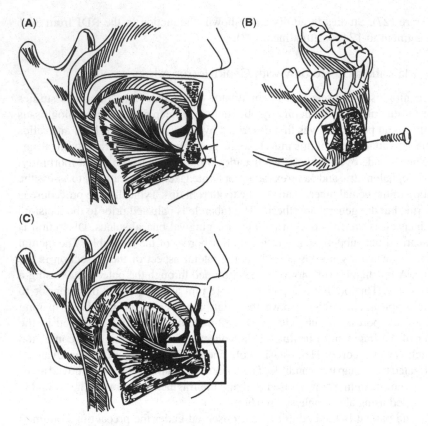

Figure 3 (**A**) Identification of the geniotubercle. (**B**) Advancement and fixation of the mandibular fragment and genioglossus. (**C**) Final position of the advancement.

using permanent sutures. The wound is then closed and a passive drain placed for 24 hours (Fig. 4).

Once again, careful monitoring of the airway is carried out post-operatively localized infection, seroma, and hematoma are infrequent but potential complications.

Maxillary-Mandibular Advancement

Anterior advancement of the maxilla and mandible provides the most aggressive and significant widening of the hypopharyngeal airway. This has led some authors to advocate this surgery as a first-step procedure (30). The stepwise approach outlined previously as our protocol provides an acceptable cure rate with a less invasive technique. However, in those individuals who fail Phase I surgery and still have significant disease, or in those with craniofacial disorders in whom advancement of the midface will improve occlusion or aesthetics, bimaxillary advancement is an extremely effective treatment.

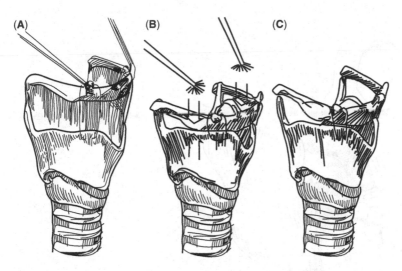

Figure 4 (**A**) Isolation of the hyoid and thyroid cartilage. (**B**) Advancement of the hyoid. (**C**) Fixation of the hyoid to the superior aspect of the thyroid cartilage.

Careful attention is paid to the patient's pre-existing occlusion in addition to the standard preoperative evaluation outlined previously. Although the goal is to maintain the existing occlusion, in those patients with class II occlusion (over-bite), the lower jaw is corrected more aggressively to obtain normal occlusion.

Generally, two units of autologous-packed red blood cells are available prior to surgery. The patient is nasally intubated with the surgical team in attendance. Arch bars are placed if orthodontic bands were not placed preoperatively. These provide stabilizing points during the surgery to maintain occlusion. The maxilla is addressed primarily. The Le Fort I osteotomy is performed using a sagittal saw. The neurovascular bundle is maintained, but other soft tissue attachments are dissected free to allow aggressive mobilization of the maxilla. Rigid fixation is then accomplished with wires and titanium plates.

Sagittal split osteotomies are then performed taking great care to preserve the inferior alveolar nerve. The anterior segment of the mandible is then advanced to match the maxilla. The mandible is then fixated with titanium plates and screws.

With current plating techniques, rigid intermaxillary fixation is generally not required but can be used at the surgeon's discretion (Fig. 5).

The patient is admitted to the intensive care unit for hemodynamic monitoring as well as airway observation. Careful blood pressure maintenance helps reduce postoperative edema and the chance of hemorrhage. Other potential complications such as malocclusion or malunion are reduced by the use of meticulous fixation techniques and the maintenance of a soft diet postoperatively for six weeks.

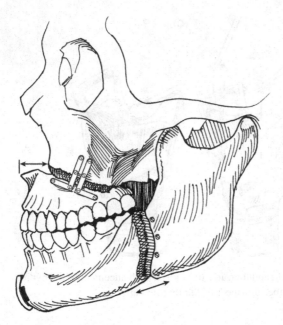

Figure 5 Postoperative view of maxillary–mandibular advancement with rigid fixation in place.

CONCLUSION

As the awareness of sleep apnea in the pediatric population and its associated morbidities grow, the need to successfully treat those patients who have persistent disease after traditional tonsillectomy and adenoidectomy will be paramount. A careful and stepwise technique to identify the levels of obstruction and treat them with minimal morbidity should be the goal of the physician. The application of the above-described procedures, which have shown their safety and success in the adult population, should be applied judiciously to the pediatric population.

REFERENCES

1. Gozal D, Pope DW. Snoring during early childhood and academic performance at ages thirteen to fourteen years. Pediatr 2001; 107:1394–1399.
2. Chervin RD, Archbold KH, Dillon IE, et al. Inattention, hyperactivity, and symptoms of sleep-disoriented breathing. Pediatr 2002; 109:449–456.
3. Chiba S, Ashikawa T, Moriwaki H, Tokunaga M, Miyazaki H, Moriyama H. The influence of sleep breathing disorder on growth hormone secretion in children with tonsil hypertrophy. Nippon Jibiinkoka Gakkai Kaiho 1998; 101:873–888.
4. Clinical practice guideline: diagnosis and management of childhood obstructive sleep apnea syndrome. Pediatr 2002; 109:704–712.

5. Hill W. On some causes of backwardness and stupidity in children and the relief of the symptoms in some instances by nasopharyngeal scarifications. BMJ 1889; 2:711–712.

6. Suen JS, Arnold JE, Brooks LJ. Adenotonsillectomy for treatment of obstructive sleep apnea in children. Arch Otolaryngol Head Neck Surg 1995; 121:525–530.

7. Hultcrantz E, Larson M, Hellqist R, Ahlquist-Rostad J, Svanholm H, Jakobsson OP. The influence of tonsillar obstruction and tonsillectomy on facial growth and dental arch morphology. Int J Ped Otorhinolaryngol 1991; 22:125–134.

8. de Serres LM, Derkay C, Sie K, et al. Impact of adenotonsillectomy on quality of life in children with obstructive sleep disorders. Arch Otolaryngol Head Neck Surg 2002; 128:489–496.

9. Guilleminault C, Li K, Quo S, Inouye R. A prospective study on the surgical outcomes of children with sleep disordered breathing. Sleep 2004; 27:95–100.

10. Riley RW, Powell NB, Guilleminault C. Obstructive sleep apnea syndrome: a review of 306 consecutively treated surgical patients. Otolaryngol Head Neck Surg 1993; 108:117–125.

11. Goldstein NA, Pugazhendhi V, Rao SM, et al. Clinical assessment of pediatric obstructive sleep apnea. Pediatr 200; 114:33–43.

12. Gorur K, Doven O, Unal M, Akkus N, Ozcan C. Preoperative and postoperative cardiac and clinical findings of patients with adenotonsillar hypertrophy. Int J Pediatr Otorhinolaryngol 2001; 59:41–46.

13. Li K, Riley R, Powell N, Zonato A, Troell R, Ouilleminault C. Postoperative airway findings after maxillomandibular advancement for obstructive sleep apnea syndrome. Laryngoscope. 2000; 110: 325–327.

14. Burgess L, Deraerian S. Morin G, Gonzalez C, Zajtchuk JT. Postoperative risk following uvulopalatopharyngoplasty for obstructive sleep apnea. Otolaryngol Head Neck Surg 1992; 106:81–86.

15. Powell N, Riley R, Guilleminault C. Obstructive sleep apnea, continuous positive airway pressure, and surgery. Otolaryngol Head Neck Surg 1998; 99:362–369.

16. Guilleminault C, Partinen M, Praud J-P, Quera-Salva MA, Powell NB, Riley R. Morphometric facial changes and obstructive sleep apnea in adolescence. J Pediatr 1989; 114:997–999.

17. Li K, Powell N, Riley R, Troell R. Radiofrequency volumetric tissue reduction for treatment of turbinate hypertrophy: a pilot study. Otolaryngol Head Neck Surg 1998; 119:569–577.

18. Fischer Y, Gosepath J, Amedee R, Mann WJ. Radiofrequency volumetric tissue reduction (RFVTR) of inferior turbinates: a new method in the treatment of chronic nasal obstruction. Amer J Rhinol 2000; 21:355–360.

19. Ikematsu T. Study of snoring, fourth report: therapy (in Japanese). Jpn Otorhinolaryngol 1964; 64:434–435.

20. Fujita S. UPPP for sleep apnea and snoring. Ear Nose Throat J 1984; 64:74.

21. Sher AE, Schechtman KB, Piccirillo JF. The efficacy of surgical modification of the upper airway in adults with obstructive sleep apnea syndrome. Sleep 1996; 19: 156–177.

22. Powell N, Riley R, Guilleminault C, Troell R. A reversible uvulopalatal flap for snoring and obstructive sleep. Sleep 1996; 19:593–599.

23. Powell N, Riley R, Troell R, Li K, Blumen MB, Guilleminault C. Radiofrequency volumetric tissue reduction of the palate in subject with sleep-disordered breathing. Chest 1998; 113:1163–1174.

24. Terris D, Chen V. Occult mucosal injuries with radiofrequency ablation of the palate. Otolaryngol Head Neck Surg 2001; 125:468–472.
25. Blumen M, Dahan S, Fleury B, Hausser-Hauw C, Chabolle F. Radiofrequency ablation for the treatment of mild to moderate sleep apnea. Laryngoscope 2002; 112:2086–2092.
26. Powell N, Riley R, Troell R, Blumen MB, Guilleminault C. Radiofrequency volumetric reduction of the tongue: a porcine pilot study for the treatment of obstructive sleep apnea syndrome. Chest 1997; 111:1348–1355.
27. Pazos G, Mair E. Complications of radiofrequency albation in the treatment of sleep-disordered breathing. Otolaryngol Head Neck Surg 2001; 125:462–467.
28. Powell N, Riley R, Guilleminault C. Radiofrequency tongue base reduction in sleep-disordered breathing: a pilot study. Otolaryngol Head Neck Sur 1999; 120:656–664.
29. Riley R, Guilleminault C, Powell N, Derman S. Mandibular osteotomy and hyoid bone advancement for obstructive sleep apnea: a case report. Sleep 1984; 7:79.
30. Hochban W, Conradt R, Brandenburg V, Heltmann J, Peter JH. Surgical maxillofacial treatment of obstructive sleep apnea. Plas Reconstr Surg 1997; 99:619–626.

10

Nonsurgical Management of Sleep-Disordered Breathing

Holger Link

*Pediatric Sleep Lab, Pediatrics and Pulmonary Medicine,
Oregon Health & Science University, Portland, Oregon, U.S.A.*

CHAPTER HIGHLIGHTS

- A thorough assessment of sleep-disordered breathing (SDB) should include an evaluation of the effects of sleep disruption on the child's daytime functioning and health in addition to a polysomnography.
- As most nonsurgical treatments for SDB demand a long-term commitment, the parents and child need to understand the goals and reason for therapy from the beginning.
- Children require careful preparation for their first continuous positive airway pressure (CPAP) trial.
- Children with SDB need ongoing positive encouragement to help them adhere to their therapies.
- Children on CPAP should be closely followed for changes in their SDB and complications.
- Weight loss should be a goal for all obese children with SDB.
- Co-existing diseases that interfere with sleep quality should be treated aggressively.

INTRODUCTION

Sleep-disordered breathing (SDB) is associated with significant physical, cognitive, and behavioral health problems (1). Children are particularly vulnerable to the effects of SDB (2). They suffer from disrupted sleep, and in more severe cases, intermittent hypoxia, while going through critical phases of growth. The resulting significant behavior and learning problems have been well documented in children with SDB. It is therefore important to treat SDB in children aggressively.

Many children with SDB are treated successfully with adenotonsillectomy (3,4). A few require more invasive surgery on their upper airway. However, there is a group of children that requires nonsurgical treatment for SDB. This group includes patients that have failed surgery, have congenital upper-airway abnormalities, are too young for corrective surgery, or have a high operative risk, muscular weakness, or rare storage disease.

This chapter will discuss options for the nonsurgical treatment of SDB. Continuous positive airway pressure (CPAP) is the most common nonsurgical treatment for SDB and will therefore be discussed in detail.

GENERAL PRINCIPLES

Who Needs Treatment?

A number of variables must be taken into account when making a decision to treat or not treat a child who has documented SDB. The choice should not be based solely on the apnea-hypopnea index (AHI). While it is usually fairly easy to make a treatment decision in patients that have documented moderate to severe SDB on a polysomnogram, it is more difficult to determine the benefit of treating children whose polysomnograms show only mild abnormalities. In these cases, it can be helpful to include an assessment of the child's daytime functioning. For example, it might be hard to convince the parents of a four-year-old child with a mildly abnormal AHI and no behavioral or sleepiness symptoms to start treatment with CPAP.

Treatment Goals

The primary goals of treating SDB in children are to improve the patient's quality of life and neurocognitive development while reducing daytime somnolence and behavior problems. It is vital that the treatment goals are clear to both parents and child, and that they understand the importance of treatment. Most children will require treatment for many years and the intervention is likely to fail if the parents and the child do not commit to the treatment from the beginning. Likewise, it is essential to follow the patients after initiation of treatment to determine whether or not they are meeting these goals. Patients who realize the most benefit from treatment are the ones most likely to continue it on an ongoing basis.

> Most children will require treatment for many years and the intervention is likely to fail if the parents and the child do not commit to the treatment from the beginning.

Age Considerations

Treatment of younger children with CPAP can be very challenging. They may have a hard time tolerating the equipment and it may be difficult to find a mask that fits well. Very young children with SDB tend to have other comorbidities (5). These patients need to be managed in a team approach that includes close collaboration between the sleep physicians and craniofacial surgeons. Despite these challenges, CPAP can be used successfully in very young children (6,7). It must also be born in mind that, unlike adults, children with SDB go through periods of growth that change the anatomy and physiology of their upper airway. Careful follow-up is therefore critical in order to detect changes in the severity of the SDB.

Special Populations

Patients with Down syndrome require particular attention. A recent study showed that 65% of male patients with Down syndrome also had SDB (8), yet the daytime consequences of SDB are sometimes not fully appreciated, as behavioral problems are common in this population. These patients also often have low muscle tone and a large tongue that contribute to upper-airway collapse (9). They are therefore at risk for having residual SDB after surgical adenotonsillectomy. Due to their behavioral problems, however, they are a very challenging group to treat with CPAP. They usually require intensive preparation for the first trial of CPAP and are more likely to need complex surgery on their upper airway in case of CPAP failure.

> A recent study showed that 65% of male patients with Down syndrome also had SDB.

CONTINUOUS POSITIVE AIRWAY PRESSURE

Indications

CPAP is often used as the sole treatment of SDB. However, it can also be very effective in improving a patient's quality of sleep and daytime functioning while the patient is undergoing other treatments for SDB such as weight loss or staged upper-airway surgeries.

Preparing the Child for Continuous Positive Airway Pressure

The success of CPAP treatment stands or falls with the preparation of the child and family for the first night of CPAP (10). There are several models for preparing the child, depending on the child's age and developmental status. The general approach should be positive and encouraging (11). Most younger children and those with anxiety and behavior problems require at least one outpatient preparatory session prior to a CPAP trial in the sleep laboratory. Challenging patients may require many weeks of intense preparation. It is extremely important to educate both the parents and the patient about the indication for CPAP and specific treatment goals. Full involvement of the parents in the process is critical. If the parents have doubts about the need for CPAP, it will be very difficult to convince the child.

The success of CPAP treatment stands or falls with the preparation of the child and family for the first night of CPAP.

Sleep centers that treat children with CPAP should ideally have a dedicated CPAP team that includes child life specialists or staff trained in preparing children for procedures. All staff involved in preparing the child for the first night of CPAP should be sensitive to the individual child's needs and preferences. They should inquire about the child's previous medical experiences and ask the patient and family what things were helpful in the past. Playing with a doll can be very useful in demonstrating the setup for CPAP titration and may help alleviate anxiety.

The child's initial visit should be conducted with a qualified staff member in a comfortable setting. During that visit, the child should be introduced to the concept of CPAP and have a chance to explore the equipment in a safe environment. The child should be given as much time as is needed to examine the equipment. The emphasis should be on age-appropriate explanations.

Younger children and those with significant anxiety can take the mask and ideally a CPAP machine home, and practice with their parents' help. The parents should be instructed to take a very positive approach to the training, giving frequent positive feedback to the child. Written stepwise instructions can also be helpful. Once the child can fall asleep with the mask on at a low pressure, he or she is ready for a trial of CPAP.

This basic approach will work for most children, but not all. Some children tolerate the mask very quickly, while others may take a long time or refuse to wear it entirely. Fortunately, additional preparatory work with such children can be very effective. A recent study at a large pediatric sleep center is encouraging: approximately 10% of patients who needed CPAP failed the standard approach and went on to further intervention. The intervention consisted of a targeted 1.5-hour consultation and recommendation session or an intensive course of behavioral therapy. The overall success rate of the intervention in this challenging population was 75% (12). This demonstrates that most children will tolerate CPAP with appropriate preparation.

Interface

The interface between the CPAP machine and the patient is probably the most critical technical component of successful CPAP therapy. Finding the right mask for the child is essential, as it can mean the difference between a successful CPAP trial and failure. Comfort, of course, is paramount, although older children might base their choice not just on the feel but also the look of the mask.

> Finding the right mask for the child is essential, as it can mean the difference between a successful CPAP trial and failure.

The number of available masks and cannulas has increased substantially over the past few years, though the availability of masks in pediatric sizes can vary regionally and from country to country. Most children will be served with a small adult or pediatric-sized mask or a nasal pillow. Children with predominant mouth breathing often require a full-face mask to achieve adequate ventilation, as most of the air would leak out through the mouth with a nasal mask. Adult patients with SDB use chinstraps but children do not tolerate them very well.

Very young children and those with craniofacial abnormalities pose a particular challenge. They often have to try many different masks, which then need to be carefully fitted and modified. On occasion, they may require a custom-made mask.

Air Humidification

Because of the high CPAP airflow, the patients cannot properly humidify the inhaled air through the nose and, consequently, they often experience nasal discomfort and complain of dryness in their mouth. This discomfort can make it harder for the patients to adhere to the therapy. The use of a heated humidifier can help alleviate dryness of the mouth and pharynx (13). The ultimate choice, however, is with the patient. A common complication of air humidification is the collection of condensation water in the CPAP hose, but this can be remedied by insulating the hose with a cloth cover.

Titrating Continuous Positive Airway Pressure

In current practice, children stay in the sleep laboratory for their first night of CPAP, both to help accustom the child to the CPAP and to assure adequate titration of CPAP pressure. A well-trained pediatric sleep technician and good preparation are essential to success. It is very important to take time and not rush the child. The setup for children usually takes longer than for adults and the schedule should be set accordingly. The laboratory room should provide a welcoming, child-friendly environment. Children should be encouraged to bring a favorite video or something used in their daily bedtime routine at home. One strategy to relieve anxiety is to involve the child through play in the study setup. Every step of the setup should be explained in advance. Once the child is comfortably settled, the actual CPAP trial may begin. A typical study would start with a low pressure around 4 cm H_2O, which is gradually increased as tolerated until respiratory events are relieved.

A well-trained pediatric sleep technician and good preparation are essential to success.

CPAP titration in the sleep laboratory is relatively expensive, and less time-consuming alternatives are being explored. Some adult patients now use an auto-CPAP device that they can start at home. The device has sensors that automatically adjust the inhalation pressure depending on the degree of upper-airway obstruction. The device keeps a record of the pressure settings and number of obstructive events that later can be reviewed by the treating physician.

A recent study evaluated the use of auto-CPAP in a sleep laboratory in a small group of children (14). Most of the patients had significant improvements in their respiratory disturbance index and oxygen saturations. No studies have looked at home auto-CPAP titration in children. More studies are needed to evaluate the usefulness and safety of auto-CPAP in children.

Complications

CPAP is generally a safe treatment for SDB. Most side effects are minor and can be relieved easily. Dry mouth and nasal congestion can occur if the patient does not use a humidifier. A poorly fitting mask can lead to skin irritation or break-down, as well as dry, irritated eyes, when a leak exists. Patients on high CPAP pressure can experience aerophagia, and nosebleeds and hoarseness have been documented. A more serious potential side effect, midface hypoplasia, has been described in a case report (15). This clearly highlights the importance of fitting the mask just tight enough to eliminate air leak, but not tighter. In addition, children should be assessed for changes in their midface structure during routine follow-ups.

Full-face masks present a risk of aspiration in the event of emesis during sleep. They should not be used in children with uncontrolled gastroesophageal reflux disease (GERD) or during acute gastrointestinal illness. Caution also must be exercised in children with altered mental status, as they might not be able to protect their airway during sleep.

Duration of Continuous Positive Airway Pressure Treatment and Follow-Up

The need for CPAP can change depending on comorbidities, weight loss, and the growth of the child's upper airway. Studies in children show that a substantial number of patients can come off their CPAP over time (6). It is therefore crucial to follow CPAP-treated children on a regular basis in clinic and with repeat sleep studies, in order to make note of any changes in sleep quality, daytime functioning, and recurrence of snoring. Follow-up visits also provide an opportunity to explore barriers to CPAP adherence and discover any treatment complications the patient may be experiencing. In addition, such visits can provide vital positive encouragement to the family and patient.

It is crucial to follow CPAP-treated children on a regular basis in clinic and with repeat sleep studies, in order to make note of any changes in sleep quality, daytime functioning, and recurrence of snoring.

ALTERNATIVES AND COMPLEMENTARY TREATMENTS TO CONTINUOUS POSITIVE AIRWAY PRESSURE

Weight Loss

The textbook child with SDB is thin with large tonsils and/or adenoids. This picture, however, is changing. The number of overweight and obese children in the U.S.A. and worldwide is growing at a very rapid pace (16). As obesity is a risk factor for SDB, we can anticipate seeing an increase in the number of children who present with SDB who are also obese (17).

These patients are at increased risk for cardiovascular and endocrine complications, as well as asthma and obesity-hypoventilation. Furthermore, recent studies have suggested a possible link between obesity, SDB, and systemic inflammation (18).

Obese children are at higher risk for residual SDB after adenotonsillectomy (19). Weight loss is a strategy associated with improvements in SDB and is an essential component of treatment for overweight or obese children. Weight loss is desirable because it not only helps alleviate SDB, but also reduces overall risk for obesity-related comorbidities. It therefore should also be a goal for overweight or obese children who are treated successfully with CPAP alone. Though studies in children are not available, a study in adults showed a 26% decrease in AHI with a 10% weight loss (20). However, individual improvements may vary substantially from patient to patient.

Weight loss is desirable because it not only helps alleviate SDB, but also reduces overall risk for obesity-related comorbidities.

Unfortunately, it is often extremely difficult for obese patients to lose weight or to maintain the lower weight. Overweight children with SDB may suffer from poor sleep and experience significant daytime sleepiness and lack of energy. In addition, sleepiness and fatigue may prevent the child from doing more vigorous physical exercise, which in turn makes weight loss more difficult. To have the best chance for success, weight management should be undertaken in close cooperation with a dedicated team of weight loss specialists that includes endocrinologists, nutritionists, and psychologists (16).

Some patients have a clear genetic predisposition and come from a family where all members are morbidly obese. These children might be candidates for bariatric surgery as late adolescents, if they are otherwise unable to achieve sustained significant weight loss (21).

Nasal Steroids

Nasal congestion and allergic rhinitis can narrow the size of nasal airways and thereby contribute to the severity of SDB. Nasal steroids are an attractive adjunct treatment for SDB as they might help improve nasal airflow and alleviate SDB.

A randomized study compared a six-week course of nasal fluticasone versus placebo in a small group of children three to four years of age with mild-to-moderate SDB. The patients in the fluticasone group experienced a significant decline in the AHI and the desaturation index, though there was no difference in the obstructive sleep apnea symptom score (22). Another study looked at the short-term effect of four weeks of intranasal Budesonide in children 2 to 14 years of age. The AHI and symptom score were significantly decreased two weeks after finishing a course of budesonide (23).

Nasal steroids appear to be inferior to surgical treatment but might be helpful as a bridge while the patient with mild-to-moderate SDB is waiting for surgery. Inhaled nasal steroids also may be indicated and beneficial in patients with severe allergic rhinitis. On a cautionary note, nasal steroids have not been well studied in children who already had an adenotonsillectomy. In addition, there are safety concerns with regard to administration to very young children and prolonged use.

> Nasal steroids appear to be inferior to surgical treatment, but might be helpful as a bridge while the patient with mild-to-moderate SDB is waiting for surgery.

Orthodontics

Some children have significant SDB because of a constricted maxillary arch and associated narrowing of the nasal airway. Recent studies have evaluated the effect of rapid maxillary expansion on nasal airway patency and severity of SDB.

The procedure employs an appliance that is fixed to anchor teeth and rapidly expanded over three weeks followed by a stabilization period of 6 to 12 months. The procedure appears to be generally well tolerated. Studies in selected groups of children who were treated with rapid maxillary expansion have shown very encouraging improvements in SDB (24). The method has not been studied as an alternative to adenotonsillectomy or in overweight and obese children. Rapid maxillary expansion should be considered in select older children who have failed other treatments. It might be particularly attractive in children with Down syndrome who are resisting CPAP treatment (25).

> Rapid maxillary expansion should be considered in select older children who have failed other treatments.

Body Positioning

Upper-airway patency can change with body position. Certain patients' polysomnography shows a higher number of obstructive events in a particular body position. If the difference in the sleep disturbance is significant, the patient can benefit from sleeping in the position that is associated with the lowest number of apneas. Positioning has not been studied systematically in children, but a variety of methods have been used in adults. For example, a tennis ball can be sewn into a pocket on the back of the pajamas to prevent back-sleeping and the patient can try supportive pillows. This therapy may be prohibitively uncomfortable and challenging for children.

TREATMENT OF COEXISTING DISEASES

Asthma

A recent study showed an association between obesity, SDB, and wheezing (26). Obese children are more likely to have both asthma and SDB than children with normal weight. Poorly controlled asthma with nocturnal symptoms can contribute to sleep disruption and frequent arousals through cough or increased work of breathing. This in turn may increase daytime sleepiness and cognitive and behavioral problems. It is therefore very important to aim for optimal asthma control in patients with SDB.

Sleep Hygiene

The use of alcohol and sedative medications such as benzodiazepines have been associated with increased upper-airway collapse and worsening SDB that can be complicated further by a blunted arousal response (27). Teenagers should therefore be counseled on the risk of worsening their SDB when drinking alcohol. Benzodiazepines should be avoided if at all possible in children with SDB.

Chronic Sinusitis

Chronic sinusitis can contribute to chronic nasal and pharyngeal inflammation and result in narrowing of the nasal airway. Some patients may therefore benefit from aggressive treatment with antibiotics, decongestants, and possibly surgery.

OTHER TREATMENTS

Oxygen

Oxygen alone is not recommended for the treatment of SDB. It may occasionally be indicated as adjunct therapy in children that do not otherwise respond to maximum treatment. A previous study in children with SDB showed hypoventilation in response to oxygen therapy in some patients. Oxygen should therefore be used with caution and children that are started on it should be evaluated for their pCO_2 response (28).

Stimulant Medication

Recent studies in adults have shown that the use of alerting medications may be useful in patients that experience residual daytime fatigue after airway surgery or CPAP treatment (29). The benefit of alerting medications in children with SDB has not been studied. The routine use should therefore be discouraged.

Oral Appliances

Oral appliances that work by either moving the tongue forward or advancing the jaw have been used by adults with predominantly mild SDB who preferred not to wear a CPAP mask during sleep. Success in adults is comparable to some of the airway surgeries (30). Most of the oral devices are initially uncomfortable to wear and require a great deal of motivation and tolerance from patients. The use of oral appliances has not been studied in children, as there is serious concern that these devices will lead to abnormal tooth and jaw development.

REFERENCES

1. Guilleminault C, Lee JH, Chan A. Pediatric obstructive sleep apnea syndrome. Arch Pediatr Adolesc Med, 2005; 159(8):775–785.
2. Bass JL, Corwin M, Gozal D, et al. The effect of chronic or intermittent hypoxia on cognition in childhood: a review of the evidence. Pediatrics 2004; 114(3):805–816.
3. Stewart MG, Glaze DG, Friedman EM, Smith EO, Bautista M. Quality of life and sleep study findings after adenotonsillectomy in children with obstructive sleep apnea. Arch Otolaryngol Head Neck Surg 2005; 131(4):308–314.

4. Mitchell RB, Kelley J, Call E, Yao N. Quality of life after adenotonsillectomy for obstructive sleep apnea in children. Arch Otolaryngol Head Neck Surg 2004; 130(2):190–194.

5. Mitchell RB, Kelly J. Outcome of adenotonsillectomy for obstructive sleep apnea in children under 3 years. Otolaryngol Head Neck Surg 2005; 132(5):681–684.

6. McNamara, F. and C.E. Sullivan. Obstructive sleep apnea in infants and its management with nasal continuous positive airway pressure. Chest 1999; 116(1):10 16.

7. Downey R 3rd, Perkin RM, MacQuarrie J. Nasal continuous positive airway pressure use in children with obstructive sleep apnea younger than 2 years of age. Chest 2000; 117(6):1608–1612.

8. de Miguel-Diez J, Villa-Asensi JR, Alvarez-Sala JL. Prevalence of sleep-disordered breathing in children with Down syndrome: polygraphic findings in 108 children. Sleep 2003. 26(8):1006–1009.

9. Donnelly LF, Shott SR, LaRose CR, Chini BA, Amin RS. Causes of persistent obstructive sleep apnea despite previous tonsillectomy and adenoidectomy in children with Down syndrome as depicted on static and dynamic cine MRI. AJR Am J Roentgenol 2004; 183(1):175–181.

10. Massa F, Gonsalez S, Laverty A, Wallis C, Lane R. The use of nasal continuous positive airway pressure to treat obstructive sleep apnoea. Arch Dis Child 2002; 87(5):438–443.

11. Zaremba E, Barkey M, Mesa C, Sanniti K, Rosen C. Making polysomnography more "child friendly": a family-centered care approach. J Sleep Med 2005; 1(2):189–198.

12. Koontz KL, Slifer KJ, Cataldo MD, Marcus CL. Improving pediatric compliance with positive airway pressure therapy: the impact of behavioral intervention. Sleep 2003; 26(8):1010–1015.

13. Massie CA, Hart RW, Peralez K, Richards GN. Effects of humidification on nasal symptoms and compliance in sleep apnea patients using continuous positive airway pressure. Chest 1999; 116(2):403–408.

14. Palombini L, Pelayo R, Guilleminault C. Efficacy of automated continuous positive airway pressure in children with sleep-related breathing disorders in an attended setting. Pediatrics 2004; 113(5):e412–e417.

15. Li KK, Riley RW, Guilleminault C. An unreported risk in the use of home nasal continuous positive airway pressure and home nasal ventilation in children: midface hypoplasia. Chest 2000; 117(3):916–918.

16. Baker S, Barlow S, Cochran W, et al. Overweight children and adolescents: a clinical report of the North American Society for Pediatric Gastroenterology Hepatology and Nutrition. J Pediatr Gastroenterol Nutr 2005; 40(5):533–543.

17. Wing YK, Hui SH, Pak WM, et al. A controlled study of sleep related disordered breathing in obese children. Arch Dis Child 2003; 88(12):1043–1047.

18. Kelly A, Marcus CL. Childhood obesity, inflammation, and apnea: what is the future for our children? Am J Respir Crit Care Med 2005; 171(3):202–203.

19. Mitchell RB, Kelly J. Adenotonsillectomy for obstructive sleep apnea in obese children. Otolaryngol Head Neck Surg 2004; 131(1):104–108.

20. Peppard PE, Young T, Palta M, Dempsey J, Skatrud J. Longitudinal study of moderate weight change and sleep-disordered breathing. JAMA 2000; 284(23):3015–3021.

21. Sugerman HJ, Sugerman EL, DeMaria EJ, et al. Bariatric surgery for severely obese adolescents. J Gastrointest Surg 2003; 7(1):102–107; discussion 107–108.

22. Brouillette RT, Manoukian JJ, Ducharme FM, et al. Efficacy of fluticasone nasal spray for pediatric obstructive sleep apnea. J Pediatr 2001; 138(6):838–844.
23. Alexopoulos EI, Kaditis AG, Kalampouka E, et al. Nasal corticosteroids for children with snoring. Pediatr Pulmonol 2004; 38(2):161–167.
24. Pirelli P, Saponara M, Attanasio G. Obstructive sleep apnoea syndrome (OSAS) and rhino-tubaric disfunction in children: therapeutic effects of RME therapy. Prog Orthod 2005; 6(1):48–61.
25. de Moura CP, Vales F, Andrade D, et al. Rapid maxillary expansion and nasal patency in children with Down syndrome. Rhinology 2005; 43(2):138–142.
26. Sulit LG, Storfer-Isser A, Rosen CL, Kirchner HL, Redline S. Associations of obesity, sleep-disordered breathing, and wheezing in children. Am J Respir Crit Care Med 2005; 171(6):659–664.
27. Montravers P, Dureuil B, Desmonts JM. Effects of i.v. midazolam on upper airway resistance. Br J Anaesth 1992; 68(1):27–31.
28. Marcus CL, Carroll JL, Bamford O, Pyzik P, Loughlin GM. Supplemental oxygen during sleep in children with sleep-disordered breathing. Am J Respir Crit Care Med 1995; 152(4 Pt 1):1297–1301.
29. Pack AI, Black JE, Schwartz JR, Matheson JK. Modafinil as adjunct therapy for daytime sleepiness in obstructive sleep apnea. Am J Respir Crit Care Med 2001; 164(9):1675–1681.
30. Lim J, Lasserson TJ, Fleetham J, Wright J. Oral appliances for obstructive sleep apnoea. Cochrane Database Syst Rev 2006; 1:Art. No. CD004435.

11

Psychiatric Illness and Sleep in Children and Adolescents

Kyle P. Johnson

Division of Child and Adolescent Psychiatry, Departments of Psychiatry and Pediatrics, Oregon Health & Science University, Portland, Oregon, U.S.A.

CHAPTER HIGHLIGHTS

- Children with mental illness have higher rates of sleep problems.
- Sleep disruption from primary sleep disorders can cause mood, behavioral, and neurocognitive sequelae.
- Sleep disturbances frequently occur in traumatized children, particularly if they subsequently develop posttraumatic stress disorder (PTSD).
- Approximately 75–90% of children and adolescents with a major depressive disorder complain of sleep problems, with one-third to two-thirds of patients experiencing insomnia and approximately one-fourth of patients experiencing hypersomnia.
- It has been estimated that between 44% and 83% of children with autism have sleep problems. These sleep problems are primarily comprised of difficulties initiating and maintaining sleep.
- An issue complicating the assessment of sleep complaints in children with psychiatric conditions is the impact of psychotropic medicines on sleep architecture. Many psychotropic medications may cause or exacerbate sleep disturbances.

INTRODUCTION

It has been suggested that mental illnesses are the chronic diseases of the young (1). The 12-month prevalence of mental disorders in the U.S. population is estimated at 26% with half of all cases reporting onset prior to age 14 (2). The majority of mental illnesses in children and adolescents go unrecognized for years, and when treatment is initiated, it is often inadequate. Given that childhood psychiatric illness is often recurrent or chronic, persisting into adulthood, the societal costs of unrecognized and undertreated mental illness in the young are enormous.

Children and adolescents with psychiatric illness often present with sleep complaints. In fact, sleep complaints are considered part of the criteria for many psychiatric illnesses presenting in childhood, such as mood and anxiety disorders (3). The clinician assessing sleep complaints in children and adolescents is well situated not only to treat the sleep problem, but also to recognize psychiatric illness and make appropriate referral.

A bi-directional relationship exists between psychiatric illness and sleep problems in children (4). Children with mental illness have higher rates of sleep problems and, conversely, experimentally induced sleep deprivation or sleep disruption from primary sleep disorders can cause mood, behavioral, and neurocognitive sequelae. The treatment of primary sleep disorders may in fact prevent the development of psychiatric illnesses such as major depressive disorder (MDD) (5).

It is important for the clinician who sees children and adolescents with sleep complaints, whether a primary care provider or sleep specialist, to be versed in screening for and recognizing comorbid psychiatric illness. Therefore, this chapter will review the associations between psychiatric illnesses commonly seen in the pediatric population and sleep. Additionally, recommendations will be outlined for the assessment and treatment of sleep complaints in children with psychiatric conditions.

ANXIETY DISORDERS

Anxiety disorders, as a class, are the most common psychiatric disorders in adults and children with a lifetime prevalence estimate of 28.8% (2). Undoubtedly, the clinician evaluating children with sleep complaints will see children with these common disorders. Although many children experience some fears at bedtime or in the middle of the night, children with clinical anxiety disorders experience frequent, intense, and impairing anxiety that usually spills over into the daytime. Anxiety disorders in children frequently associated with sleep problems include separation anxiety disorder, generalized anxiety disorder, and posttraumatic stress disorder (PTSD). Initial insomnia is the primary sleep complaint often associated with hyperarousal, hypervigilance, obsessive ruminations, and somatic tension. Sleep maintenance problems are also common.

Children with separation anxiety disorder experience excessive anxiety when separated from home or from those to whom they feel attached, typically parents (Table 1). The disturbance must last for at least four weeks and cause significant distress or impairment. The prevalence rate is estimated to be about 4% in children and young adolescents, with decreasing prevalence from childhood through adolescence. Children with separation anxiety disorder often need to know the whereabouts of their parents. They frequently are desperate to stay in touch with attachment figures, often making phone calls to parents at work or when traveling. Children may have difficulties being away from home, such as on sleepovers with peers. Children with separation anxiety disorder may ruminate about their attachment figures or themselves being involved in accidents or suffering illnesses. School refusal is often part of this disorder, as is "clinging" behavior. Frequently, children have difficulty initiating sleep without the attachment figure

Table 1 DSM-IV-TR Diagnostic Criteria for Separation Anxiety Disorder

Diagnostic criteria for 309.21 separation anxiety disorder
A. Developmentally inappropriate and excessive anxiety concerning separation from home or from those to whom the individual is attached, as evidenced by three (or more) of the following:
    1. Recurrent excessive distress when separation from home or major attachment figures occurs or is anticipated
    2. Persistent and excessive worry about losing, or about possible harm befalling, major attachment figures
    3. Persistent and excessive worry that an untoward event will lead to separation from a major attachment figure (e.g., getting lost or being kidnapped)
    4. Persistent reluctance or refusal to go to school or elsewhere because of fear of separation
    5. Persistently and excessively fearful or reluctant to be alone or without major attachment figures at home or without significant adults in other settings
    6. Persistent reluctance or refusal to go to sleep without being near a major attachment figure or to sleep away from home
    7. Repeated nightmares involving the theme of separation
    8. Repeated complaints of physical symptoms (such as headaches, stomach aches, nausea, or vomiting) when separation from major attachment figures occurs or is anticipated
B. Duration of the disturbance is at least four weeks.
C. Onset is before 18 years of age.
D. The disturbance causes clinically significant distress or impairment in social, academic (occupational), or other important areas of functioning.
E. The disturbance does not occur exclusively during the course of a pervasive developmental disorder, schizophrenia, or other psychotic disorder and, in adolescents and adults, is not better accounted for by panic disorder with agoraphobia.

Source: Diagnostic and Statistical Manual of Mental Disorders, Fourth Edition-Text Revision (DSM-IV-TR).

present, and often insist on sleeping in the parental bed or bedroom. If they are not allowed to enter the parental bedroom, they may sleep in the hallway, outside the door. Additionally, nightmares that express the child's fears may be present (6).

Generalized anxiety disorder, as defined by the DSM, is synonymous with over-anxious disorder of childhood (Table 2). Children with this condition experience excessive anxiety and worry for at least six months, occurring more days than not. They worry about a number of activities or events and the worry is very difficult to control. In children, this anxiety and worry is accompanied by at least one additional symptom such as irritability, muscle tension, difficulty concentrating, or disturbed sleep. Children with generalized anxiety disorder often ruminate at night while trying to initiate sleep. They suffer with hyperarousal and hypervigilance, which makes falling asleep very difficult. Less commonly, they may experience middle-of-the-night insomnia (6).

Table 2 DSM-IV-TR Diagnostic Criteria for Generalized Anxiety Disorder

---

Diagnostic criteria for 300.02 generalized anxiety disorder

A. Excessive anxiety and worry (apprehensive expectation), occurring more days than not for at least six months, about a number of events or activities (such as work or school performance).

B. The person finds it difficult to control the worry.

C. The anxiety and worry are associated with three (or more) of the following six symptoms (with at least some symptoms present for more days than not for the past six months). Note: Only one item is required in children.
1. Restlessness or feeling keyed up or on edge
2. Being easily fatigued
3. Difficulty concentrating or mind going blank
4. Irritability
5. Muscle tension
6. Sleep disturbance (difficulty falling or staying asleep, or restless unsatisfying sleep)

D. The focus of the anxiety and worry is not confined to features of an Axis I disorder, for example, the anxiety or worry is not about having a panic attack (as in panic disorder), being embarrassed in public (as in social phobia), being contaminated (as in obsessive-compulsive disorder), being away from home or close relatives (as in separation anxiety disorder), gaining weight (as in anorexia nervosa), having multiple physical complaints (as in somatization disorder), or having a serious illness (as in hypochondriasis), and the anxiety and worry do not occur exclusively during PTSD.

E. The anxiety, worry, or physical symptoms cause clinically significant distress or impairment in social, occupational, or other important areas of functioning.

F. The disturbance is not due to the direct physiological effects of a substance (e.g., a drug of abuse, a medication) or a general medical condition (e.g., hyperthyroidism) and does not occur exclusively during a mood disorder, a psychotic disorder, or a pervasive developmental disorder.

Abbreviation: PTSD, posttraumatic stress disorder.
Source: Diagnostic and Statistical Manual of Mental Disorders, Fourth Edition-Text Revision (DSM-IV-TR).

Sleep disturbances frequently occur in traumatized children, particularly if they subsequently develop PTSD. Children confronted with an event that threatens their life or physical integrity and causes intense fear and feelings of helplessness may develop PTSD (Table 3). The trauma is often either a man-made or natural disaster, abuse, or observation of domestic violence. Children with PTSD suffer with distressing recurrent and intrusive recollections of the event(s), increased arousal, and avoidance behavior (6). The sleep disturbances include initial and maintenance insomnia and nightmares. The nightmares may be directly related to the trauma, although more often they are nonspecific and recurrent, involving frightening themes. Children with PTSD may demonstrate intense fear at bedtime, unable to separate from parents.

MOOD DISORDERS

Mood disorders, particularly MDD, are fairly common in children and especially adolescents. It is estimated that approximately 2% of children and up to 8% of adolescents suffer from MDD. The lifetime prevalence rate in adolescents is estimated to be as high as 20% (7). Bipolar affective disorder has a prevalence rate in the general population of 1%. Approximately 25% of prepubescent children who experience a major depressive episode will eventually meet criteria for bipolar affective disorder. Mood disorders are often recurrent, with evidence of higher recurrence rates in individuals with earlier onset of illness, particularly prepubertal onset.

The diagnosis of MDD is based on the same DSM criteria used in adults with some important concessions (Table 4). Youth with MDD often present with irritability rather than dysphoria, boredom, and social withdrawal. Somatic symptoms such as headaches, fatigue, and abdominal pain are common. Children with MDD may lose weight, gain weight, or fail to make expected weight gains. Psychomotor agitation or retardation may be present as well as easy tearfulness. Low self-esteem and feelings of worthlessness are frequently experienced as well as obsessions with death and thoughts of suicide. If psychotic symptoms occur, they are typically mood-congruent auditory hallucinations.

It is important to recognize and treat MDD in youth for several reasons. First and foremost is the real risk of completed suicide. It has been estimated that 90% of adolescent completed suicides are associated with a psychiatric illness, most commonly MDD, conduct disorder, and substance-use disorders. Additionally, youth with MDD frequently fail to achieve their potential academically and occupationally and are at high risk for developing comorbid substance abuse or dependence. Because MDD is typically a recurrent illness, early recognition and treatment may change the course of the illness, leading to fewer recurrences over a lifetime.

It has long been recognized that there are specific sleep disturbances associated with mood disorders in adults. Sleep abnormalities in adults with MDD include prolonged sleep latency, maintenance insomnia, early-morning awakenings with an inability to return to sleep, reduced sleep efficiency, and decreased

Table 3 DSM-IV-TR Diagnostic Criteria for PTSD

Diagnostic criteria for 309.81 PTSD

A. The person has been exposed to a traumatic event in which both of the following were present:
  1. The person experienced, witnessed, or was confronted with an event or events that involved actual or threatened death or serious injury, or a threat to the physical integrity of self or others
  2. The person's response involved intense fear, helplessness, or horror. Note: In children, this may be experienced as disorganized or agitated behavior.
B. The traumatic event is persistently reexperienced in one (or more) of the following ways:
  1. Recurrent and intrusive distressing recollections of the event, including images, thoughts, or perceptions. Note: In young children, repetitive play may occur in which themes or aspects of the trauma are expressed
  2. Recurrent distressing dreams of the event. Note: In children, there may be frightening dreams without recognizable content.
  3. Acting or feeling as if the traumatic event were recurring (includes a sense of reliving the experience, illusions, hallucinations, and dissociative flashback episodes, including those that occur on awakening or when intoxicated). Note: In young children, trauma-specific reenactment may occur
  4. Intense psychological distress at exposure to internal or external cues that symbolize or resemble an aspect of the traumatic event
  5. Physiological reactivity on exposure to internal or external cues that symbolize or resemble an aspect of the traumatic event
C. Persistent avoidance of stimuli associated with the trauma and numbing of general responsiveness (not present before the trauma), as indicated by three (or more) of the following:
  1. Efforts to avoid thoughts, feelings, or conversations associated with the trauma
  2. Efforts to avoid activities, places, or people that arouse recollections of the trauma
  3. Inability to recall an important aspect of the trauma
  4. Markedly diminished interest or participation in significant activities
  5. Feeling of detachment or estrangement from others
  6. Restricted range of affection (e.g., unable to have loving feelings)
  7. Sense of a foreshortened future (e.g., does not expect to have a career, marriage, children, or a normal life span)
D. Persistent symptoms of increased arousal (not present before the trauma), as indicated by two (or more) of the following:
  1. Difficulty falling or staying asleep
  2. Irritability or outbursts of anger
  3. Difficulty concentrating
  4. Hypervigilance
  5. Exaggerated startle response
E. Duration of the disturbance (symptoms in Criteria B, C, and D) is more than one month.
F. The disturbance causes clinically significant distress or impairment in social, occupational, or other important areas of functioning.

Specify if:
  Acute: if duration of symptoms is less than three months
  Chronic: if duration of symptoms is three months or more

Specify if:
  With delayed onset: if onset of symptoms is at least six months after the stressor

Abbreviation: PTSD, posttraumatic stress disorder.
Source: Diagnostic and Statistical Manual of Mental Disorders, Fourth Edition-Text Revision (DSM-IV-TR).

Table 4 DSM-IV-TR Diagnostic Criteria for Major Depressive Episode

Criteria for major depressive episode
A. Five (or more) of the following symptoms have been present during the same two-
    week period and represent a change from previous functioning. At least one of the
    symptoms is either depressed mood or loss of interest or pleasure. Note: Do not
    include symptoms that are clearly due to a general medical condition or mood-
    incongruent delusions or hallucinations.
    1. Depressed mood most of the day, nearly every day, as indicated by either subjective
       report (e.g., feels sad or empty) or observation made by others (e.g., appears
       tearful). Note: In children and adolescents, can be irritable mood
    2. Markedly diminished interest or pleasure in all, or almost all, activities most of the
       day, nearly every day (as indicated by either subjective account or observation
       made by others)
    3. Significant weight loss when not dieting or weight gain (e.g., a change of more than
       5% of body weight in a month), or decrease or increase in appetite nearly every day.
       Note: In children, consider failure to make expected weight gains
    4. Insomnia or hypersomnia nearly every day
    5. Psychomotor agitation or retardation nearly every day (observable by others, not
       merely subjective feelings of restlessness or being slowed down)
    6. Fatigue or loss of energy nearly every day
    7. Feelings of worthlessness or excessive or inappropriate guilt (which may be
       delusional) nearly every day (not merely self-reproach or guilt about being sick)
    8. Diminished ability to think or concentrate, or indecisiveness, nearly every day
       (either by subjective account or as observed by others)
    9. Recurrent thoughts about death (not just fear of dying), recurrent suicidal ideation
       without a specific plan, or a suicide attempt or a specific plan for committing
       suicide
B. The symptoms do not meet criteria for a mixed episode.
C. The symptoms cause clinically significant distress or impairment in social,
    occupational, or other important areas of functioning.
D. The symptoms are not due to the direct psychological effects of a substance (e.g., a
    drug of abuse, a medication) or a general medical condition (e.g., hypothyroidism).
E. The symptoms are not better accounted for by bereavement, i.e., after the loss of a
    loved one, the symptoms persist for longer than two months or are characterized by
    marked functional impairment, morbid preoccupation with worthlessness, suicidal
    ideation, psychotic symptoms, or psychomotor retardation.

Source: Diagnostic and Statistical Manual of Mental Disorders, Fourth Edition-Text Revision
(DSM-IV-TR).

total sleep time. Additionally, adults experience abnormalities in sleep architecture including the amount and distribution of nonrapid eye movement (nonREM)
sleep stages across the night and reductions in the amount of slow-wave sleep.
Adults with MDD have REM sleep disturbances including a short latency to
the first rapid eye movement (REM) sleep, an increased total REM sleep time,
and a prolonged first REM sleep period (8). Lastly, insomnia may be an independent predictor of suicidal behavior in depressed patients (9).

The associations between MDD and sleep disturbances in children and adolescents, although less strong than those seen in adults, are nevertheless present. Approximately 75–90% of children and adolescents with MDD complain of sleep problems (10,11), with one-third to two-thirds of patients experiencing insomnia and approximately one-fourth of patients experiencing hypersomnia (10,12). Studies using actigraphy have shown poor sleep quality and irregular sleep–wake rhythms (13,14). A recent study using actigraphy in outpatients with MDD (ages 7–18 years) and healthy controls demonstrated that the youth with MDD had lower light exposure and less time in bright light (15). The adolescents with MDD had lower daytime activity levels and dampened circadian amplitude compared with normal controls. Sleep electroencephalogram (EEG) studies have demonstrated less consistency than adult EEG studies. Only one of several studies has demonstrated shortened REM latency in prepubertal children with MDD (16). Adolescents, especially inpatients with more severe depression, have demonstrated increased sleep latency and decreased REM latency (17). There is some evidence that sleep disturbance present at initial diagnosis may predict risk of relapse of MDD (18).

There are two primary types of bipolar disorder, Bipolar I disorder and Bipolar II disorder. The clinical course of Bipolar I disorder is characterized by the occurrence of one or more episodes of mania. Bipolar II disorder is characterized by one or more episodes of hypomania. Mania and hypomania differ by degree, with mania associated with marked impairment in functioning, need for hospitalization, and often psychosis (6). Otherwise, the diagnostic criteria are the same (Table 5). Decreased need for sleep (e.g., feeling rested after only two to three hours of sleep) is a major symptom of mania and hypomania and is one of the primary symptoms suggested to best discriminate bipolar disorder from attention-deficit/hyperactivity disorder (ADHD) in prepubertal children and early adolescents. One study found approximately 40% of children with mania presenting with a dramatically decreased need for sleep (19). Children and adolescents who are manic, much like manic adults, will not show evidence of tiredness or fatigue during the day, despite decreased or absent sleep. On the contrary, manic individuals will demonstrate increased energy and goal-directed behavior during the day. In some individuals, decreased need for sleep can be the first symptom to signal an episode of mania (3). Recognition and treatment of this decreased need for sleep may subvert the development of a full-blown episode of mania and the associated sequelae such as psychosis, danger to self or others, and hospitalization.

AUTISM SPECTRUM DISORDER

The term autism spectrum disorder (ASD) refers to a group of developmental disorders of brain function with a broad range of behavioral consequences and severity. The DSM refers to this spectrum as pervasive developmental disorder (6). The main symptoms of ASD are impaired social interaction, deficits in

Table 5 DSM-IV-TR Diagnostic Criteria for Manic Episode

Criteria for manic episode

A. A distinct period of abnormally and persistently elevated, expansive, or irritable mood, lasting at least one week (or any duration if hospitalization is necessary).

B. During the period of mood disturbance, three (or more) of the following symptoms have persisted (four if the mood is only irritable) and have been present to a significant degree:
   1. Inflated self-esteem or grandiosity
   2. Decreased need for sleep (e.g., feels rested after only three hours of sleep)
   3. More talkative than usual or pressure to keep talking
   4. Flight of ideas or subjective experience that thoughts are racing
   5. Distractibility (i.e., attention too easily drawn to unimportant or irrelevant external stimuli)
   6. Increase in goal-directed activity (either socially, at work or school, or sexually) or psychomotor agitation
   7. Excessive involvement in pleasurable activities that have a high potential for painful consequences (e.g., engaging in unrestrained buying sprees, sexual indiscretions, or foolish business investments)

C. The symptoms do not meet criteria for a mixed episode.

D. The mood disturbance is sufficiently severe to cause marked impairment in occupational functioning or in usual social activities, or relationships with others, or to necessitate hospitalization to prevent harm to self or others, or there are psychotic features.

E. The symptoms are not due to the direct physiological effects of a substance (e.g., a drug of abuse, a medication, or other treatment) or a general medical condition (e.g., hypothyroidism). Note: Manic-like episodes that are clearly caused by somatic antidepressant treatment (e.g., medication, electroconvulsive therapy, light therapy) should not counted toward a diagnosis of Bipolar I disorder.

Source: Diagnostic and Statistical Manual of Mental Disorders, Fourth Edition-Text Revision (DSM-IV-TR).

reciprocal, nonverbal, and verbal communication, stereotyped behaviors, and a narrow range of interests (20). Other features include impaired imagination, lack of cognitive flexibility, rigidity, preservation, and often disabling anxiety. Onset occurs during the first years of life with an average prevalence estimate of 1 per 1000 (21). Approximately 75% of individuals with "classic autism," as defined by the label autistic disorder in the DSM have intellectual deficits. Asperger's disorder, another form of ASD, by definition does not have intellectual deficits or significant language delays.

It has been estimated that between 44% and 83% of children with autism have sleep problems (22). These sleep problems are primarily comprised of difficulties initiating and maintaining sleep. Additionally, these children suffer with irregular sleep–wake patterns, early-morning awakenings, and poor sleep routines. Since the majority of this research has been done with subjects diagnosed with classic autism, these prevalence rates need to be evaluated in the context of the prevalence of sleep problems in patients with intellectual deficits. Attempts have been made to separate sleeping problems due to autism from those due to intellectual deficits, and it appears that ASD is an independent risk factor for sleep problems (23,24). A recent study specifically looked at parental perception of sleep problems in children of normal intelligence with ASD compared with age-matched controls. The prevalence of sleep problems in the ASD group was significantly higher than in the comparison group (78% and 26%, respectively, $P < 0.002$), as was the severity (25).

The prevalence rates for sleeping problems in children with autism mentioned above are from parental surveys. More recent research has used objective measures of sleep such as actigraphy and polysomnography (PSG), and there are discrepancies between parental reports of sleeping problems and these objective measures. In one study using actigraphy, the only parameter found to be significantly different between children with autism and normal controls was early-morning awakening (26). In another study using actigraphy, children aged 5–16 were divided into two groups, those with sleeplessness and those without sleeplessness. The children in both groups wore an actigraph for five weekdays and nights. Actigraphically-determined sleep patterns of children with sleeplessness did not differ from those without reported sleeplessness (27). Research using PSG in the autistic population has been limited in large part to adolescents and adults. One interesting study of children, however, demonstrated higher rates of REM sleep behavior disorder (28). Five of the 11 children in this study demonstrated REM sleep behavior disorder, with the majority of them responding well to low-dose clonazepam (0.25–0.5 mg at bedtime).

There have been numerous studies of sleep–wake rhythms in individuals with ASD. There appear to be abnormalities in the sleep–wake rhythms including late bedtimes and early final awakenings (29,30). Several studies have demonstrated significantly lower nocturnal melatonin in subjects with autism compared with controls (31,32). In one very recent study, urinary 6-sulfatoxymelatonin was studied in children and adolescents with confirmed autism and age- and sex-matched controls. The nocturnal 6-sulfatoxymelatonin excretion rate was significantly lower in the autistic group and most marked in the prepubertal children (33).

ASSESSMENT

The assessment of a child or adolescent presenting with sleep complaints in the context of psychiatric disturbance, either previously diagnosed or suspected, is rather complex. The clinician is obligated to first assess whether there may be sleep disruptors at play, which if properly diagnosed and treated may lead to substantial improvement in sleep and daytime functioning. An overnight polysomnogram should be ordered if indicated, especially if sleep apnea or periodic limb movement disorder is suspected. If one of these sleep disruptors is present, treatment of that condition should be the priority with follow-up to determine if sleep problems persist despite adequate treatment. If sleep disruptors such as sleep apnea or periodic limb movement disorder are not suspected or have been ruled out, the clinician should assess whether active psychiatric illness is the cause of the sleep complaint. Interviewing the patient alone and possibly the parent(s) alone is important, especially adolescents, as youth may be less comfortable talking about certain topics with parents present. Seeing the youth alone will also allow for a more accurate assessment of comorbid substance use. Conversely, parents may be more willing to share important historical data (e.g., family psychiatric history, trauma history) when not in the presence of their child. There are a number of reliable and valid psychiatric screening instruments that can be used efficiently in a clinic setting (Table 6).

When a child with ASD presents with sleep complaints, another level of complexity is added, particularly if the child is nonverbal. Children with ASD are at risk for behavioral insomnia, so special attention needs to be given to the sleep environment and psychosocial stressors. Although children with ASD do not appear to be at increased risk for sleep-disordered breathing (SDB), this condition must be screened for in this population. Patients with classic autism are at higher risk for epilepsy, therefore nocturnal seizures must be considered in the differential diagnosis for any child presenting with unusual behavior at night. PSG should be used in the same circumstances that it is used in the typically developing population, such as when SDB, periodic limb movement disorder, or nocturnal seizures are suspected. Given the reported increased risk of REM sleep behavior disorder, PSG may be indicated in children with ASD who present with unusual behaviors at night.

An issue complicating the assessment of sleep complaints in children with psychiatric conditions is the impact of psychotropic medicines on sleep architecture. Many psychotropic medications may cause or exacerbate sleep disturbances (Table 7). Stimulant medicines, especially if given too late in the day, may cause

Table 6 Screening Instruments for Psychiatric Illness in Children and Adolescents

---

CDI is a self-report measure of symptoms of depression in children and adolescents aged 7–17 yr (Multi-Health Systems, Inc., www.mhs.com).

CRS-R assesses symptoms of ADHD in children and adolescents aged 3–17 yr. Parent and teacher rating scales as well as an adolescent self-report form are available (Multi-Health Systems, Inc., www.mhs.com).

The MASC is a self-report scale designed to assess a wide range of anxiety symptoms in youth aged 8–19 yr (Multi-Health Systems, Inc., www.mhs.com).

The CBCL/1.5–5 and CBCL/6–18 and TRF/6–18 are screening instruments for a wide range of psychopathology (ASEBA Products, www.aseba.org).

Abbreviations: ADHD, attention-deficit/hyperactivity disorder; CDI, children's depression inventory; CRS-R, Conner's rating scale-revised; MASC, multidimensional anxiety scale for children; CBCL, child behavior checklist; TRF, teacher's report form.

Table 7 Psychotropic Medications that Cause or Exacerbate Sleep Disturbances

Drug	Class	Indication	Sedating	TST	Effect on sleep SWS	Effect on sleep REM	Other
Amitriptyline	Tertiary TCA	Antidepressant	Yes	Increase	None	Decrease	May increase PLMs May increase upper motor tone
Fluoxetine	SSRI	Antidepressant	No	Decrease	Decrease	Decrease	May increase PLMs
Lithium	Mood stabilizer	Bipolar disorder	Yes/no	Increase	Increase	Decrease	
Valproate	Mood stabilizer	Bipolar disorder	Yes	Increase	Increase	Decrease	
Clonidine	Alpha agonist	Anxiety	Yes	Increase	Increase	Decrease	
Clonazepam	Benzo	Anxiety	Yes	Increase	Decrease	Decrease	
MPH	Stimulant	ADHD	No	Decrease	Decrease	Decrease	Impact on sleep depends on timing of dose

Note: Indication listed above is clinical indication, not necessarily FDA-labeled indication.
Abbreviations: MPH, methylphenidate; ADHD, attention-deficit/hyperactivity disorder; REM, rapid eye movement; SSRI, serotonin reuptake inhibitor; TCA, tricyclic antidepressant; TST, total sleep time; SWS, slow wave sleep; PLMs, periodic limb movements.

initial insomnia. Selective serotonin reuptake inhibitors (SSRIs) are known to suppress REM sleep and may cause or worsen insomnia or periodic limb movements. Atypical antipsychotics such as risperidone are often used to treat aggression or self-injurious behavior in autistic children and may impact sleep architecture.

TREATMENT

Treatment, of course, depends upon the diagnosis. Clinicians assessing children with sleep complaints should refer the children and adolescents with psychiatric disturbances to mental health professionals if they are not comfortable treating the youths themselves. Cognitive behavioral therapy or interpersonal psychotherapy may be all that is needed to treat the underlying psychiatric disturbance and thus improve the sleep complaint. Pharmacology may be indicated in some cases and should be tailored to the underlying psychiatric disturbance. SSRIs are helpful for both anxiety disorders and MDD in children and adolescents. When insomnia persists despite psychotherapy and potential pharmacotherapy, soporific medications may need to be prescribed. Unfortunately, there are no Food and Drug Administration (FDA)-approved medications for treating pediatric insomnia. "Off-label" prescribing may be necessary, using standard hypnotics or potentially sedating antidepressants.

Treatment of sleep problems in children with ASD should be multifaceted. Since many of the sleep problems reported in children with ASD appear to be behavioral in origin, behavioral treatments are of utmost importance. Alternative interventions may be needed for older, verbal children such as relaxation techniques and cognitive behavioral therapy. Massage therapy has also been studied in children with insomnia associated with ASD, with 15 minutes of massage before bedtime improving not only sleep, but also daytime behavior at home and school (34). Sleep hygiene should be assessed as well and improved upon when indicated. Children with ASD may be taking psychotropic medications to help with aggressive behavior and anxiety, which may impact sleep.

Because of the studies demonstrating abnormalities in melatonin levels, research has turned to the use of exogenous melatonin in children with ASD and insomnia. In one open-label, twenty-four-month trial with controlled release melatonin, a dose of 3 mg at bedtime improved bedtime resistance, sleep duration, and number and duration of night awakenings with no adverse side effects (35). Another study of children and adolescents with Asperger's disorder demonstrated both subjective and objective improvements in sleep with the use of 3 mg melatonin at bedtime (36). Daytime behaviors also improved with the use of melatonin. Risperidone, an atypical antipsychotic, has been used to treat aggression in children with ASD. In one case series, older adolescents with autism and intellectual deficits demonstrated improvements in sleep onset and maintenance with the use of risperidone 0.5 mg twice a day (37).

Table 8   Signs of Potential Psychiatric Illness in Need of Referral

Younger children
   Marked decrease in school performance
   School refusal
   Persistent nightmares
   Persistent disobedience or aggression
   Provocative opposition to authority figures
   Frequent, unexplainable tantrums
Preadolescents and adolescents
   Marked change in school performance
   Frequent physical complaints
   Sexual acting out
   Inability to cope with problems and daily activities
   Threats of self-harm or harm to others
   Self-injury or self-destructive behavior
   Threats to run away
   Frequent outbursts of anger or aggression
   Unusual behaviors or strange thoughts or beliefs

Source: Your Child: what every parent needs to know about childhood development from birth to preadolescence and Your Adolescent: what every parent needs to know: what's normal, what's not, and when to seek help, 1999, The American Academy of Child and Adolescent Psychiatry.

SUMMARY

The clinician assessing children and adolescents with sleep complaints will see children with previously unrecognized psychiatric disturbance. This clinical encounter is an opportunity to screen for psychiatric illness (Table 8) and make appropriate referrals when indicated. Additionally, the clinician will be asked to assess the sleep problems of children already diagnosed with psychiatric illness, thus it is important to understand what sleep disturbances may be attributed to the underlying psychiatric condition or its treatment. Sleep disorders such as sleep apnea and periodic limb movement disorder may be comorbid with psychiatric illness. When this occurs, treatment of both conditions is needed.

Resources for parents:
The American Academy of Child & Adolescent Psychiatry (AACAP) website
   (www.aacap.org) is an in-depth and reliable resource for parents. "The
   Facts for Families" section is particularly useful.
The following are useful books for parents of children with psychiatric illness:
   Your Child, American Academy of Child & Adolescent Psychiatry
   Your Adolescent, American Academy of Child & Adolescent Psychiatry
   Helping Your Anxious Child, Ronald Rapee, Susan Spence, Vanessa
      Cobham, and Ann Wignall
   More than Moody: Recognizing and Treating Adolescent Depression,
      Harold Koplewicz

REFERENCES

1. Demyttenaere K, Bruffaerts R, Posada-Villa J, et al. Prevalence, severity, and unmet need for treatment of mental disorders in the World Health Organization World Mental Health Surveys. J Am Med Assoc 2004; 291(21):2581–2590.
2. Kessler RC, Berglund P, Demler O, et al. Lifetime prevalence and age-of-onset distributions of DSM-IV disorders in the National Comorbidity Survey Replication. Arch Gen Psych 2005; 62(6):593–602.
3. Ivanenko A, Crabtree VM, Gozal, D. Sleep in children with psychiatric disorders. Pediatr Clin North Am 2004; 51(1):51–68.
4. Dahl RE, Ryan ND. The psychobiology of adolescent depression. In: Cicchetti D, Toth SL, eds. Adolescence: Opportunities and Challenges. Rochester, NY: University of Rochester Press, 1996:197–232.
5. McCracken JT. The search for vulnerability signatures for depression in high-risk adolescents: mechanisms and significance. In: Carskadon MA, ed. Adolescent Sleep Patterns: Biological, Social, and Psychological Influences. Cambridge, UK: Cambridge University Press, 2002:254–268.
6. American Psychiatric Association. Diagnostic and Statistical Manual of Mental Disorders, 4th ed. Washington, DC: American Psychiatric Association, 1994.
7. Lewinsohn PM, Hops H, Roberts RE, et al. Adolescent psychopathology, I: prevalence and incidence of depression and DSM-III-R disorders in high school students. J Abnorm Psychol 1993; 102:133–144.
8. Brunello N, Armitage R, Feinberg I, et al. Depression and sleep disorders: clinical relevance, economic burden and pharmacological treatment. Neuropsychobiology 2000; 42(3):107–119.
9. Agargun MY, Kara H, Solmaz M. Sleep disturbances and suicidal behavior in patients with major depression. J Clin Psychiatry 1997; 58(6):249–251.
10. Ryan ND, Puig-Antich J, Ambrosini P, et al. The clinical picture of major depression in children and adolescents. Arch Gen Psychiatry 1987; 44(10):854–861.
11. Roberts RE, Lewinsohn PM, Seeley JR. Symptoms of DSM-III-R major depression in adolescence: evidence from an epidemiological survey. J Am Acad Child Adolesc Psychiatry 1995; 34(12):1608–1617.
12. Puig-Antich J, Goetz R, Hanlon C, et al. Sleep architecture and REM sleep measures in prepubertal children with major depression: a controlled study. Arch Gen Psychiatry 1982; 39(8):932–939.
13. Teicher MH, Glod CA, Harper D, et al. Locomotor activity in depressed children and adolescents: I. Circadian dysregulation. J Am Acad Child Adolesc Psychiatry 1993; 32(4):760–769.
14. Sadeh A, McGuire JP, Sachs H, et al. Sleep and psychological characteristics of children on a psychiatric inpatient unit. J Am Acad Child Adolesc Psychiatry 1995; 34(6):813–819.
15. Armitage R, Hoffman R, Emslie G, et al. Rest-activity cycles in childhood and adolescent depression. J Am Acad Child Adolesc Psychiatry 2004; 43(6):761–769.
16. Emslie GJ, Rush AJ, Weinberg WA, et al. Children with major depression show reduced rapid eye movement latencies. Arch Gen Psychiatry 1990; 47(2):119–124.
17. Dahl RE, Ryan ND, Matty MK, et al. Sleep onset abnormalities in depressed adolescents. Biol Psychiatry 1996; 39:400–410.

18. Emslie GJ, Armitage R, Weinberg WA. Sleep polysomnography as a predictor of recurrence in children and adolescents with major depressive disorder. Int J Neuropsychopharmacol 2001; 4(2):159–168.

19. Geller B, Zimerman B, Williams M, et al. Phenomenology of prepubertal and early adolescent bipolar disorder: examples of elated mood, grandiose behaviors, decreased need for sleep, racing thoughts and hypersexuality. J Child Adolesc Psychopharmacol 2002; 12(1):3–9.

20. Rapin I. Autism. N Engl J Med 1997; 337(2):97–104.

21. Tanguay PE. Pervasive developmental disorders: a 10-year review. J Am Acad Child Adolesc Psychiatry 2000; 39(9):1079–1095.

22. Richdale A. Sleep problems in autism: prevalence, cause, and intervention. Dev Med Child Neurol 1999; 41:60–66.

23. Bradley EA, Summers JA, Wood HL, et al. Comparing rates of psychiatric and behavior disorders in adolescents and young adults with severe intellectual disability with and without autism. J Autism Dev Disord 2004; 34(2):151–161.

24. Richdale AL, Prior MR. The sleep/wake rhythm in children with autism. Eur Child Adolesc Psychiatry 1995; 4(3):175–186.

25. Couturier JL, Speechley KN, Steele M, et al. Parental perception of sleep problems in children of normal intelligence with pervasive developmental disorders: prevalence, severity, and pattern. J Am Acad Child Adolesc Psychiatry 2005; 44(8): 815–822.

26. Hering E, Epstein R, Elroy S, et al. Sleep patterns in autistic children. J Autism Dev Disord 1999; 29(2):143–147.

27. Wiggs L, Stores, G. Sleep patterns and sleep disorders in children with autistic spectrum disorders: insights using parent report and actigraphy. Dev Med Child Neurol 2004; 46(6):372–380.

28. Thirumalai SS, Shubin RA, Robinson R. Rapid eye movement sleep behavior disorder in children with autism. J Child Neurol 2002; 17(3):173–178.

29. Segawa M. Circadian rhythm in early infantile autism. Adv Neurol Sci (Tokyo) 1985; 29:140–153.

30. Takase M, Taira M, Sasaki H. Sleep-wake rhythm of autistic children. Psychiatry Clin Neurosci 1999; 52(2):181–182.

31. Nir I, Meir D, Zilber N, et al. Brief report: circadian melatonin, thyroid-stimulating hormone, prolactin, and cortisol levels in serum of young adults with autism. J Autism Dev Disord 1995; 25(6):641–654.

32. Kulman G, Lissoni P, Rovelli F, et al. Evidence of pineal endocrine hypofunction in autistic children. Neuroendocrinol Lett 2000; 21(1):31–34.

33. Tordjman S, Anderson GM, Pichard N, et al. Nocturnal excretion of 6-sulphatoxymelatonin in children and adolescents with autistic disorder. Biol Psychiatry 2005; 57:134–138.

34. Escalona A, Field T, Singer-Strunck R, et al. Brief report: improvements in the behavior of children with autism following massage therapy. J Autism Dev Disord 2001; 31(5):513–516.

35. Giannotti F, Cortesi F, Antonella C, et al. Long-term melatonin treatment for sleep disorders in autistic children: a two-year follow-up study. Sleep 2004; 27(abstract supplement):A94.

36. Paavonen EJ, Nieminen-von Wendt T, Vanhala R, et al. Effectiveness of melatonin in the treatment of sleep disturbances in children with Asperger disorder. J Child Adolesc Psychopharmacol 2003; 13(1):83–95.
37. Horrigan JP, Barnhill LJ. Risperidone and explosive aggressive autism. J Autism Dev Disord 1997; 27(3):313–323.

12

Neurobehavioral Morbidity in Children with Sleep-Disordered Breathing

David Gozal

Departments of Pediatrics, Pharmacology and Toxicology, Psychology, and Brain Sciences, Kosair Children's Hospital Research Institute, University of Louisville School of Medicine, Louisville, Kentucky, U.S.A.

Leila Kheirandish-Gozal

Division of Pediatric Sleep Medicine, Department of Pediatrics, University of Louisville School of Medicine, Louisville, Kentucky, U.S.A.

CHAPTER HIGHLIGHTS

- The consequences of respiratory sleep disturbances on neurocognitive function in children have impelled increased research efforts, which thus far suggest a strong causal association between the episodic hypoxia and sleep fragmentation that characterize the disease and the development of diminished memory, attention, and intelligence.
- Problematic and hyperactive behaviors and mood disturbances also seem to originate as a consequence of sleep disordered breathing.
- Infants, toddlers, and school-age children who are reported as poor sleepers by their parents display increased incidence and severity of behavioral issues compared to children without sleep problems.
- Thirty percent or so of all children with frequent, loud snoring or obstructive sleep apnea (OSA) manifest parentally-reported hyperactivity and inattentive symptoms, with improvements being noted following surgical treatment of sleep-disordered breathing (SDB).

SLEEP DISTURBANCES IN CHILDREN

Inappropriate sleep habits in children have increased in developed countries over the most recent decades and have now become a major public health concern. Indeed, the impositions of daily life in technologically advanced societies on sleep and wake schedules have markedly shortened the total duration of sleep that children obtain these days. As a corollary of such alterations in sleep hygiene and duration, awareness of the existence of daytime sleepiness as a frequent problem in children and adolescents and its consequences for behavior and academic performance have recently drawn more focused investigations. One should notice that the term "sleepiness" is rather ambiguous and may be perceived differently by different people or even by different professionals. One potential approach to the quantification of sleepiness involves the multiple sleep latency test (MSLT). This rather simple method involves a series of polysomnographically assessed daytime "nap" opportunities in which subjects are allowed 20 to 30 minutes to fall asleep in a "sleep-promoting environment" (i.e., darkened and quiet room and comfortable bed and temperature). Under such standardized circumstances, the shorter the sleep latency during these nap opportunities, the higher the degree of sleepiness. Although very few studies have objectively measured daytime sleepiness in children, it is quite clear that both homeostatic influences (e.g., the time elapsed since the previous sleep period and circadian clock regulatory systems) and individual differences (e.g., motivation to fall asleep and psychological tension or anxiety) will affect daytime sleepiness. Extensive work by Carskadon et al. (1,2) has shown that pubertal development was associated with increased daytime sleepiness, hence postpubertal adolescents actually require more sleep to retain prepubertal levels of alertness. Despite this physiological evidence, school start times in the U.S.A. and in many other countries around the world dictate that high school students have to wake up earlier than elementary school students, a decision that appears to be in clear conflict with the biological preferences for later bedtimes and later wake-up times during the more advanced stages of puberty (3). In addition to the developmental aspects of daytime sleepiness in children and adolescents, circumstances that lead to either inadequate or fragmented sleep have the potential to adversely affect daytime functioning. This is of substantial concern, particularly when considering the high prevalence of objectively measured sleep fragmentation among school children (4).

Studies on the behavioral and neurocognitive sequelae of sleep disruption in children have thus far addressed the daytime effects of sleep restriction, deprivation, and sleep-related breathing disorders, for example, snoring and OSA, which may be associated with sleep fragmentation. In addition, recently developed animal models have also allowed us to further explore the potential mechanisms underlying such neurobehavioral consequences. In this review, we will therefore examine the potential neurobehavioral and cognitive consequences of disrupted sleep.

BEHAVIORAL CONSEQUENCES OF SLEEP DISTURBANCE

When sleep fragmentation is conducted in healthy adults using auditory stimuli to elicit arousals throughout the night, detriments in performance are clearly apparent the following day (5–7). In this context, cognitive functions requiring concentration and dexterity are more readily affected by the excessive daytime sleepiness (EDS) which results from sleep fragmentation, and often confusion and disorientation occur, which have led to the term "sleep drunkenness." Aggressive outbursts, irritability, anxiety, and depression are known manifestations of EDS in adults and appear to be fully reversed once sleep is allowed and recovery occurs. Similar to adult findings, Sadeh et al. (4) reported a high prevalence of sleep fragmentation in children; however, the effects of sleep fragmentation on daytime functioning have yet to be examined in more detail among pediatric populations.

It is important to note that infants, toddlers, and school-age children who are reported as poor sleepers by their parents display increased incidence and severity of behavioral issues when compared with children without sleep problems (8–13). These observations have been further confirmed by objective sleep assessments, in which the degree of disturbance in sleep measures and the severity of behavioral alterations were strongly associated (14–19). Furthermore, 36% of young children with global reports of sleep problems presented with significant behavioral problems (20); daytime hyperactivity and anxiety and depressive symptoms were associated with global sleep problems, such as prolonged sleep latency (13,20). Preschool children with shorter total sleep time exhibited more behavioral problems (21), and the reciprocal of this observation holds true as well, as improvements in sleep are associated with improvement in daytime behavior (15,22). Thus, sleep and behavior exhibit a complex array of interactions that may either interfere with each other or synergistically enhance each other in children. In order to further understand the potential impact of hypoxia on cognitive and behavioral daytime functioning in the context of SDB, awareness that hypoxia is unlikely to occur in isolation and may impact sleep integrity is necessary. Therefore, a short review on the effects of sleep restriction on higher level functioning in children seems appropriate.

Sleep Restriction

Acute sleep restriction for one night in children has been shown to increase inattentive behavior the following day, although no changes were observed in hyperactive or impulsive behaviors (23). Similarly, extended sleep restriction for seven nights led to increased parent-reported oppositional and inattentive behaviors, but no increases in teacher-reported behavioral problems (24). Notwithstanding such observations, total sleep time does not appear to be the major determinant of daytime behavior problems in children; disruption of the sleep process, rather than total amount of sleep, may be the key factor underlying the behavioral alterations that are vulnerable to sleep disruption (25). Thus, fragmentation by multiple arousals such as is observed in OSA or in periodic limb-movement disorder of sleep would be expected to be associated with neurobehavioral disturbances. To corroborate this assumption, a recent study from our laboratory found significant relationships between arousals associated with periodic limb movements during sleep and attention-deficit/hyperactivity disorder (ADHD) (26). Thus, an associative and possibly causative link appears to be present between fragmented sleep and hyperactive behaviors.

Snoring and Obstructive Sleep Apnea

OSA is a more severe form of SDB and is a common occurrence in both adults and children, with up to 3% of young children being affected (9,27–30). OSA is characterized by repeated events of partial or complete upper airway obstruction during sleep. These upper airway changes will induce disruption of normal alveolar ventilation and sleep structure and lead to blood gas abnormalities and sleep fragmentation (31) (Figs. 1 and 2). Despite the fact that OSA and its associated manifestations were first described over 120 years ago (32,33), it was only in

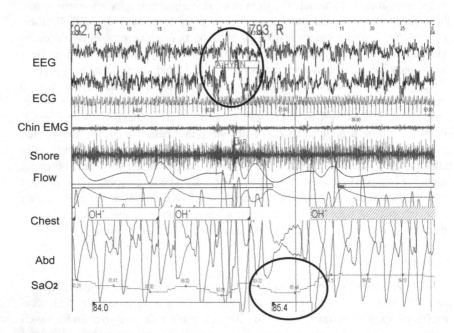

Figure 1 Illustrative example of a partial upper airway obstruction (hypopnea), with reduction (OH) of oronasal airflow in the presence of respiratory efforts, oxyhemoglobin desaturation, and sleep arousal (circles). These events occurred during rapid eye movement sleep (R). *Abbreviations*: EEG, electroencephalogram; ECG, electrocardiogram; EMG, electromyogram; Snore, sound channel; AF, airflow; SaO$_2$, oxyhemoglobin saturation.

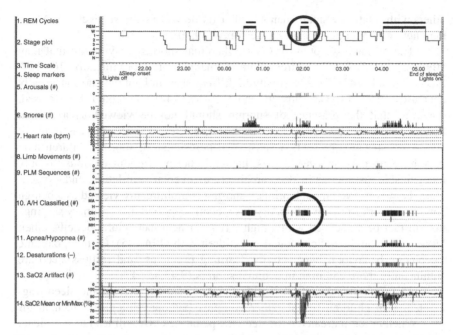

Figure 2 Overnight hypnogram of an eight-year-old child with mild-to-moderate obstructive sleep apnea illustrating the clustering of respiratory events during rapid eye movement sleep (circles). *Abbreviation*: REM, rapid eye movement.

1976 that Guilleminault (34) reported on OSA as a clinically relevant entity in children. Furthermore, Osler (33) reported that children with "loud and snorting" respirations with "prolonged pauses" were often "stupid looking" and slow to respond to questions, and yet it took our "fast paced scientific community" a century before Osler's observations on neurocognitive decrements in pediatric OSA were actually investigated using scientific methodology. Of particular emphasis is the fact that OSA in children is radically distinct from the OSA that occurs in adults, and such differences are particularly striking in relation to gender distribution, clinical manifestations, and treatment (35,36). In children, OSA is frequently diagnosed in association with adenotonsillar hypertrophy and is also common in children with craniofacial abnormalities and neurological disorders affecting upper airway patency during sleep. In earlier reports, Guilleminault (34) suggested that removal of the enlarged adenotonsillar tissue would lead to complete resolution of clinical symptoms and cure of OSA. However, although enlarged tonsils and adenoids are by far the most important contributor to the pathophysiology of OSA in children, children with OSA also demonstrate the presence of increased upper airway collapsibility (37,38). Thus, adenotonsillar hypertrophy alone is usually not sufficient to cause OSA, and in fact, some children with "kissing tonsils" will not have OSA, whereas others with relatively small adenotonsillar tissue will manifest severe OSA and may not be cured after adenotonsillectomy (39,40).

The primary symptom of OSA is habitual snoring, a symptom that may affect up to 27% of children, with a median of approximately 10–12% (9,19,28, 29,41–43). This relatively high frequency in habitual snoring usually decreases in 9–14-year olds to about 3–5% (44). It should be stressed, however, that the presence of snoring should not be viewed as a normal feature of sleeping children and in fact indicates that the increased upper airway resistance is present. A substantial percentage of snoring children may only have primary snoring, that is, habitual snoring without obvious visually recognizable disruptions in sleep architecture, alveolar ventilation, and oxygenation. However, even though primary snoring is traditionally viewed as a benign condition, work from our laboratory has recently reported that "primary snoring" may in fact be associated with a higher risk for neurobehavioral deficits, albeit less severe than the deficits found in children with OSA (45). Of note, daytime sleepiness, behavioral hyperactivity, learning problems, and restless sleep are significantly more common in habitual snorers (9,43,45–47).

The consequences of OSA with its associated hypoxemia and sleep fragmentation in children reveal rather complex pathophysiological mechanisms (48). Whether left untreated or treated late, pediatric OSA will lead to significant morbidity affecting multiple target organs and systems, and such injurious consequences may, under certain circumstances, be partially irreversible despite appropriate therapy. The thus-far-known morbid consequences of OSA in children include behavioral disturbances and learning deficits (9,12,14, 47–53), pulmonary hypertension (54), systemic hypertension and other cardiovascular disturbances such as left ventricular hypertrophy (55–58), and compromised somatic growth (59). In addition, pediatric OSA is associated with poor quality of life (60,61), depressed mood (61), and increased healthcare utilization (62,63).

Schooling problems have been reported in multiple case-series of children with OSA, and in fact, such findings may underscore more extensive behavioral disturbances such as restlessness, aggressive behavior, EDS, and poor test performances (9,12,14,15,18,64–66). Improvements in behavior emerge following treatment for OSA in children (15,50,67), suggesting that at least some of the deficits may be reversible (see subsequent sections for additional considerations).

Obstructive Sleep Apnea and Behavioral Disturbances

Both habitual snoring and OSA are associated with behavioral problems, particularly hyperactivity and ADHD (9,15,68). Hyperactive and inattentive behaviors occur frequently in children with OSA (14,34,47,50) and in children with habitual snoring (9,12,18,45–47,65). Furthermore, ~30% of all children with frequent, loud snoring or OSA manifest parentally reported hyperactivity and inattentive symptoms (9), with improvements being noted following the surgical treatment of SDB (15,69). Interestingly, although children with ADHD appear to exhibit more sleep disturbances than normal children (70,71), we found that despite parental reports of sleep disturbances in >70% of children with ADHD, only 20% of these children had sleep disturbances when assessed by objective polysomnographic criteria (19). Interestingly, SDB was not more likely to occur among children with true ADHD (i.e., diagnoses following the stringent criteria recommended by the Academy of Pediatrics and the Academy of Psychiatry), yet SDB was significantly more prevalent among children with hyperactive behaviors that do not fulfill strict ADHD criteria, suggesting that the subtle disruptions of sleep elicited by the presence of SDB can be associated with significant behavioral effects. As mentioned earlier, sleep fragmentation associated with periodic limb jerks is more frequent in children with ADHD, thus supporting the notion that restless sleep is indeed more common in ADHD patients.

NEUROCOGNITIVE CONSEQUENCES OF SLEEP DISRUPTION IN SLEEP-DISORDERED BREATHING

In adult patients, substantial cumulative evidence indicates that neurocognitive deficits emanate from sleep disruption induced by SDB. These deficits may include deficits in attention, concentration, memory, and verbal and non-verbal intelligence (72–77). Sleep deprivation exerts profound effects on cognitive function in adults, with complex tasks being more susceptible to such deprivation when compared with simpler or automatic tasks (78). Adult patients with OSA exhibit a wide range of neurocognitive deficits, particularly those underlying executive functioning, that is, the brain processes mediating the planning, initiation, and self-regulation of goal-oriented behaviors (79). The literature is not as extensive in children. Similar deficits in neurocognitive function emerge as a result of sleep disruption.

In the context of SDB, the magnitude and probability of neurocognitive dysfunction in children with OSA is more profound than those associated with primary snoring (45,47,53), thereby suggesting a dose-dependent response. Furthermore, hypoxemia is closely correlated with deficits in executive function, whereas sleepiness is preferentially associated with attention loss (73,74). The frequently reported deficits in executive performance in adults with SDB could emanate from hypoxemia-induced frontal lobe dysfunction (80). Several groups of investigators have posited that sleep disturbances are associated with dysfunction of the prefrontal cortex (PFC) in adults, and the same principles should be applicable to children (81). Furthermore, we have recently proposed a theoretical model, in which sleep apnea induces daytime cognitive deficits via disruption of PFC-dependent processes (80). These processes will be described separately as follows.

Attention

The ability to remain focused on task and appropriately respond to extraneous stimuli in the environment plays an important role in learning and, consequently, in social and academic development. Using acute sleep restriction and sleep deprivation, Carskadon et al. (82,83) showed that despite increased sleep propensity, as measured by the MSLT, no impairments could be found in an auditory attention task or in a visual test of sustained attention and inhibition (23). These findings in the laboratory are therefore in contradiction with parental reports of impaired attention following acute sleep restriction in these children. For example, children with early school-starting times have reported more difficulty than their later starting peers when requested to rate attention and concentration ability during school hours (84). Sadeh et al. (85) found no correlations between sleep schedules or sleep duration and neurobehavioral functioning, and Meijer et al. (86) found no significant relationships between subjective sleep variables, such as time in bed, quality of sleep, feeling rested, and difficulty getting up in the morning, and performance on a task of selective attention. Thus, the cumulative evidence would suggest that sleep deprivation rather than sleep restriction appears to be associated with more important effects on intellectual performance.

Inattentive behavior has also been reported in children with OSA (14,49) and in children with habitual snoring (9,12,46). Furthermore, Owens-Stively et al. (87) suggested a dose–response in the scores obtained using attention–impulsivity scales in the presence of OSA in children. Blunden et al. (47) also reported that children with mild SDB demonstrated diminished selective and sustained attention when compared with control children. Studies from our laboratory further buttress the concept that children with primary snoring (45) as well as those with OSA (88,89) are at higher risk for deficits in attention, compared with control children when measured on parental report scales, and that such deficits will be substantially improved after adenotonsillectomy (15,49,51).

Memory

Following acute sleep restriction, no deficits are usually apparent in word memory tasks (82), yet such deficits emerge following 38 hours of sleep deprivation in a sample of similar-aged children (83). Performance of a verbal memory task was unaffected by acute sleep restriction (90), and three nights of restricted sleep in children aged 10 to 14 did not suggest the presence of any deficits on a working memory task (91). However, in children with OSA, memory performance on standardized psychometric tests is significantly affected when compared with control children (47,66) and children with higher respiratory disturbance indices showing greater memory deficits (66). These findings are not consistently reported, as Owens-Stively et al. (87) and O'Brien et al. (19,45,88) did not find any differences in memory performance in children with varying degrees of OSA severity when compared with control children. The limited number of studies in this area and the contradictory results will clearly require further investigation.

Intelligence

Cognitive ability is unaffected by acute sleep restriction but will be impaired on abstract problem-solving tests and verbal fluency (90,91). Neither acute sleep restriction (82), sleep restriction for three nights (91), nor total sleep deprivation for 38 hours (83) will lead to significant shortfalls in computational accuracy, although computational speed will decline after total sleep deprivation. Thus, cognitive functions that require verbal creativity and abstract thinking may be more sensitive to sleep restriction in children than their visual/imagery counterparts.

In children with OSA, several studies have documented significantly reduced IQ scores (obtained from the Wechsler Intelligence Scale for Children—WISC-III), compared with control children (47,66,92). In these studies, the probability for lower normal or borderline range performance was much higher in children with SDB. More recently, we have clearly documented significantly impaired General Conceptual Ability scores [a measure of IQ obtained from the Differential Ability Scales (DAS)] in children with OSA (88) when compared with control children. However, Ali et al. (15) failed to detect any differences in the short-form version of the WISC-III. Interestingly, Lewin et al. (53) found an inverse relationship between the severity of OSA and verbal ability (obtained from the DAS). These investigators suggested that only severe OSA is a risk factor for disruption of verbal abilities. However, this issue merits further investigation because in our rather extensive study, the majority of children had an apnea/hypopnea index between 5 and 10, that is, not severe OSA, and despite relatively modest levels of SDB severity, the verbal abilities and overall language scores were adversely affected (88). In a more recent study in toddlers with OSA who were prospectively screened through parental questionnaires, we were further able to show complete reversibility of cognitive deficits following timely treatment (93). Thus, these studies suggest that early SDB diagnosis and intervention may lead to overall favorable outcomes (94).

Learning and School Performance

Epidemiological surveys in which the total amount of sleep is assessed with questionnaires have indicated that children with later, irregular bedtimes, short sleep duration, and increased daytime sleepiness have lower academic achievements than other children (95,96), although such findings have not been consistent (97). Lower school performance has also been described in children with OSA (14,34,49,67,98,99) and the reciprocal has also been shown to be true, that is, children with poor academic performance are more likely to have sleep disturbances such as snoring and breathing difficulties (50,65). Indeed, we found a 6–9-fold increase in the expected incidence of OSA among first-grade children who ranked in the lowest 10th percentile of their class (50), and significant improvements emerged in school grades after those children with OSA were effectively treated. However, as the optimal intellectual ability and academic performance for these children were unknown, we cannot exclude the possibility that long-term residual deficits may be present after treatment.

To further examine this possibility, Gozal and Pope (100) investigated the history of snoring during early childhood in two groups of 13–14-year-old children who were matched for age, gender, race, school being attended, and socioeconomic status, but whose performance was either in the upper or lower quartile of their class. We found that children who snored frequently and loudly during early childhood were at greater risk for lower academic performance in later years, well after snoring had resolved. These findings suggest that even if the major portion of OSA-induced learning deficits is reversible, there may be long-lasting residual deficits in learning capability. The latter could represent either a "learning debt," that is, the decreased learning capacity during OSA may have led to such a delay in learned skills that recuperation is only possible with additional teaching assistance, or may suggest that OSA may have irreversibly altered the performance characteristics of the neuronal circuitry responsible for learning particular skills.

As indicated earlier, executive dysfunction can markedly alter the functional recruitment of cognitive abilities and therefore result in problematic daytime behaviors such as hyperactivity, impulsivity, poor planning, and difficulty maintaining attention (101). Therefore, poor executive function will associate with dysfunction of other cognitive skills. For example, children with primary language deficits may perform poorly on tasks of executive function that incidentally require language processing (80).

SUMMARY

Sleep disturbance in children, whether due to poor sleep habits or to SDB, is accompanied by marked and obvious behavioral and neurocognitive deficits. Both sleep fragmentation and intermittent hypoxia contribute to neurobehavioral morbidity in pediatric SDB. Although the long-term outcome for children with untreated SDB is currently unknown, reversibility of neurobehavioral morbidities following treatment has been reported. Increased awareness by physicians and parents and early identification and treatment of conditions leading to altered sleep and nocturnal oxygenation should lead to improved neurocognitive outcomes in pediatric SDB.

ACKNOWLEDGMENT

This work was supported by grants from the National Institutes of Health (HL65270 and HL69932), The Children's Foundation Endowment for Sleep Research, and The Commonwealth of Kentucky Research Challenge Trust Fund.

REFERENCES

1. Carskadon MA, Dement WC. Sleepiness in the normal adolescent. In: Guilleminault C, ed. Sleep and Its Disorders in Children. New York: Raven Press, 1987:53–66.
2. Carskadon MA, Harvey K, Duke P, Anders TF, Litt IF, Dement WC. Pubertal changes in daytime sleepiness. Sleep 1980; 2:453–460.
3. Carskadon MA, Viera C, Acebo C. Association between puberty and delayed phase preference. Sleep 1993; 16:258–262.
4. Sadeh A, Raviv A, Gruber R. Sleep patterns and sleep disruptions in school age children. Dev Psychol 2000; 36:291–301.
5. Stepansky EJ, Lamphere P, Badia P. Sleep fragmentation and daytime sleepiness. Sleep 1984; 7:18–26.
6. Stepansky EJ, Lamphere J, Roehrs T. Experimental sleep fragmentation in normal subjects. Int J Neurosci 1987; 33:207–214.
7. Chugh DK, Weaver TE, Dinges DF. Neurobehavioral consequences of arousals. Sleep 1996; 19:S198–S201.
8. Zuckerman B, Stevenson J, Bailey V. Sleep problems in early childhood: continuities, predictive factors, and behavioral correlates. Pediatrics 1987; 80:664–671.
9. Ali NJ, Pitson DJ, Stradling JR. Snoring, sleep disturbance, and behaviour in 4–5 year olds. Arch Dis Child 1993; 68:360–366.
10. Minde K, Popiel K, Leos N, Falkner S, Parker K, Handley-Derry M. The evaluation and treatment of sleep disorders in young children. J Child Psychol Psychiatry 1993; 34:521–533.
11. Ali NJ, Pitson DJ, Stradling JR. Natural history of snoring and related behaviour problems between the ages of 4 and 7 years. Arch Dis Child 1994; 71:74–76.
12. Chervin R, Dillon J, Bassetti C, Ganoczy D, Pituch K. Symptoms of sleep disorders, inattention, and hyperactivity in children. Sleep 1997; 20:1185–1192.
13. Stein MA, Mendelsohn J, Obermeyer WH, Amomin J, Benca R. Sleep and behavior problems in school-aged children. Pediatrics 2001; 107:e60.
14. Guilleminault C, Korobkin R, Winkle R. A review of 50 children with obstructive sleep apnea syndrome. Lung 1981; 159:275–287.
15. Ali NJ, Pitson D, Stradling JR. Sleep disordered breathing: effects of adenotonsillectomy on behaviour and psychological functioning. Eur J Pediatr 1996; 155:56–62.
16. Aronen ET, Paavonen EJ, Fjallberg M, Soininen M, Torronen J. Sleep and psychiatric symptoms in school-age children. J Am Acad Child Adolesc Psychiatry 2000; 39:502–508.
17. Chervin RD, Hedger K, Dillon JE, Pituch KJ. Pediatric sleep questionnaire (PSQ): validity and reliability of scales for sleep-disordered breathing, snoring, sleepiness, and behavioral problems. Sleep Med 2000; 1:21–32.
18. Chervin RD, Archbold KH. Hyperactivity and polysomnographic findings in children evaluated for sleep-disordered breathing. Sleep 2001; 24:313–320.
19. O'Brien LM, Holbrook CR, Mervis CB, et al. Sleep and neurobehavioral characteristics in 5–7 year old hyperactive children. Pediatrics 2003; 111.
20. Smedje H, Broman JE, Hetta J. Associations between disturbed sleep and behavioural difficulties in 635 children aged six to eight years: a study based on parents' perceptions. Eur Child Adolesc Psychiatry 2001; 10:1–9.
21. Lavigne JV, Arend R, Rosenbaum D, Smith A. Sleep and behaviour problems among preschoolers. Dev Behav Pediatr 1999; 20:164–169.

22. Minde K, Faucon A, Falkner S. Sleep problems in toddlers: effects of treatment on their daytime behavior. J Child Adolesc Psychiatry 1994; 33:1114–1121.
23. Fallone G, Acebo C, Arnedt TA, Seifer R, Carskadon MA. Effects of acute sleep restriction on behavior, sustained attention, and response inhibition in children. Percept Mot Skills 2001; 93:213–229.
24. Fallone G, Seifer R, Acebo C, Carskadon MA. Prolonged sleep restriction in 11- and 12-year-old children: effects on behavior, sleepiness, and mood. Sleep 2000; 23 (suppl 2):A28.
25. Stores G. Practitioner review: assessment and treatment of sleep disorders in children and adolescents. J Child Adolesc Psychol Psychiatry 1996; 37:907–925.
26. Crabtree VM, Ivanenko A, O'Brien LM, Gozal D. Periodic limb movement disorder of sleep in children. J Sleep Res 2003; 12:73–81.
27. Brouillette R, Hanson D, David R, Klemka L, Szatowski A, Fernbach S, Hunt C. A diagnostic approach to suspected obstructive sleep apnea in children. J Pediatr 1984; 105:10–14.
28. Gislason T, Benediktsdottir B. Snoring, apneic episodes, and nocturnal hypoxemia among children 6 months to 6-years-old. Chest 1995; 107:963–966.
29. Hulcrantz E, Lofstarnd TB, Ahlquist RJ. The epidemiology of sleep related breathing disorders in children. Int J Pediatr Otorhinolaryngol 1995; 6(suppl):S63–S66.
30. Young T, Peppard PE, Gottlieb DJ. Epidemiology of obstructive sleep apnea: a population health perspective. Am J Respir Crit Care Med 2002; 165:1217–1239.
31. American Thoracic Society. Standards and indications for cardiopulmonary sleep studies in children. Am J Respir Crit Care Med 1995; 153:866–878.
32. McKenzie M. A Manual of Diseases of the Throat and Nose, including the Pharynx, Larynx, Trachea Oesophagus, Nasal Cavities, and Neck. London: Churchill, 1880.
33. Osler W. The Principles and Practice of Medicine. New York: Appleton and Co., 1892:335–339.
34. Guilleminault C, Eldridge F, Simmons FB, Dement WC. Sleep apnea in eight children. Pediatrics 1976; 58:28–31.
35. Carroll JL, McLoughlin GM. Diagnostic criteria for obstructive sleep apnea in children. Pediatr Pulmonol 1992; 14:71–74.
36. Rosen CL, D'Andrea L, Haddad GG. Adult criteria for obstructive sleep apnea do not identify children with serious obstruction. Am Rev Respir Dis 1992; 146: 1231–1234.
37. Isono S, Shimada A, Utsugi M, Konno A, Nishino T. Comparison of static mechanical properties of the passive pharynx between normal children and children with sleep-disordered breathing. Am J Respir Crit Care Med 1998; 157:1201–1212.
38. Gozal D, Burnside MM. Increased upper airway collapsibility in awake children with obstructive sleep apnea. Am J Resp Crit Care Med 2004; 169:163–167.
39. Suen JS, Arnold JE, Brooks LJ. Adenotonsillectomy for treatment of obstructive sleep apnea in children. Arch Otolaryngol Head Neck Surg 1995; 121:525–530.
40. Lipton AJ, Gozal D. Treatment of obstructive sleep apnea in children: do we really know how? Sleep Med Rev 2003; 7:61–80.
41. Teculescu DB, Caillier I, Perrin P, Rebstock E, Rauch A. Snoring in French preschool children. Pediatric Pulmonol 1992; 13:239–244.
42. Owen GO, Canter RJ, Robinson A. Snoring, apnea and ENT symptoms in the paediatric community. Clin Otolaryngol Allied Sci 1996; 21:130–134.

43. Ferreira AM, Clemente V, Gozal D, et al. Snoring in Portuguese primary school children. Pediatrics 2000; 106:5:e64.
44. Corbo GM, Forastiere F, Agabiti N, Pistelli R, Dell'Orco V, Perucci CA, Valente S. Snoring in 9- to 15-year-old children: risk factors and clinical relevance. Pediatrics 2001; 180:1149–1154.
45. O'Brien LM, Mervis CB, Holbrook CR, et al. Neurobehavioral implications of habitual snoring in children. Pediatrics 2004; 114:44–49.
46. Chervin RD, Archbold KH, Dillon JE, et al. Inattention, hyperactivity, and symptoms of sleep disordered breathing. Pediatrics 2002; 109:449–456.
47. Blunden S, Lushington K, Kennedy D, Martin J, Dawson D. Behavior and neurocognitive performance in children aged 5–10 years who snore compared to controls. J Clin Exp Neuropsychol 2000; 22:554–568.
48. Bass JL, Corwin M, Gozal D, et al. The effect of chronic or intermittent hypoxia on cognition in childhood: a systematic review of the literature. Pediatrics 2004; 114:805–816.
49. Guilleminault C, Winkle R, Korobkin R, Simmons B. Children and nocturnal snoring—evaluation of the effects of sleep related respiratory resistive load and daytime functioning. Eur J Pediatr 1982; 139:165–171.
50. Gozal D. Sleep-disordered breathing and school performance in children. Pediatrics 1998; 102:616–620.
51. Owens JA, Spiritio A, Marcotte A, McGuinn M, Berkelhamer L. Neuropsychological and behavioral correlates of obstructive sleep apnea in children: a preliminary study. Sleep Breath 2000; 2:67–78.
52. Blunden S, Lushington K, Kennedy D. Cognitive and behavioral performance in children with sleep-related obstructive breathing disorders. Sleep Med Rev 2001; 5:447–461.
53. Lewin DS, Rosen RC, England SJ, Dahl RE. Preliminary evidence of behavioral and cognitive sequelae of obstructive sleep apnea in children. Sleep Med 2002; 3:5–13.
54. Shiomi T, Guilleminault C, Stoohs R, Schnittger I. Obstructed breathing in children during sleep monitored by echocardiography. Acta Paediatr 1993; 82:863–871.
55. Marcus CL, Greene MG, Carroll JL. Blood pressure in children with obstructive sleep apnea. Am J Respir Crit Care Med 1998; 157:1098–1103.
56. Amin RS, Kimball TR, Bean JA, et al. Left ventricular hypertrophy and abnormal ventricular geometry in children and adolescents with obstructive sleep apnea. Am J Respir Crit Care Med 2002; 165:1395–1399.
57. O'Brien LM, Gozal D. Autonomic dysfunction in children with sleep-disordered breathing. Sleep 2005; 28:747–752.
58. Amin RS, Kimball TR, Kalra M, et al. Left ventricular function in children with sleep-disordered breathing. Am J Cardiol 2005; 95:801–804.
59. Everett AD, Koch WC, Saulsbury FT. Failure to thrive due to obstructive sleep apnea. Clin Pediatr 1987; 26:90–92.
60. Rosen CL, Palermo TM, Larkin EK, Redline S. Health-related quality of life and sleep-disordered breathing in children. Sleep 2002; 25:648–657.
61. Crabtree V, Varni JW, Gozal D. Quality of life and depressive symptoms in children with suspected sleep-disordered breathing. Sleep 2004; 27:1131–1138.
62. Reuveni H, Simon T, Tal A, Elhayany A, Tarasiuk A. Healthcare services utilization in children with obstructive sleep apnea syndrome. Pediatrics 2002; 110:68–72.

63. Tarasiuk A, Simon T, Tal A, Reuveni H. Adenotonsillectomy in children with obstructive sleep apnea syndrome reduces health care utilization. Pediatrics 2004; 113:351–356.
64. Owens J, Opipari L, Nobile C, Spirito A. Sleep and daytime behavior in children with obstructive sleep apnea and behavioral sleep disorders. Pediatrics 1998; 102:1178–1184.
65. Weissbluth M, Davis A, Poncher J, Reiff J. Signs of airway obstruction during sleep and behavioral, developmental and academic problems. Dev Behav Pediatr 1983; 4:119–121.
66. Rhodes SK, Shimoda KC, Wald LR, et al. Neurocognitive deficits in morbidly obese children with obstructive sleep apnea. J Pediatr 1995; 127:741–744.
67. Stradling JR, Thomas G, Warley ARH, Williams P, Freeland A. Effect of adenotonsillectomy on nocturnal hypoxaemia, sleep disturbance, and symptoms in snoring children. Lancet 1990; 335:249–253.
68. Chervin RD, Archbold KH. Hyperactivity and polysomnographic findings in children evaluated for sleep-disordered breathing. Sleep 2001; 24:313–320.
69. Dagan-Friedman B, Hendeles-Amitay A, Kozminzki E, et al. Impaired cognitive performance in children with obstructive sleep apnea syndrome. Am J Resp Crit Care Med 2002; 165:A263.
70. Trommer BL, Hoeppner JB, Rosenberg RS, Armstrong KJ, Rothstein JA. Sleep disturbance in children with attention deficit disorder. Ann Neurol 1988; 24:322.
71. Berry DTR, Webb WB, Block AJ, Bauer RM, Switzer DA. Nocturnal hypoxia and neuropsychological variables. J Clin Exp Neuropsychol 1986; 8:229–238.
72. Greenberg GD, Watson RK, Deptula D. Neuropsychological dysfunction in sleep apnea. Sleep 1987; 10:254–262.
73. Bedard MA, Montplasir J, Richer F, Rouleau I, Malo J. Obstructive sleep apnea syndrome: pathogenesis of neuropsychological deficits. J Clin Exp Neuropsychol 1991; 13:950–964.
74. Naegele B, Thouvard V, Pepin JL, et al. Deficits of cognitive executive functions in patients with sleep apnea syndrome. Sleep 1995; 18:43–52.
75. Kim HC, Young T, Matthews CG, Weber SM, Woodward AR, Palta M. Sleep disordered breathing and neuropsychological deficits. Am J Respir Crit Care Med 1997; 156:1813–1819.
76. Engleman H, Joffe D. Neuropsychological function in obstructive sleep apnea. Sleep Med Rev 1999; 3:59–78.
77. Lee MM, Strauss ME, Adams N, Redline S. Executive functions in persons with sleep apnea. Sleep Breath 1999; 3:13–16.
78. Harrison Y, Horne JA. Sleep loss impairs short and novel language tasks having a prefrontal focus. J Sleep Res 1998; 7:95–100.
79. Lezak MD. Neuropsychological Assessment. 3rd ed. New York: Oxford University Press, 1995.
80. Beebe DW, Gozal D. Obstructive sleep apnea and the prefrontal cortex: towards a comprehensive model linking nocturnal upper airway obstruction to daytime cognitive and behavioral deficits. J Sleep Res 2002; 11:1–16.
81. Dahl RE. The impact of inadequate sleep on children's daytime and cognitive function. Semin Pediatr Neurol 1996; 3:44–50.
82. Carskadon MA, Harvey K, Dement WC. Sleep loss in young adolescents. Sleep 1981; 4:299–312.

83. Carskadon MA, Harvey K, Dement WC. Acute restriction of nocturnal sleep in children. Percept Mot Skills 1981; 53:103–112.
84. Epstein R, Chillag N, Lavie P. Starting times of school: effects on daytime functioning of fifth-grade children in Israel. Sleep 1998; 21:250–256.
85. Sadeh A, Gruber R, Raviv A. Sleep, neurobehavioral functioning, and behavior problems in school-age children. Child Dev 2002; 73:405–417.
86. Meijer AM, Habekothe HT, Van Den Wittenboer GL. Time in bed, quality of sleep and school functioning of children. J Sleep Res 2000; 9:145–153.
87. Owens-Stively J, McGuinn M, Berkelhammer L, Marcotte A, Nobile C, Spirito A. Neuropsychological and behavioral correlates of obstructive sleep apnea in children. Sleep Res 1997; 26(suppl):452.
88. O'Brien LM, Mervis CB, Holbrook CR, et al. Neurobehavioral correlates of sleep disordered breathing in children. J Sleep Res 2004; 13:165–172.
89. O'Brien LM, Tauman R, Gozal D. Sleep pressure correlates of cognitive and behavioral morbidity in snoring children. Sleep 2004; 27:279–282.
90. Randazzo AC, Muehlbach MJ, Schweitzer PK, Walsh JK. Cognitive function following acute sleep restriction in children ages 10–14. Sleep 1998; 21:861–868.
91. Randazzo AC, Schweitzer PK, Walsh JK. Cognitive function following 3 nights of sleep restriction in children ages 10–14. Sleep 1998; 21:s249.
92. Beebe DW, Wells CT, Jeffries J, Chini B, Kalra M, Amin R. Neuropsychological effects of pediatric obstructive sleep apnea. J Int Neuropsychol Soc 2004; 10:962–975.
93. Montgomery-Downs HE, Crabtree VM, Gozal D. Cognition sleep and respiration in at-risk children treated for obstructive sleep apnea. Eur J Resp Dis 2005; 25: 336–342.
94. Friedman BC, Hendeles-Amitai A, Kozminsky E, et al. Adenotonsillectomy improves neurocognitive function in children with obstructive sleep apnea syndrome. Sleep 2003; 26:999–1005.
95. Kahn A, Van de Merckt C, Rebuffat E, Mozin MJ, Sottiaux M, Blum D. Sleep problems in healthy preadolescents. Pediatrics 1989; 84:542–546.
96. Wolfson AR, Carskadon MA. Sleep schedules and daytime functioning in adolescents. Child Dev 1998; 69:875–887.
97. Eliasson A, Eliasson A, King J, Gould B, Eliasson A. Association of sleep and academic performance. Sleep Breath 2002; 6:45–48.
98. Guilleminault C, Pelayo R, Ledger D, Clerk A, Bocian RCZ. Recognition of sleep disordered breathing in children. Pediatrics 1996; 98:871–882.
99. Richards W, Ferdman RM. Prolonged morbidity due to delays in the diagnosis and treatment of obstructive sleep apnea in children. Clin Pediatr 2000; 39:103–108.
100. Gozal D, Pope DW. Snoring during early childhood and academic performance at age thirteen to fourteen years. Pediatrics 2001; 107:1394–1399.
101. Goldberg E. The Executive Brain: Frontal Lobes and the Civilized Mind. Oxford University Press: Oxford, 2001.

13

Evidence-Based Approach to Therapy

Nira A. Goldstein and Richard M. Rosenfeld

Division of Pediatric Otolaryngology, Department of Otolaryngology, State University of New York, Downstate Medical Center, Brooklyn, New York, U.S.A.

CHAPTER HIGHLIGHTS

- Despite the large body of literature evaluating treatment of pediatric sleep-disordered breathing (SDB), most of the studies suffer from methodologic problems including the lack of controls and randomization and nonuniform definitions of disease and outcome measures. There are no studies evaluating long-term effects or possible resolution of SDB in untreated children.
- The published studies, which largely consist of nonrandomized, uncontrolled trials and outcomes studies, suggest that tonsillectomy and adenoidectomy (T&A) is effective as a first-line therapy in most children. Secondary to ethical concerns, one cannot perform a randomized control study to determine the efficacy of a T&A for the treatment of SDB.
- Based on a few retrospective case series and small cohort studies, nasal continuous positive airway pressure (CPAP) and bilevel positive airway pressure (BiPAP), uvulopalatopharyngoplasty (UPPP), and craniofacial surgery appear to have a role in the treatment of selected patients with comorbid conditions or who fail T&A.

- Preliminary studies on the use of topical nasal steroids, oral steroids, and oral antibiotics suggest that the above therapies are not indicated for children with severe OSA, but may have a role in the treatment of milder SDB or for temporary relief of symptoms.
- The natural history of pediatric SDB needs to be elucidated as well as the significance of minor polysomnography (PSG) abnormalities. This will allow complete evaluation of the efficacy of the various treatment options.

INTRODUCTION

Childhood obstructive SDB used to be neatly categorized into obstructive sleep-apnea syndrome (OSAS), which required therapy, and benign primary snoring, which was believed to be clinically insignificant. PSG was considered the "gold standard" diagnostic test to separate the two entities. With the recognition of upper airway resistance syndrome (UARS), SDB is now viewed as a continuum of sleep-related airway obstruction with snoring on one end and complete upper airway obstruction and obstructive hypoventilation on the other.

The relationship between sleep-related upper airway obstruction and its consequences is not straightforward because children with snoring may exhibit severe nighttime and daytime symptoms, whereas children with severe apnea may exhibit few daytime symptoms. Treatment has traditionally been recommended for children who exceeded a threshold for respiratory disturbance index (RDI), degree of oxygen saturation, and other normative criteria in order to relieve the nighttime obstructive symptoms and daytime symptoms and prevent future morbidity. Yet, PSG remains a poorly validated test that has not been shown to predict future morbidity. In addition, children with milder degrees of sleep-related upper airway obstruction may also require therapy.

LIMITATIONS OF POLYSOMNOGRAPHY

Standards for positive PSG in children have been based on studies of their normative values. On the basis of the recommendations of the American Thoracic Society, OSAS is diagnosed when the RDI is greater than five, the obstructive apnea index (AI) is greater than one, the peak end-tidal CO_2 is >50 mmHg for $>10\%$ of the total sleep time, or the minimum SpO_2 is $<92\%$ (1). However, few studies have documented the relationship between PSG abnormalities and daytime sleepiness, impaired neurocognitive function, behavioral abnormalities, or other adverse outcomes of pediatric SDB. It is unclear whether children with mild PSG abnormalities, although outside of the normative range, require therapy. In addition, sleep laboratories around the world use different testing procedures and diagnostic criteria. PSG focuses heavily on breathing with minimal measures of sleep quality. Normative data are limited to classic OSA and are not available for many PSG measures (2).

There are no diagnostic standards for UARS, as few laboratories perform esophageal pressure monitoring since the monitoring is poorly tolerated (3). Some laboratories, based on experience, will consider a PSG suggestive of UARS based on thresholds of nocturnal awakenings (>1/hr), arousal index (>10/hr), or sleep efficiency ($<80\%$) (4). Nasal pressure monitoring which measures inspiratory and expiratory airflows may suggest UARS (5). Currently, UARS remains a subjective diagnosis based on individual judgment and experience.

NATURAL HISTORY

Little is known about the natural history of untreated SDB. As children with OSAS and clinically significant SDB are routinely treated, there are no studies evaluating long-term effects or possible resolution of SDB. Two studies have evaluated children with untreated primary snoring and found that only 8–10% progressed to mild OSAS at one- to three-year follow-up (6,7). Although infantile and childhood OSAS may predispose individuals to adult OSAS because of anatomical and familial factors, there is no current evidence that adults with OSAS had SDB during infancy and childhood (8).

TONSILLECTOMY AND ADENOIDECTOMY

Treatment of SDB aims to reverse or prevent the morbidities associated with the disease, including growth disturbance, neurobehavioral consequences, and cardiovascular effects. The mainstay of therapy is T&A. A review of the published studies evaluating the efficacy of T&A in the treatment of SDB is presented in Table 1. Articles were identified by the use of an English-language MEDLINE Search (search words pediatric sleep-apnea treatment and pediatric T&A, from the 1950s through June 2005, inclusive). Search results were limited to human subjects and supplemented with articles from bibliographies of textbooks, review articles, source articles, and discussion with experts. Most studies included only otherwise healthy children and excluded children with neuromuscular disorders and craniofacial syndromes, and some excluded children with obesity. The studies were graded as to their level of evidence as found on the web site of the Centre for Evidence-Based Medicine in Oxford (http://www.cebm.net/levels_of_evidence.asp) which are listed as follows (9):

1. Level 1a, systematic reviews of randomized, controlled trials
2. Level 1b, individual randomized, controlled trials
3. Level 1c, all-or-none studies
4. Level 2a, systematic reviews of cohort studies with controls
5. Level 2b, individual cohort studies with controls
6. Level 3a, systematic reviews of case–control studies
7. Level 3b, individual case–control studies
8. Level 4, case series, including reviews and uncontrolled cohort studies
9. Level 5, expert opinion

Table 1 Efficacy of Tonsillectomy and Adenoidectomy for the Treatment of Pediatric Sleep-Disordered Breathing

Author	Study design	n	Age (yrs)	Procedure	Follow-up (mo)	Clinical cure (%)	PSG cure (%)	Level of evidence
Mitchell and Kelly (11)	Prospective cohort	20	2.2 (1.1–3)	T&A	7.2	—	35	4
Mitchell and Kelly (12)	Prospective cohort	29	7.1 (1.4–17.0)	T&A	5.8	—	31	4
Shatz (13)	Retrospective case series	24	<1	A	—	100	—	4
Goldstein et al. (14)	Prospective cohort	21	7.0 (3.6)	T&A	7.9 (3.4)	90	90	4
Tauman et al. (15)	Prospective cohort	70	6.6 (4.3)	T&A	4.3 (3.2)	—	75.7	4
Guilleminault et al. (16)	Prospective cohort	56	5.1 (3.1)	T&A in 36	3–6	77.7	77.7	4
Sorin et al. (17)	Retrospective case series	278	4.7 (1.8)	PITA	1–12	99.3 (of T&A)	—	4
Guilleminault et al. (18)	Retrospective case series	400	6.5 (4)	T&A in 251	3	83.5	85.5	4
Lipton and Gozal (19)	Systematic review	401	—	T&A	—	80	80	4
		251	—	T&A	—	97	—	4
Greenfeld et al. (20)	Prospective cohort	29	1.0 (0.33)	T&A in 27 A in 2	48	74	—	4
Nieminen et al. (21)	Prospective cohort	21	5.6 (2.1)	T&A	6	100	90.5	4
Elsherif and Kareemullah (22)	Retrospective case series	52	5–10	T&A	1.5	95–100	—	4
Hultcrantz et al. (23)	Prospective randomized to treatment	21	6 (1.5)	TT	12	90.5–100	—	4
		20		T		100		

Study	Design	N	Age	Procedure				
Agren et al. (24)	Prospective cohort	20	6	T&A in 16 T in 3 A in 1	12	100	75	4
Shintani et al. (25)	Prospective cohort	134	4.4 (1.5)	T&A in 114 A in 13 AMT in 4 T in 3	2	—	77.6	4
Kudoh and Sanai (26)	Prospective cohort	31	7.9	T&A	0.17	—	100	4
Nishimura et al. (27)	Retrospective case series	55	2–10	T&A in 46 AMT in 5 A in 3 Epipharyngeal tumor resection in 1	—	87	86	4
Suen et al. (28)	Prospective cohort	26	1–14	T&A	1.5	—	85	4
Freezer et al. (29)	Retrospective case series	29	1.1 0.5–1.4	T&A	6	—	86 in healthy 79 overall	4
Marcus et al. (30)	Prospective cohort	14	4 (1)	T&A	5 (2)	100	100	4
Zucconi et al. (31)	Prospective cohort	34	3.5 (1.6)	T&A in 10 AMT in 19 A in 5	2–15	93	93	4
Stradling et al. (32)	Prospective cohort	61	4.7 (1.7)	T&A	6	—	78.4	4
Ahlqvist-Rastad et al. (33)	Prospective cohort	85	1.5–14	T in 76 T&A in 9	Within 12	100	—	4
Potsic et al. (34)	Prospective cohort	100	5.8	T&A	1.5	99	—	4

(Continued)

Table 1 Efficacy of Tonsillectomy and Adenoidectomy for the Treatment of Pediatric Sleep-Disordered Breathing (*Continued*)

Author	Study design	n	Age (yrs)	Procedure	Follow-up (mo)	Clinical cure (%)	PSG cure (%)	Level of evidence
Frank et al. (35)	Retrospective case series	17	2–14	T&A in 14 Trach in 2 Incision of nasal septal hematoma	1–1.5	100	—	4
Brouillette et al. (36)	Retrospective case series	22	—	T&A in 8 A in 2 T in 1 Trach and T&A in 2 Trach and A in 1 Trach in 8	6–21	91	—	4

Abbreviations: T&A, tonsillectomy and adenoidectomy; PITA, powered intracapsular tonsillectomy and adenoidectomy; TT, tonsillotomy; AMT, adenomonoton-sillectomy; Trach, tracheotomy; PSG, polysomnography.

Review of the published literature reveals evidence levels of only four or five, limited to prospective, observational, uncontrolled studies and retrospective case series. There are no randomized, controlled trials comparing T&A to no treatment. An attempted systematic review by the Cochrane Collaboration on the efficacy of T&A for SDB could not be completed because no trials met entry criteria (10). Owing to ethical concerns, it is unlikely that a randomized, controlled study will ever be performed.

Except for two recent studies by Mitchell and Kelly (11,12), published studies (Table 1) uniformly report a success rate for resolution of PSG abnormalities of 75–100% in otherwise healthy children. Most of the studies had very short follow-up, some only a few months and nearly all less than one year. The longest follow-up reported was 21 (36) and 48 months (20). There are no studies evaluating long-term outcome after T&A. The meta-analysis by Lipton and Gozal (19) reported a success rate of 80%. Studies evaluating clinical resolution of obstructive symptoms after T&A report higher cure rates in the range of 90–100%, highlighting the need for further evaluation of the validity of PSG abnormalities in predicting future morbidity.

Few studies analyzed the subgroups of patients most at risk for surgical failure. Only four studies addressed the relationship between preoperative sleep-study indices and the risk of surgical failure. Suen et al. (28), in a study of 26 patients, found that children with a preoperative RDI >19.1 were at higher risk. Mitchell and Kelly (12), in a study of 29 children with severe OSA (mean RDI of 63.9), found that only 31% had resolution of OSA as measured by a postoperative RDI of less than five. However, Shintani et al., (25) in a study of 134 patients, found no relationship between preoperative RDI and surgical failure, but a lower preoperative SaO_2 in children with residual OSA. Guilleminault et al. (18), in a study of 400 patients, found no relationship between preoperative sleep-study indices and surgical results. Other risk factors identified included age under three (11,20), obesity (16), maxillomandibular deficiency (16,25), and a smaller epipharyngeal airspace, as demonstrated by cephalometric studies (25).

There are few studies that compare traditional T&A with adenoidectomy alone or variations of the traditional tonsillectomy. Shatz (13) found that adenoidectomy alone resulted in a 100% clinical cure in 24 infants. Nieminen et al. (21) reported that 16 of 21 (73%) of their patients aged 3 to 10 had undergone previous adenoidectomy and were cured by T&A and residual adenoid tissue was not found at reoperation. Shintani et al. (25) found equal success in improvement in PSG parameters in 114 children who had undergone T&A, 13 with small tonsils who had undergone adenoidectomy alone, four who had undergone monotonsillectomy, and three who had undergone tonsillectomy alone. Four children (two in the adenoidectomy group and two in the monotonsillectomy group) needed reoperation because of recurrence of obstructive sleep apnea (OSA) and regrowth of the tonsil and adenoid tissue. In their retrospective review of 400 children, Guilleminault et al. (18) found a higher rate of failure in patients who had undergone adenoidectomy or tonsillectomy alone as compared to T&A. Of the 58 with residual OSA, 26 had undergone isolated adenoidectomy and 17 isolated tonsillectomy. The authors also found better results in the children who had undergone T&A with suturing of the tonsillar pillars to tighten and enlarge the upper airway than traditional T&A.

Recent studies have evaluated the partial or intracapsular tonsillectomy as compared to the traditional total tonsillectomy. Although preliminary studies have demonstrated that partial tonsillectomy is less painful and results in a more rapid recovery (17,23,37,38), only two studies have evaluated the efficacy of the procedure. Hultcrantz et al. (23) found that there was no recurrence of sleep-apnea symptoms in 21 children who underwent tonsillotomy performed with the CO_2 laser and 20 children who underwent traditional tonsillectomy at one-year follow-up, although two children who underwent tonsillotomy still snored. Sorin et al. (17) found that two of 278 (0.7%) children who had undergone powered intracapsular tonsillectomy and adenoidectomy (PITA) required complete tonsillectomy because of recurrence of OSA symptoms. PSG was not performed in either of these studies.

There are a few studies evaluating the efficacy of T&A in treating the neurobehavioral, cardiac, and growth effects of SDB. Pulmonary hypertension is a rare complication of SDB. There have been a few case reports and case series documenting resolution after T&A. Goldstein et al. (14,39) in two prospective studies evaluating the clinical diagnosis of SDB performed echocardiograms on all study participants. Pulmonary hypertension was found in 0/30 (0%) and 1/56 (2%) patients and resolved in the one patient after T&A. Miman et al. (40) identified 17 children with obstructive symptoms and adenotonsillar hypertrophy who had mild pulmonary hypertension by echocardiography. The pulmonary hypertension resolved in all patients after T&A, adenomonotonsillectomy, or adenoidectomy. In the studies by Goldstein et al. (14,39), systemic hypertension was also found in 5/30 (16.7%) and 8/59 (20%) patients. It resolved in all patients after T&A (14).

Failure to thrive has been reported to occur in approximately 10% of children (41,42) and 42–56% of infants with OSA (20,29,43). There have been several case reports, case series, and retrospective cohort studies documenting improvement in growth in children with failure to thrive and OSA after T&A (29,32,36,43–48). Several prospective cohort studies of children with SDB not selected for poor growth prior to surgery have demonstrated significant improvement in weight and height standard deviation (z) scores after T&A (41,42,49,50). The z-scores represent the variance from the population median at a given age and assess changes in height or weight for age over time. Greenfeld et al. (20) found that 14/29 (48%) infants with OSA dropped two or more percentiles for weight before treatment, and a significant weight gain was observed after surgery.

Behavioral and neurocognitive difficulties have been found in 8.5–63% of children with SDB (51–55). The few studies that have evaluated improvement after T&A are presented in Table 2. Children were diagnosed with SDB by

Table 2 Impact of Tonsillectomy and Adenoidectomy on Child Behavior and Academic Performance

Author	Design	n	Age (yrs) Mean (SD or range)	Instrument	Follow-up (mo)	Results	Level of evidence
Tran et al. (54)	Prospective cohort, control group underwent unrelated surgery	42 study (RDI > 5) 41 control	5.8 (2.5) 7.3 (3.8)	CBCL	5.4 (1.9) 5.3 (1.4)	Change in mean total problem *T*-score and change in total *T*-score classification significantly greater in OSA group than controls	2b
Avior et al. (51)	Prospective cohort	19	7.8 (5–14)	TOVA CBCL	2	Significant improvement in CBCL total score and TOVA score, all children but one showed significant improvement in TOVA score	4
Goldstein et al. (52)	Prospective cohort	64 with clinical history of SDB	5.8 (3.1)	CBCL	3	Significant improvement in mean total problem *T*-score, internalizing, externalizing, and most individual syndrome scales; significant improvement in *T*-score classification for total problem score, anxious/depressed,	4

(Continued)

Table 2 Impact of Tonsillectomy and Adenoidectomy on Child Behavior and Academic Performance (*Continued*)

Author	Design	n	Age (yrs) Mean (SD or range)	Instrument	Follow-up (mo)	Results	Level of evidence
						thought problems, sleep problems; CBCL scores demonstrated significant correlation with scores on validated quality-of-life instrument (OSA-18)	
Goldstein et al. (56)	Prospective cohort	15 with clinical history of SDB	4.6 (2–10)	CBCL	3	Significant improvement in mean total problem *T*-score, internalizing, and most individual syndrome scales; changes in *T*-score classification not significant	4
Gozal (57)	Prospective cohort, control group refused surgery	24 study 30 control	First grade	—	12	Of 297 children whose school performance was in the lowest 10th percentile of class, study and control patients demonstrated	2b

| Ali et al. (58) | Prospective cohort, control group underwent unrelated surgery or recruited from the community | 12 SDB 11 snorers 10 control | 7.5 (5.8–12.5) | Conners behavior rating | 3–4 | SDB identified by overnight video recording and pulse oximetry. SBD showed significant reduction in aggression, inattention, and hyperactivity on Conners scale and improvement in vigilance on Continuous Performance Test. Snorer group also improved, but no change for control group | 2b |
| | | | | Continuous performance test | | sleep-associated gas exchange abnormalities, mean grades in second grade increased significantly in study patients but not controls | |

Abbreviations: RDI, respiratory disturbance index; CBCL, child behavior checklist; TOVA, test of variables of attention; SDB, sleep-disordered breathing; OSA, obstructive sleep apnea.

PSG in one study (54), by pulse oximetry, end-tidal CO_2 capnography, or video recording in two studies (57,58), and by clinical assessment alone in three studies (51,52,56). Five of the studies used standardized behavioral assessments, the child behavior checklist (CBCL) (51,52,54,56), the Test of Variables of Attention (TOVA) (51), the Conners Behavior Rating (58), or the Continuous Performance Test (58), whereas one evaluated the children's school performance (57). Only one study had an untreated control group of children whose families refused surgical intervention (57). Despite these limitations, all the studies demonstrated significant improvements in assessment scores after T&A.

Although the improvements are statistically significant, it is not known whether they are clinically significant. The CBCL is divided into normal (<95th percentile), borderline (≥95th percentile but <98th percentile), and abnormal (≥98th percentile) ranges based on scores of children in normative samples. Two of the three studies using the CBCL demonstrated significant improvements in the CBCL score classification after T&A (52,54). Avior et al. (51) found that 63% of children with SDB scored in the abnormal range on the TOVA preoperatively, whereas only 21% of children scored in the abnormal range after T&A. Although these findings suggest that the behavioral and neurodevelopmental improvements are clinically relevant, these studies do not demonstrate actual improvement in the children's school performance. The best evidence that the improvements are clinically relevant is the significant improvement in academic performance found by Gozal in children with SDB who underwent T&A as compared to the children whose parents refused surgery (57).

OUTCOMES RESEARCH

Outcomes research utilizes patient-based assessments to evaluate health-related quality-of-life (HRQL). An HRQL survey focuses on the physical problems, functional limitations, and emotional consequences of a disease. Surveys are self-administered questionnaires composed of items grouped into domains that reflect a particular focus of attention. A survey is designed to discriminate among individuals who have a better quality of life from those who have a worse quality of life and/or to evaluate how much quality of life has changed after a particular intervention. Two disease-specific HRLQ surveys, the Obstructive Sleep Apnea-18 (OSA-18) and the Obstructive Sleep Disorders-6 (OSD-6), have been found to be psychometrically reliable, valid, and responsive to longitudinal change (56,59–62). The OSA-18 has been validated against nap PSG and has been widely used and accepted by other investigators.

Change scores of <0.5 indicate trivial change, 0.5 to 0.9 indicate small change, 1.0 to 1.4 indicate moderate change, and ≥1.5 indicate large change. The OSA-18 consists of 18 items divided into five domains: sleep disturbance, physical suffering, emotional distress, daytime problems, and caregiver concerns. The OSD-6 consists of six domains represented by a single question designed to reflect the global impact of the symptom cluster. The domains are physical suffering, sleep disturbance, speech and swallowing difficulties, emotional distress, activity limitations, and caregiver concerns. Another disease-specific HRLQ survey, the Tonsil and Adenoid Health Status Instrument, is also fully validated and is divided into subscales based on different types of problems caused by tonsil and adenoid disease: infection, airway and breathing, behavior, swallowing, healthcare utilization, and cost of care (63).

Eleven outcomes studies evaluated disease-specific quality-of-life in children with SDB (Table 3). In five studies, the diagnosis of SDB was made clinically (52,59,60,62,67), whereas in six studies, the children were diagnosed by PSG (12,54,61,64–66). In general, the impact of the children's SDB was moderate or large for 70% of the children. The domains most affected were sleep disturbance, physical symptoms, and caregiver concerns.

Eight studies have evaluated disease-specific improvements in the quality of life of children with SDB after T&A using the OSA-18 or the OSD-6. A large improvement in quality of life was found in seven studies, whereas a moderate improvement was found in one study. Significant improvements were found for the total score and all the individual domains. In seven of the studies, the improvements were demonstrated in the short term, six months or less. Mitchell et al. (65) found that the improvements persisted at 12-month follow-up, although some symptoms recurred. Stewart et al. (64) administered the Tonsil and Adenoid Health Status Instrument to 47 children, 31 of whom had positive PSG, at enrollment and six months later. There was a significant improvement in the airway and breathing subscale in the 24 children who underwent T&A as compared to the five children whose parents refused surgery. There were also significant improvements in the infections, swallowing, and behavior subscales.

There have been three studies on global quality of life in children with SDB. Rosen et al. (68) administered the Child Health Questionnaire Parent Form-50 (CHQ-PF50) and performed overnight home sleep studies on 298 children of index families identified because one member had laboratory-confirmed sleep apnea, and a community of control families. Significant differences were found in overall physical health and complaints of bodily pain in children with generally mild levels of SDB as compared to control children. Flanary (67) evaluated global quality of life using the CHQ-PF28 before and after T&A. Although there were significant improvements in the Physical Summary parameter, there was no significant improvement in the Psychosocial scores. Stewart et al. (64) also administered the CHQ-PF28 in their study. There were significant improvements in the behavior and parental impact-emotional subscales in the T&A children as compared to the control children, but there were no significant improvements in the physical functioning subscale or the remainder of the psychosocial scores.

None of the studies were randomized to T&A versus no surgery, as ethical considerations precluded the performance of such a study. Only Stewart et al. (64) had a control group of children with SDB who did not undergo T&A, but

Table 3 Impact of Tonsillectomy and Adenoidectomy on Quality of Life in Children

Author	Design	n	Age (yrs) Mean (SD or range)	Instrument	Follow-up (mo)	Initial survey score, mean (SD or CI)[a]	Change score, mean (SD or CI)[b]	P-value for change
Tran et al. (54)	Prospective cohort, control group underwent unrelated surgery	42 study 41 control	5.8 (2.5) 7.3 (3.8)	OSA-18	5.4 (1.9) 5.3 (1.4)	4.0 (1.2) 1.5 (0.5)	2.5 (1.2) −0.07 (0.62)	<0.001
Stewart et al. (64)	Prospective cohort, control group of children whose parents refused T&A	24 study 5 control	8.1 6–12	T&A health status— airway subscale[c]	6	58.8 (23.4) for all patients	51.9 study −3.8 control	0.002
				CHQ-PF28[d]		92.8 (18.3) for all patients	5.6 study −8.0 control	0.10
Mitchell et al. (65)	Prospective cohort	34	6.7 (3.0–16.8)	OSA-18	12.4	4.3 (2.5–4.6)	2.3 (2.0–2.6)	<0.001
Mitchell et al. (66)	Prospective cohort	60	7.1 (3–12)	OSA-18	4.2	4.0	2.0 (1.6–2.4)	<0.002
Mitchell and Kelly (12)	Prospective cohort	29	7.1 (1.4–17.0)	OSA-18	1.8	4.3 (4.0–5.3)	2.5	<0.0001

Study	Design	N		Instrument		Preop mean (SD)	Change score	p-value
Flanary (67)	Prospective cohort	55	6 (1–16)	CHQ-PF28[e] OSA-18	6 1	41.7 (13.9) 4.22 (0.95)	9.4 2.14	0.002 <0.001
Sohn and Rosenfeld (62)	Prospective cohort	69	6.1 (0.6–13)	OSA-18	1	3.1 (0.9)	1.14 (0.71)	<0.001
Goldstein et al. (52)	Prospective cohort	64	5.8 (3.1)	OSA-18	3	3.9 (1.5)	2.3 (1.9–2.7)	<0.001
de Serres et al. (60)	Prospective cohort	101	6.2 (2.5)	OSD-6	1.2 (0.49)	3.6 (1.0)	2.3 (2.1–2.6)	<0.001
Rosen et al. (68)	Observational	20 severe SDB 25 moderate SDB 50 obstructive symptoms 203 control	11.1 (3.5)	CHQ-PF50[f]	—	76.8 (6.2) 85.2 (6.1) 80.7 (16.1) 88.3 (14.5)	—	—
de Serres et al. (59)	Prospective cohort	100	6.2 (2.1–12.9)	OSD-6	1	4.5 (median)	3.0 (2.7–3.4)	—
Franco et al. (61)	Prospective cohort	61	4 (1–12)	OSA-18	—	3.9 (median)	—	—

[a]The items on the OSA-18 and OSD-6 are both scored on a seven point ordinal scale: the OSA-18 from 1 to 7 assessing the frequency of the specific symptom, whereas the OSD-6 is scored from 0 to 6 assessing the severity of the symptom.

[b]Change scores for the OSA-18 and OSD-6 are calculated by subtracting the postoperative mean survey score from the preoperative mean survey score. Change scores range from −7.0 to 7.0, with negative numbers indicating deterioration and positive numbers indicating improvement in quality of life. Change scores of <0.5 indicate trivial change, 0.5–0.9 indicate small change, 1.0–1.4 indicate moderate change, and ≥1.5 indicate large change.

[c]The Tonsil and Adenoid Health Status Instrument airway and breathing subscale.

[d]CHQ-PF28 physical functioning subscale.

[e]The CHQ-PF28 Physical Summary Score.

[f]CHQ-PF50 global general health score.

Abbreviations: T&A, tonsillectomy and adenoidectomy; OSA, obstructive sleep apnea; OSD, obstructive sleep disorders; CHQ-PF, Child Health Questionnaire Parent Form; SDB, sleep-disordered breathing; SD, standard deviation; CI, confidence interval.

the numbers were small. Tran et al. (54) included a control group of children without a history of snoring or SDB who were undergoing unrelated elective surgery, and the improvements in the OSA-18 survey scores were significant for the OSA children as compared to the control children.

MEDICAL THERAPIES

Although the majority of studies have focused on T&A for the treatment of SDB, a few studies have evaluated topical nasal steroids, oral steroids, and oral antibiotics. Demain and Goetz (69) performed an eight-week, double-blind, placebo-controlled crossover study of aqueous nasal beclomethasone in the treatment of 20 children with adenoidal hypertrophy followed by a 16-week open-label, follow-on study. Improvements in the mean adenoidal obstruction of the choanae and the mean nasal obstruction symptom score were significantly greater in the study group as compared to the placebo group, and a significant carryover effect was found. The findings were enhanced over the 16-week open-label study. The study did not evaluate SDB, and PSG was not performed. Brouillette et al. (70) performed a randomized, triple-blind, placebo-controlled trial of six weeks of nasal fluticasone proprionate in 25 children with SDB. There was a significant reduction in the mixed/obstructive apnea/hypopnea index in the study patients from 10.7 ± 2.6 to 5.8 ± 2.2 as compared to the placebo group, although there was no significant change in symptom score and tonsil and adenoid size between groups. Although this study demonstrated a moderate reduction in the AI, an index of 5.8 is still abnormal, and patients continued to have episodes of desaturation (71). In addition, patients with severe OSA, 4+ tonsils, craniofacial conditions, and infants were excluded. The study also did not address the duration of therapy, so it is unclear whether the topical nasal steroids need to be continued for a continued response.

Al-Ghamdi et al. (72) performed an open-label pilot study of five days of oral prednisone on nine children with OSA. There was no improvement in symptomatology, sleep-study indices or tonsil and adenoid size. There have been two studies evaluating oral antibiotics. Sclafani et al. (73) performed a prospective, randomized, double-blind, placebo-controlled trial of 30 days of amoxicillin/clavulanate potassium in 168 children with obstructive symptoms. Sleep studies were not performed. Treatment with the antibiotic significantly reduced the need for T&A at one-month follow-up as compared to placebo (37.5% vs. 62.7%). By 24 months, most of the children in both groups had undergone T&A (83.3% of the study group vs. 98.0% of the placebo group). Don et al. (74) performed a randomized, double-blind, placebo-controlled trial of 30 days of azithromycin in 22 children with OSA documented by PSG. There were no significant differences in sleep-study indices, tonsil size, or symptoms in the azithromycin group as compared to the placebo group. These preliminary studies suggest that these therapies are not indicated for children with severe OSA, but may have a role in the treatment of milder SDB or for temporary relief of symptoms.

Nasal CPAP or BiPAP is used in children with predisposing factors for OSA including craniofacial anomalies, neuromuscular weakness, or obesity in whom T&A is ineffective or not indicated and for children with idiopathic OSA after T&A. In addition to case reports, six retrospective studies including one multicenter study have reported efficacies of 86–100% in normalizing the PSG indices with long-term compliance rates of 80% (75–80). Two prospective cohort studies, one involving 24 infants with OSA with either craniofacial anomalies or a history of apparent life-threatening events (81) and one involving four children with craniofacial anomalies (82), reported similar results. Neither of these studies was controlled. McNamara and Sullivan (83) studied eight term infants with OSA and age-matched symptomatic and normal controls. Treatment with CPAP normalized the obstructive AI, sleep architecture, and arousals during REM as compared to nontreated patients. Supplemental oxygen has been used as a temporary measure to improve oxygenation in children with OSA. Two studies have demonstrated efficacy, although end-tidal CO_2 must be monitored as alveolar hypoventilation occurred in two children (84,85). There has been no reported use of supplemental oxygen as the sole treatment modality for OSA.

OTHER SURGICAL THERAPIES

Most studies on surgical modalities other than T&A have evaluated children with comorbid conditions. As the experience of individual institutions with this group of patients is small, available studies only consist of case series and retrospective chart reviews. Four studies have evaluated UPPP in neurologically impaired patients (86–89). Sample sizes were small with each study evaluating between 10 and 15 patients. Success rates as measured by clinical and/or PSG criteria ranged from 80% to 87%. Mandibular distraction osteogenesis has been described in children with micrognathia and respiratory obstruction from Pierre Robin sequence, Treacher Collins syndrome, Nager syndrome, and hemifacial microsomia. The procedure has been used successfully to prevent tracheotomy in affected infants, treat OSA in older nontracheotomized children, and allow decannulation (90–95). In the largest of the published retrospective series, seven of eight (88%) infants avoided tracheostomy and five of six (83%) older micrognathic children were cured of OSA, but only 2 of 12 (17%) tracheotomized children with complex congenital syndromes were successfully decannulated (93). Sidman et al. (96) prospectively performed mandibular distraction on 11 infants and children, each serving as his own control. Prior to distraction, none could be decannulated or extubated, but after distraction, all were successfully decannulated.

Cohen and Burstein (97–99) have published several case series describing their use of skeletal expansion combined with soft-tissue reduction in their children with craniofacial syndromes or cerebral palsy and refractory obstructive sleep apnea. In addition to T&A and UPPP, soft-tissue procedures included sep-toplasty and turbinectomy, tongue reduction, and tongue hyoid suspension. Skeletal expansion procedures included mandibular advancement, costochondral grafts, mandibular distraction, temporomandibular joint arthroplasty, and Le Fort procedures. Tracheotomy was avoided in 90% of their patients, whereas 80% of their tracheotomized children were successfully decannulated. Supplemental oxygen therapy or CPAP was still required by 8% of the patients. The mean apnea–hypopnea index decreased from 25.9 to 4.4 after surgery, whereas the mean lowest oxygen saturation increased from 61% to 92%. Based on a few pub-lished case series, tracheotomy is considered curative in complicated children with refractory OSA and severe upper airway obstruction (100,101).

REFERENCES

1. American Thoracic Society. Standards and indications for cardiopulmonary sleep studies in children. Am J Respir Crit Care Med 1996; 153(2):866–878.
2. Schechter MS. Technical report: diagnosis and management of childhood obstruc-tive sleep apnea. Pediatrics 2002; 109(4):e69.
3. Chervin RD, Ruzicka DL, Wiebelhaus JL, et al. Tolerance of esophageal pressure monitoring during polysomnography in children. Sleep 2003; 26(8):1022–1026.
4. Carroll JL. Obstructive sleep-disordered breathing in children: new controversies, new directions. Clin Chest Med 2003; 24:261–282.
5. Serebrisky D, Cordero R, Mandeli J, et al. Assessment of inspiratory flow limitation in children with sleep-disordered breathing by nasal cannula pressure transducer system. Pediatr Pulmonol 2002; 33(5):380–387.
6. Marcus CE, Hamer A, Loughlin GM. Natural history of primary snoring in children. Pediatr Pulmonol 1998; 26(1):6–11.
7. Topol HI, Brooks LJ. Follow-up of primary snoring in children. J Pediatr 2001; 138(2):291–293.
8. McNamara F, Sullivan CE. The genesis of adult sleep apnoae in childhood. Thorax 2000; 55(11):964–969.
9. Oxford Centre for Evidence-Based Medicine. Levels of Evidence (May 2001). Avail-able at http://www.cebm.net/levles_of_evidence.asp (accessed July 18, 2005).
10. Lim J, McKean M. Adenotonsillectomy for obstructive sleep apnoae in children. The Cochrane Database of Systematic Reviews 2001, Issue 3. Art. No.: CD003136. DOI: 10.1002/14651858.CD003136.
11. Mitchell RB, Kelly J. Outcome of adenotonsillectomy for obstructive sleep apnea in children under 3 years. Arch Otolaryngol Head Neck Surg 2005; 132(5):681–684.
12. Mitchell RB, Kelly J. Outcome of adenotonsillectomy for severe obstructive sleep apnea syndrome. Int J Pediatr Otorhinolaryngol 2004; 68(11):1375–1379.
13. Shatz A. Indications and outcomes of adenoidectomy in infancy. Ann Otol Rhinol Laryngol 2004; 113(10):835–838.
14. Goldstein NA, Pugazhendhi V, Rao SM, et al. Clinical assessment of pediatric obstructive sleep apnea. Pediatrics 2004; 114(1):33–43.
15. Tauman R, Montgomery-Downs JE, Ivanenko A, et al. Changes in sleep architecture and respiratory function following adenotonsillectomy in children with obstructive sleep apnea syndrome. Sleep 2004; 27(suppl):A100.

16. Guilleminault C, Li K, Quo S, et al. A prospective study on the surgical outcomes of children with sleep-disordered breathing. Sleep 2004; 27(1):95–100.
17. Sorin A, Bent JP, April MM. Complications of microdebrider-assisted powered intracapsular tonsillectomy and adenoidectomy. Laryngoscope 2004; 114(2):297–300.
18. Guilleminault C, Li KK, Khramtsov A, et al. Sleep disordered breathing: surgical outcomes in prepubertal children. Laryngoscope 2004; 114(1):132–137.
19. Lipton AJ, Gozal D. Treatment of obstructive sleep apnea in children: do we really know how? Sleep Med Rev 2003; 7(1):61–80.
20. Greenfeld M, Tauman R, DeRowe A, et al. Obstructive sleep apnea syndrome due to adenotonsillar hypertrophy in infants. Int J Pediatr Otorhinolaryngol 2003; 67(10):1055–1060.
21. Nieminen P, Tolonen U, Löppönen H. Snoring and obstructive sleep apnea in children: a 6-month follow-up study. Arch Otolaryngol Head Neck Surg 2000; 126(4):481–486.
22. Elsherif I, Kareemullah C. Tonsil and adenoid surgery for upper airway obstruction in children. Ear Nose Throat J 1999; 78(8):617–620.
23. Hultcrantz E, Linder A, Markström A. Tonsillectomy or tonsillotomy? A randomized study comparing postoperative pain and long-term effects. Int J Pediatr Otorhinolaryngol 1999; 51(3):171–176.
24. Agren K, Nordlander B, Linder-Aronsson S, et al. Children with nocturnal upper airway obstruction: postoperative orthodontic and respiratory improvement. Acta Otolaryngol (Stockh) 1998; 118(4):581–587.
25. Shintani T, Asakura K, Kataura A. The effect of adenotonsillectomy in children with OSA. Int J Pediatr Otorhinolaryngol 1998; 44(1):51–58.
26. Kudoh F, Sanai A. Effect of tonsillectomy and adenoidectomy on obese children with sleep-associated breathing disorders. Acta Otolaryngol (Stockh) 1996; 523(suppl):216–218.
27. Nishimura T, Morishima N, Hasegawa S, et al. Effect of surgery on obstructive sleep apnea. Acta Otolaryngol (Stockh) 1996; 523(suppl):231–233.
28. Suen JS, Arnold JE, Brooks LJ. Adenotonsillectomy for treatment of obstructive sleep apnea in children. Arch Otolaryngol Head Neck Surg 1995; 121(5): 525–530.
29. Freezer NJ, Bucenss IK, Robertson CF. Obstructive sleep apnoea presenting as failure to thrive in infancy. J Paediatr Child Health 1995; 31(3):172–175.
30. Marcus CL, Carroll JL, Koerner CB, et al. Determinants of growth in children with the obstructive sleep apnea syndrome. J Pediatr 1994; 125(4):556–562.
31. Zucconi M, Strambi LF, Pestalozza G, et al. Habitual snoring and obstructive sleep apnea syndrome in children: effects of early tonsil surgery. Int J Pediatr Otorhinolaryngol 1993; 26(3):235–243.
32. Stradling JR, Thomas G, Warley ARH, et al. Effect of adenotonsillectomy on nocturnal hypoxaemia, sleep disturbance, and symptoms in snoring children. Lancet 1990; 335:249–253.
33. Ahlqvist-Rastad J, Hultcrantz E, Svanholm H. Children with tonsillar obstruction: indications for and efficacy of tonsillectomy. Acta Paediatr Scand 1988; 77(6):831–835.
34. Potsic WP, Pasquariello PS, Corso Baranak C, et al. Relief of upper airway obstruction by adenotonsillectomy. Otolaryngol Head Neck Surg 1986; 94(4):476–480.

35. Frank Y, Kravath RE, Pollak CP, et al. Obstructive sleep apnea and its therapy: clinical and polysomnographic manifestations. Pediatrics 1983; 71(5):737–742.
36. Brouillette RT, Fernbach SK, Hunt CE. Obstructive sleep apnea in infants and children. J Pediatr 1982; 100(1):31–40.
37. Koltai PJ, Solares CA, Koempel JA, et al. Intracapsular tonsillar reduction (partial tonsillectomy): reviving a historical procedure for obstructive sleep disordered breathing in children. Otolaryngol Head Neck Surg 2003; 129(5):532–538.
38. Koltai PJ, Solares A, Mascha EJ, et al. Intracapsular partial tonsillectomy for tonsillar hypertrophy in children. Laryngoscope 2002; 112(8 Pt suppl 100):17–19.
39. Goldstein NA, Sculerati N, Walsleben JA, et al. Clinical diagnosis of pediatric obstructive sleep apnea validated by polysomnography. Otolaryngol Head Neck Surg 1994; 111(5):611–617.
40. Miman MC, Kirazli T, Ozyurek R. Doppler echocardiography in adenotonsillar hypertrophy. Int J Pediatr Otorhinolaryngol 2000; 54(1):21–26.
41. Ahlqvist-Rastad J, Hultcrantz E, Melander H, et al. Body growth in relation to tonsillar enlargement and tonsillectomy. Int J Pediatr Otorhinolaryngol 1992; 24(1):55–61.
42. Selimoğlu E, Selimoğlu MA, Orbak Z. Does adenotonsillectomy improve growth in children with obstructive adenotonsillar hypertrophy? J Int Med Res 2003; 31: 84–87.
43. Williams EF, Woo P, Miller R, et al. The effects of adenotonsillectomy on growth in young children. Otolaryngol Head Neck Surg 1991; 104(4):509–516.
44. Barr GS, Osborne J. Weight gain in children following tonsillectomy. J Laryngol Otol 1988; 102(7):595–597.
45. Everett AD, Koch WC, Saulsbury FT. Failure to thrive due to obstructive sleep apnea. Clin Pediatr 1987; 26(2):90–92.
46. Guilleminault C, Korobkin R, Winkle R. A review of 50 children with obstructive sleep apnea syndrome. Lung 1981; 159(5):275–287.
47. Lind MG, Lundell BPW. Tonsillar hyperplasia in children: a cause of obstructive sleep apneas, CO_2 retention, and retarded growth. Arch Otolaryngol 1982; 108(10):650–654.
48. Soultan Z, Wadowski S, Rao M, et al. Effect of treating obstructive sleep apnea by tonsillectomy and/or adenoidectomy on obesity in children. Arch Pediatr Adolesc Med 1999; 153(1):33–37.
49. Bar A, Tarasiuk A, Segev Y, et al. The effect of adenotonsillectomy on serum insulin-like growth factor-I and growth in children with obstructive sleep apnea syndrome. J Pediatr 1999; 135(1):76–80.
50. Marcus CL, Greene MG, Carroll JL. Blood pressure in children with obstructive sleep apnea. Am J Respir Crit Care Med 1998; 157(4):1098–1103.
51. Avior G, Fishman G, Leor A, et al. The effect of tonsillectomy and adenoidectomy on inattention and impulsivity as measured by the Test of Variables of Attention (TOVA) in children with obstructive sleep apnea syndrome. Otolaryngol Head Neck Surg 2004; 131(4):367–371.
52. Goldstein NA, Fatima M, Campbell TF, et al. Child behavior and quality of life before and after tonsillectomy. Arch Otolaryngol Head Neck Surg 2002; 128(7):770–775.
53. Goodwin JL, Kaemingk KL, Fregosi RF, et al. Clinical outcomes associated with sleep-disordered breathing in Caucasian and Hispanic children—the

Tucson children's assessment of sleep apnea study (TuCASA). Sleep 2003; 26(5):587–591.

54. Tran KD, Nguyen CD, Weedon J, et al. Child behavior and quality of life in pediatric obstructive sleep apnea. Arch Otolaryngol Head Neck Surg 2005; 131(1):52–57.

55. Rosen CL, Storfer-Isser A, Taylor G, et al. Increased behavioral morbidity in school-aged children with sleep-disordered breathing. Pediatrics 2004; 114(6):1640–1648.

56. Goldstein NA, Post JC, Rosenfeld RM, et al. Impact of tonsillectomy and adenoidectomy on child behavior. Arch Otolaryngol Head Neck Surg 2000; 126(4):494–498.

57. Gozal D. Sleep-disordered breathing and school performance in children. Pediatrics 1998; 102(3):616–620.

58. Ali NJ, Pitson D, Stradling JR. Sleep disordered breathing: effects of adenotonsillectomy on behaviour and psychological functioning. Eur J Pediatr 1996; 155(1):56–62.

59. de Serres LM, Derkay C, Astley S, et al. Measuring quality of life in children with obstructive sleep disorders. Arch Otolaryngol Head Neck Surg 2000; 126(12): 1423–1429.

60. de Serres LM, Derkay C, Sie K, et al. Impact of adenotonsillectomy on quality of life in children with obstructive sleep disorders. Arch Otolaryngol Head Neck Surg 2002; 128(5):2002.

61. Franco RA, Rosenfeld RM, Rao M. Quality of life for children with obstructive sleep apnea. Otolaryngol Head Neck Surg 2000; 123(1):9–16.

62. Sohn H, Rosenfeld RM. Evaluation of sleep-disordered breathing in children. Otolaryngol Head Neck Surg 2003; 128(3):344–352.

63. Stewart MG, Friedman EF, Sulek M, et al. Validation of an outcomes instrument for tonsil and adenoid disease. Arch Otolaryngol Head Neck Surg 2001; 127(1):29–35.

64. Stewart MG, Glaze DG, Friedman EM, et al. Quality of life and sleep study findings after adenotonsillectomy in children with obstructive sleep apnea. Arch Otolaryngol Head Neck Surg 2005; 131(4):308–314.

65. Mitchell RB, Kelly J, Call E, et al. Long-term changes in quality of life after surgery for pediatric obstructive sleep apnea. Arch Otolaryngol Head Neck Surg 2004; 130(4):409–412.

66. Mitchell RB, Kelly J, Call E, et al. Quality of life after adenotonsillectomy for obstructive sleep apnea in children. Arch Otolaryngol Head Neck Surg 2004; 130(2):190–194.

67. Flanary VA. Long-term effect of adenotonsillectomy on quality of life in pediatric patients. Laryngoscope 2003; 113(10):1639–1644.

68. Rosen CL, Palermo TM, Larkin EK, et al. Health-related quality of life and sleep-disordered breathing in children. Sleep 2002; 25(6):657–666.

69. Demain JG, Goetz DW. Pediatric adenoidal hypertrophy and nasal airway obstruction with aqueous nasal beclomethasone. Pediatrics 1995; 95(3):355–364.

70. Brouillette RT, Manoukian JJ, Ducharme FM, et al. Efficacy of fluticasone nasal spray for pediatric obstructive sleep apnea. J Pediatr 2001; 138(6):838–844.

71. Marcus CL. Nasal steroids as treatment for obstructive sleep apnea: don't throw away the scalpel yet. J Pediatr 2001; 138(6):795–797.

72. Al-Ghamdi SA, Manoukian JJ, Morielli A, et al. Do systemic corticosteroids effectively treat obstructive sleep apnea secondary to adenotonsillar hypertrophy? Laryngoscope 1997; 107(10):1382–1387.

73. Sclafani AP, Ginsburg J, Shah MK. Treatment of symptomatic chronic adenotonsillar hypertrophy with amoxicillin/clavulanate potassium: short- and long-term results. Pediatrics 1998; 101(4):675–681.

74. Don DM, Goldstein NA, Crockett DM, Davidson Ward S. Antimicrobial therapy for children with adenotonsillar hypertrophy and obstructive sleep apnea: a prospective randomized trial comparing azithromycin vs. placebo. Otolaryngol Head Neck Surg 2005; 133(4):562–568.

75. Downey R III, Perkin RM, MacQuarrie J. Nasal continuous positive airway pressure use in children with obstructive sleep apnea younger than 2 years of age. Chest 2000; 117(6):1608–1612.

76. Guilleminault C, Nino-Murcia G, Heldt G, et al. Alternative treatment to tracheostomy in obstructive sleep apnea syndrome: nasal continuous positive airway pressure in young children. Pediatrics 1986; 78(5):797–802.

77. Guilleminault C, Pelayo R, Clerk A, et al. Home continuous positive airway pressure in infants with sleep-disordered breathing. J Pediatr 1995; 127(6):905–912.

78. Marcus CL, Davidson Ward SL, Mallory GB, et al. Use of nasal continuous positive airway pressure as treatment of childhood obstructive sleep apnea. J Pediatr 1995; 127(1):88–94.

79. Padman R, Hyde C, Foster P, et al. The pediatric use of bilevel positive airway pressure therapy for obstructive sleep apnea syndrome: a retrospective review with analysis of respiratory parameters. Clin Pediatr (Phila) 2002; 41(3):163–169.

80. Waters KA, Everett FM, Bruderer JW, et al. Obstructive sleep apnea: the use of nasal CPAP in 80 children. Am J Respir Crit Care Med 1995; 152(2):780–785.

81. McNamara F, Sullivan CE. Obstructive sleep apnea in infants and its management with nasal continuous positive airway pressure. Chest 1999; 116(1):10–16.

82. Rains JC. Treatment of obstructive sleep apnea in pediatric patients: behavioral intervention for compliance with nasal continuous positive airway pressure. Clin Pediatr (Phila) 1995; 34(10):535–541.

83. McNamara F, Sullivan CE. Effects of nasal CPAP therapy on respiratory and spontaneous arousals in infants with OSA. J Appl Physiol 1999; 87(3):889–896.

84. Aljadeff G, Gozal D, Bailey-Wahl SL, et al. Effects of overnight supplemental oxygen in obstructive sleep apnea in children. Am J Respir Crit Care Med 1996; 153(1):51–55.

85. Marcus CL, Carroll JL, Bamford O, et al. Supplemental oxygen during sleep in children with sleep-disordered breathing. Am J Respir Crit Care Med 1995; 152(4):1297–1301.

86. Kerschner JE, Lynch JB, Kleiner H, et al. Uvulopalatopharyngoplasty with tonsillectomy and adenoidectomy as a treatment for obstructive sleep apnea in neurologically impaired children. Int J Pediatr Otorhinolaryngol 2002; 62(3):229–235.

87. Kosko JR, Derkay CS. Uvulopalatopharyngoplasty: treatment of obstructive sleep apnea in neurologically impaired pediatric patients. Int J Pediatr Otorhinolaryngol 1995; 32(3):241–246.

88. Seid AB, Martin PJ, Pransky SM, et al. Surgical therapy of obstructive sleep apnea in children with severe mental insufficiency. Laryngoscope 1990; 100(5):507–510.

89. Wiet GJ, Bower C, Seibert R, et al. Surgical correction of obstructive sleep apnea in the complicated pediatric patient documented by polysomnography. Int J Pediatr Otorhinolaryngol 1997; 41(2):133–143.
90. Cohen SR, Simms C, Burstein FD. Mandibular distraction osteogenesis in the treatment of upper airway obstruction in children with craniofacial deformities. Plast Reconstr Surg 1998; 101(2):312–318.
91. Denny A, Kalantarian B. Mandibular distraction in neonates: a strategy to avoid tracheostomy. Plast Reconstr Surg 2002; 109(3):896–906.
92. Denny AD, Talisman R, Hanson PR, et al. Mandibular distraction osteogenesis in very young patients to correct airway obstruction. Plast Reconstr Surg 2001; 108(2):302–311.
93. Mandell DL, Yellon RF, Bradley JP, et al. Mandibular distraction for micrognathia and severe upper airway obstruction. Arch Otolaryngol Head Neck Surg 2004; 130(3):344–348.
94. Rhee ST, Buchman SR. Pediatric mandibular distraction osteogenesis: the present and the future. J Craniofac Surg 2003; 14(5):803–808.
95. Williams JK, Maull D, Grayson BH, et al. Early decannulation with bilateral mandibular distraction for tracheostomy-dependent patients. Plast Reconstr Surg 1999; 103(1):48–59.
96. Sidman JD, Sampson D, Templeton B. Distraction osteogenesis of the mandible for airway obstruction in children. Laryngoscope 2001; 111(7):1137–1146.
97. Burstein FD, Cohen SR, Scott PH, et al. Surgical therapy for severe refractory sleep apnea in infants and children: application of the airway concept zone. Plast Reconstr Surg 1995; 96(1):34–41.
98. Cohen SR, Ross DA, Burstein FD, et al. Skeletal expansion combined with soft-tissue reduction in the treatment of obstructive sleep apnea in children: physiologic results. Otolaryngol Head Neck Surg 1998; 119(5):476–485.
99. Cohen SR, Simms C, Burstein FD, et al. Alternatives to tracheostomy in infants and children with obstructive sleep apnea. J Pediatr Surg 1999; 34(1):182–187.
100. Lauritzen C, Lilja J, Jarlstedt J. Airway obstruction and sleep apnea in children with craniofacial anomalies. Plast Reconstr Surg 1986; 77(1):1–5.
101. Potsic WP. Airway obstruction and sleep apnea in children with craniofacial anomalies (discussion). Plast Reconstr Surg 1986; 77(1):6.

14

Obstructive Sleep Apnea and Anesthesia

Veronica C. Swanson and Jeffrey Koh

*Department of Anesthesia and Perioperative Medicine and Pediatrics,
Oregon Health & Science University, Portland, Oregon, U.S.A.*

CHAPTER HIGHLIGHTS

- Sleep-disordered breathing may occur after major surgery, even in patients who do not have a history of obstructive sleep apnea (OSA).
- Sedatives, anesthetics, and analgesic agents are all central depressant agents which may worsen OSA by decreasing pharyngeal tone, promoting pharyngeal collapse, and attenuating ventilatory and arousal responses to hypoxia, hypercarbia, and obstruction.
- In the setting of OSA, premedication, while useful, should be dosed judiciously, and anxiety allayed with the addition of behavioral interventions.
- The likelihood of developing negative pressure pulmonary edema increases following the administration of anesthesia due to the effects of centrally acting drugs on pharyngeal tone and ventilatory arousal response.

INTRODUCTION

Obstructive sleep apnea syndrome (OSAS) is a breathing disorder characterized by repeated collapse of the upper airway during sleep, resulting in cessation of airflow. More specifically, OSAS can be defined as cessation of airflow for more than 10 seconds, despite continuing ventilatory effort, five or more times per hour of sleep, usually associated with a decrease in arterial oxygen saturation of more than 4% (1). Given that the obese patient population represents a significant proportion of the OSA patients and that the percentage of the U.S. population that is obese continues to increase (2), it stands to reason that both the number of OSA patients and their percentage of all surgical candidates will increase. Thus, its impact on perioperative patient care is profound.

Our appreciation of OSA in medicine is relatively new within the last four decades (3,4), and our understanding of its impact continues to evolve. This disease process, with repeated arterial oxyhemoglobin desaturations, resaturations, and sleep disturbance, has the potential to place a substantial oxidative burden on many, if not all, physiologic systems, including the upper-airway soft tissues, muscles, and neural control mechanisms (5). Primary clinical sequelae of OSA include daytime hypersomnolence, changes in personality, behavior, and cognition, systemic and pulmonary arterial hypertension, cardiac arrhythmias, and cardiopulmonary failure (6,7). This chapter focuses on the perioperative implications of the disorder and its management.

ANESTHETIC CONSIDERATIONS

A great deal of research has been done on the anatomic, physiologic, and pharmacologic components of this disorder. However, in this chapter, the focus is on OSA as it pertains to anesthesiology, and four specific anesthetic implications: the systemic effects of the apneic cycle, the impact of anesthetic drugs, the dynamics of negative-pressure pulmonary edema (NPPE), and the hypoxic response.

Apneic Arousal Cycle

As the name suggests, obstructive sleep apnea is phase-specific. The patient usually has normal ventilatory patterns and arterial oxygen values during wakefulness. The cycle does not begin until the patient loses consciousness (5). Then, as upper-airway muscle tone decreases and airway resistance increases, a critical point is reached at which air exchange ceases. At this point, arterial oxygen tension decreases as a function of the initial oxygen tension, the functional residual capacity (FRC), and the duration of the apnea. Arousal eventually occurs due to carotid body response to falling PaO_2 (8,9), central nervous system response to rising $PaCO_2$ (10), increasing ventilatory effort from falling PaO_2 and rising $PaCO_2$ (11,12), and pressure-sensitive receptors in the upper

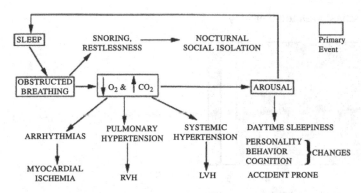

Figure 1 The systemic pathophysiology of repeated sleep → arousal → sleep cycles in obstructive sleep apnea. *Abbreviations*: RVH, right-ventricular hypertrophy; LVH, left-ventricular hypertrophy. *Source*: From Ref. 64.

airway (13). Once the patient is aroused, upper-airway muscle tone increases and air exchange resumes until the next cycle begins.

These changes in the respiratory system, with resultant hypoxia and hypercarbia, have a significant impact (Fig. 1). The cardiovascular system is particularly affected. Arrythmias including bradycardia, sinus pauses, second-degree heart block, and ventricular arrhythmias have been noted during apneic events (14,15). The greater the oxygen desaturation that occurs, the greater the severity of these arrhythmias. When the OSA is effectively treated, these arrhythmias resolve (7).

In response to these apneic/arousal cycles, elevated cardiac sympathetic activity occurs (16). A nocturnal pattern of systemic and pulmonary hypertension is thus seen in these patients. In fact, a dose-response relationship occurs between OSA and hypertension (17). Over time, these patients may develop right- and left-ventricular hypertrophy (1,18). Because of these associated medical problems, they are often classified as American Society of Anesthesiologists Physical Status III (ASA PS) and above (Fig. 2). Although ASA status was designed to provide common language between hospitals rather than to suggest anesthetic risk, it cannot be overlooked that ASA PS scores have been shown to be the predictors of both a higher incidence of cardiac arrest and of poor outcome (19,20). Thus, with increased incidence of numerous arrhythmias, pulmonary hypertension, systemic hypertension, and right- and left-ventricular hypertrophy, it follows that these patients have a significantly higher anesthetic risk than the general population.

Anesthetic Drugs

Sleep-disordered breathing may occur after major surgery, even in patients who do not have a history of OSA. However, patients with OSA are at risk for

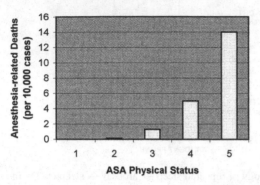

Anesthesia-related Mortality

Figure 2   Anesthesia-related mortality rates for two university-based healthcare networks are shown as a function of American Society of Anesthesiologists Physical Status ($n = 184{,}472$). Anesthesia-related mortality is defined as a perioperative death determined by peer review to be due, at least in part, to human error by an anesthesia practitioner. *Abbreviation*: ASA, American Society of Anesthesiologists. *Source*: From Ref. 19.

development of more apneas and more severe episodes of hypoxia postoperatively. This is because sedatives, anesthetics, and analgesic agents—that is, all central depressant agents—may worsen OSA by decreasing pharyngeal tone, promoting pharyngeal collapse, and attenuating ventilatory and arousal responses to hypoxia, hypercarbia, and obstruction (7,21). This tendency has been documented in propofol, thiopental sodium, benzodiazepines, nitrous oxide, and neuromuscular relaxants (7,22,23). General anesthesia also dose-dependently attenuates phasic respiratory activity of upper-airway muscles and, to a lesser extent, the activity of intercostal muscles and the diaphragm. The resulting muscle imbalance increases the propensity for the upper airway to collapse (22,23).

So, anesthetic drugs plus OSA is a bad combination: what now? After all, anesthesia is usually unavoidable. During the time that the airway is under the patient's control, such as preoperatively and postoperatively, one should minimize the amount of centrally acting agents. Careful consideration should be given to the dosing of premedications. Although intraoperatively the airway will often be secured with an endotracheal tube, thereby rendering moot the impact of the drugs on the airway, the choice of drugs will still have an impact on the postoperative period. A short-acting inhalation agent, such as sevoflurane or desflurane, and a short-acting opioid, such as fentanyl or alfentanil, are suggested to allow for more flexibility in the postoperative treatment of pain. Although it is true that pain management complicates the postoperative goals, a multimodal approach will achieve optimal analgesia and balance the amount of pain relief with minimization of respiratory side effects. Nonsteroidal anti-inflammatory drugs, acetaminophen, and corticosteroids should be maximized before using opioids. When appropriate, regional anesthetic techniques, peripheral nerve blocks, and wound infiltration with local anesthetics should be employed. More recently used adjuncts including N-methyl-D-aspartate receptor antagonists (e.g., ketamine and dextromethorphan), alpha-2 agonists (e.g., clonidine and dexmedetomidine), and anticonvulsants (e.g., gabapentin and pregabalin) also look promising, but require further investigation regarding their impact on OSA (24).

Negative-Pressure Pulmonary Edema

Pulmonary edema following an acute upper-airway obstruction is called negative-pressure pulmonary edema (NPPE) (25). Recall that the four primary forces that determine fluid movement across a capillary membrane are capillary pressure, interstitial fluid pressure, plasma colloid osmotic pressure, and interstitial fluid colloid osmotic pressure (26). When generating a respiratory effort against an obstruction, the negative intrathoracic pressure is translated across the capillary membrane, drawing fluid from the intravascular space into either the interstitial space or the alveolar space. In other words, the negative intrathoracic pressure acts as a negative interstitial fluid pressure. Although this process is usually attributed to a periglottic obstruction such as laryngospasm or epiglottitis, it can also refer to an upper-airway obstruction such as occurs in OSA. The likelihood of developing NPPE increases following the administration of anesthesia due to the effects of centrally acting drugs on pharyngeal tone and ventilatory arousal response. In particular, the effect of general anesthetics is greater on the upper airway than on the intercostals and the diaphragm, resulting in a respiratory effort against an upper-airway obstruction caused by the relaxed upper-airway musculature. NPPE usually develops within minutes of the obstruction. Similarly, it usually resolves rapidly with removal of the obstruction. In more straightforward cases, treatment often involves simply maintaining an open airway and giving supplemental oxygen. The maintenance of an open airway can be accomplished pharmacologically with reversal drugs and mechanically with patient positioning, oral or nasal airways, or intubation and administration of positive end-expiratory pressure (27), as is required in the case of more longstanding obstruction.

Hypoxic Response

In animal studies, opioid receptors are up-regulated when piglets are exposed to recurrent hypoxia (28). With this information in mind, a retrospective study was undertaken looking at morphine administration after adenotonsillectomy performed in children with OSA. It was investigated whether recurrent hypoxemia, such as occurs in OSA, alters sensitivity to opioid analgesics (29). Their results showed that the cumulative morphine dose per kilogram required for analgesia was significantly correlated with preoperative SaO_2 nadir and patient's age. The lower the nadir, the less postoperative morphine was required to achieve analgesia, confirming their hypothesis. The purported mechanism is hypoxia-induced up-regulation of the pain-related mu-opioid receptors. This has strong anesthetic implications regarding the dosing of postoperative opioid analgesics in OSA patients. Not only is a lower dose necessary to prevent apneic events, but it also provides adequate analgesia.

Perioperative Course

As most patients with OSA are undiagnosed, our first preoperative action must include considering it as a possibility. It is imperative to always take a history that differentiates those patients who are likely afflicted. Symptoms of snoring, gasping, respiratory pauses, and daytime sleepiness are certainly suggestive and should elicit further probing. At a minimum, a clinical diagnosis of OSA can be presumed if these questions are answered positively. Some degree of quantification of obstruction can come from the history, as the severity of these symptoms correlates with the severity of confirmed OSA (1,2,30–32). Further forewarning of OSA comes from a history of the comorbid conditions that develop as a result of this syndrome over time. They include developmental delay, cognitive disability, systemic and pulmonary hypertension, cardiac arrhythmias, cardiac hypertrophy, ventricular failure, stroke, inflammatory abnormalities, and increased platelet aggregation (15,33). Although OSA comorbidities are infrequently seen in children, they increase with increasing other comorbidities. For instance, clotting abnormalities would be an exceedingly rare complication of OSA by itself. However, in the pediatric patient who has undergone a Fontan procedure, the consequent polycythemia and changed flow dynamics of blood through the lungs in concert with the increased platelet aggregation from OSA may provide the tipping point at which clotting abnormalities are manifested. In like manners, these comorbid conditions of OSA increase the complexity of anesthetic planning.

In the preoperative physical exam, attention should be focussed on the anticipated site of obstruction. Most commonly, this is at the level of the oropharynx, with extension to the laryngopharynx often observed (34) (Fig. 3). More precisely, OSA has been demonstrated to be a complex process with multiple sites of both fixed and transient obstruction within the same individual. Thus, the preoperative physical exam should include a thorough airway assessment including examination of mouth opening, dentition, tongue size, Mallampati score, thyromental distance, tonsillar size, and neck range of motion (33). Neck circumference has been suggested as an independent indicator of OSA (23). Physical findings of retrognathia, mandibular hypoplasia (unilateral or bilateral), and midface anomalies are seen in conjunction with OSA and are a setup for difficult mask airway and difficult intubation. Obese patients have redundant oropharyngeal tissue, which can sometimes be seen during examination of the mouth (23,33,35,36).

The Mallampati classification relates tongue size to pharyngeal size and is used by anesthesiologists as a predictor of difficult intubations. This test is

UPPER AIRWAY ANATOMY

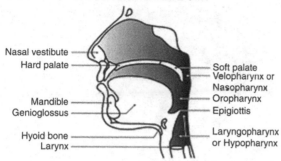

Nasal vestibule
Hard palate

Mandible
Genioglossus

Hyoid bone
Larynx

Soft palate
Velopharynx or
Nasopharynx
Oropharynx
Epiglottis

Laryngopharynx
or Hypopharynx

ACTION OF THE UPPER AIRWAY DILATOR MUSCLES

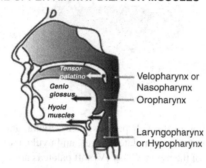

Tensor
palatino
Genio
glossus
Hyoid
muscles

Velopharynx or
Nasopharynx
Oropharynx

Laryngopharynx
or Hypopharynx

SITES OF OBSTRUCTION DURING SLEEP APNEA

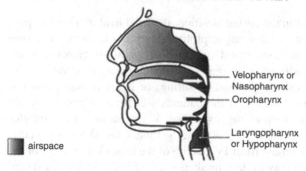

Velopharynx or
Nasopharynx
Oropharynx

Laryngopharynx
or Hypopharynx

airspace

Figure 3 The upper panel schematic shows the important upper-airway anatomy. The nasopharynx ends at the tip of the uvula; the oropharynx extends from the tip of the uvula to the epiglottis; the laryngopharynx extends from the tip of the epiglottis to the posterior cricoid cartilage. The middle panel shows the action of the most important dilator muscles of the upper airway. The tensor palatine, genioglossus, and hyoid muscles enlarge the nasopharynx, oropharynx, and the laryngopharynx, respectively. The bottom panel shows the collapse of the nasopharynx at the palatal level, the oropharynx at the glottic level, and the laryngopharynx at the epiglottic level. *Source*: From Ref. 64.

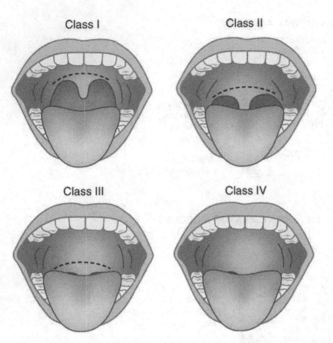

Figure 4   Class I, visualization of the soft palate, fauces, uvula, anterior, and posterior pillars. Class II, visualization of the soft palate, fauces, and uvula. Class III, visualization of the soft palate and the base of the uvula. Class IV, soft palate is not visible at all. *Source*: From Ref. 37.

performed with the patient in the sitting position, the head held in a neutral position, the mouth wide open, and the tongue protruding to the maximum. The subsequent classification is assigned based on the pharyngeal structures that are visible (Fig. 4). The classification assigned by the clinician may vary if the patient is in the supine position (instead of sitting) or if the patient phonates, which can falsely improve the view. If the patients arch their tongue, the uvula is falsely obscured. Class I view suggests ease of intubation and correlates with a laryngoscopic view grade I, 99–100% of the time. Class IV view suggests a poor laryngoscopic view (grade III or IV), 100% of the time (37). Beware of the intermediate classes which may be less predictive of difficulty in laryngoscopic visualization.

   In those patients who are determined to be at increased risk for difficult mask or intubation airway, preparation to proceed with anesthetic induction should include a plan and equipment to secure the difficult airway, including the possibility of fiberoptic intubation with the patient conscious and spontaneously breathing. Premedications should be judiciously administered, given their propensity to decrease pharyngeal tone. Topical anesthetic agents commonly used in fiberoptic intubations may cause the upper airway to relax and make the obstruction worse: this should be anticipated. As mask ventilation may also be difficult, oral or nasal airways should be available. A jaw thrust, wherein the mandible is lifted anteriorly relative to the maxilla, can successfully alleviate obstruction in the upper airway. This can be achieved by holding the mandible behind (rather than under) the angle of the mandible; in the most difficult cases, two hands are necessary to hold this mask airway and an assistant can squeeze the ventilation bag as needed. Attempts to mask the patient may prove unsuccessful and one should be prepared for rapid intubation, using the difficult airway algorithm for guidance and, if necessary, proceeding to a surgical airway (Fig. 5). For those patients who are at high risk for a difficult intubation (Mallampati III or IV, large neck circumference, small thyromental distance, poor mouth opening, craniofacial abnormalities, and poor neck range of motion), an awake intubation should be strongly considered.

In addition to history and physical examination, an overnight polysomnogram, or sleep study, is the gold standard for diagnosis of OSA (38). In its complete form, it includes electroencephalogram, electro-oculogram (EOG), oral and nasal airflow sensors, capnography, noise levels, esophageal pressure, chest and abdominal movements, submental and extremity electromyogram, oximetry, echocardiogram (ECG), and rarely pulmonary artery and radial artery pressure monitoring (7). The apneic/hypopneic index (AHI) is the final score after all the data are obtained. It represents the number of apneic and hypopneic episodes recorded per hour. In adults, a score of 5–15 suggests mild OSA, 16–30, moderate OSA, and greater than 30, severe OSA. For children, the correlation scores suggested are 1–3, 4, and 5 or more (39). An obstructive apnea index of greater than one event may be statistically significant, but whether it is clinically relevant remains unclear (40). Of adult patients who have had a sleep study, an AHI of greater than 20 has been associated with premature death (33). It remains unclear whether any such predictor is applicable to the pediatric population. Death during sleep caused by OSA in children is apparently rare, and most deaths are believed to be perioperative after adenotonsillectomy.

Although a polysomnogram provides detailed, quantitative information as to the degree of obstruction, it is expensive and inconvenient to perform. More importantly, its ability to identify children at risk and those not at risk for significant adverse clinical outcomes is unknown (41). For the purpose of preanesthetic risk assessment, overnight oximetry with digital data acquisition can be performed at home preoperatively and can provide data regarding the number of desaturations and the saturation nadir during that period. Early data suggest that a preoperative saturation nadir of ≤80% is predictive of significantly increased incidence of postoperative respiratory complications (29,39,42). Additionally, the preoperative saturation nadir identifies patients with an increased sensitivity to opioids (29) (see "Hypoxic Response"). Thus, it enables evidence-based decisions in the treatment of children with severe OSA who require adenotonsillectomy, by predicting which patients may need admission with additional monitoring following their procedure (43).

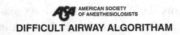

DIFFICULT AIRWAY ALGORITHAM

1. Assess the likelihood and clinical impact of basic management problems:
   A. Difficult Ventilation
   B. Difficult Incubation
   C. Difficulty with Patient Cooperation of Consent
   D. Difficult Trachoostomy

2. Actively pursue opportunities to delivery supplemental oxygen throughout the process of difficult airway management

3. Consider the relative merits and feasibility of basic management choices:

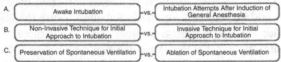

A.	Awake Intubation	–vs.–	Intubation Attempts After Induction of General Anesthesia
B.	Non-Invasive Technique for Initial Approach to Intubation	–vs.–	Invasive Technique for Initial Approach to Intubation
C.	Preservation of Spontaneous Ventilation	–vs.–	Ablation of Spontaneous Ventilation

4. Develop primary and alternative strategies:

A.

AWAKE INTUBATION

Airway Approached by Non-Invasive Intubation   Invasive Airway Access(b)*

Succeed*   FAIL

Cancel Case   Consider Feasibility of Other Options(*)   Invasive Airway Access(b)*

B.

INTUBATION ATTEMPTS AFTER INDUCTION OF GENERAL ANESTHESIA

Initial Intubation Attemts Successful*   Initial Intubation Attempts UNSUCCESSFUL

FROM THIS POINT ONWARDS CONSIDER:
1. Calling for Help
2. Returning to Spontaneous Ventilation
3. Awakening the Patient

FACE MASK VENTILATION ADEQUATE   FACE MASK VENTILATION NOT ADEQUATE

CONSIDER / ATTEMPT LMA

LMA ADEQUATE*   LMA NOT ADEQUATE OR NOT FEASIBLE

NON-EMERGENCY PATHWAY
Ventilation Adequate, Intubation Unsuccessful

EMERGENCY PATHWAY
Ventilation Not Adequate, Intubation Unsuccessful

Alternative Approaches to Intubation(*)

IF BOTH FACE MASK AND LMA VENTILATION BECOME INADEQUATE

Call for Help

Emergency Non-Invasive Airway Ventilation*)

Successful Intubation*   FAIL After Multiple Attempts   Successful Ventilation*   FAIL

Invasive Airway Access(b)*   Consider Feasibility of Other Options (*)   Awaken Patient(a)   Emergency Invasice Airway Access (b)*

* Confirm ventilation, tracheal intubation, or LMA placement with exhaled CO_2

a. Other options include (but are not limited to): surgery utilizing face mask or LMA anesthesia, local anesthesia intration or regional nerve blockade. Pursuit of these options usually imples that mask ventilation will not be problemtic. Therefore, these options may be of limited value if this step in the algorithm has been reached via the Emergency Pathway.

b. Invasive airway access includes surgical or percutaneous tracheostomy or crioothyvolomy.

c. Alternative non-invasive approaches to difficult intubation include (but are not limited to): use of different laryngoscope blades, LMA as an intubation conduit (with or without liberoptic guidance), liberoptic intubation, intubating sylet or tube changer, light want, retrograde intubation, and blind oral or nasal intubation.

d. Consider re-preparation of the patient for awake intubation or concelling surgery.

e. Options for emergency non-invasive airway ventilation include (but are not limited to): rigid bronchscope, ecphagal-tracheal combitube ventilation, or transtracheal jet ventilation.

Figure 5   Difficult airway algorithm. *Source*: Adapted from Ref. 65.

POSTOPERATIVE CONSIDERATIONS

With their obstructive airway and myriad of associated medical conditions, OSA patients are known to have an increased risk of postoperative pulmonary complications after any surgical procedure. The immediate postoperative period may be associated with hypoventilation from residual anesthetic effect and deep breathing impairment secondary to incisional pain. Duration of anesthesia is a well-established risk factor for postoperative pulmonary complications, with increasing incidence of complications as the time increases. Route of administration and type of anesthesia are also risk factors (44), as is location of surgery near the diaphragm. Use of long-acting neuromuscular blocking agents was more likely to result in postoperative hypoventilation (44). The limited evidence available regarding postoperative risks in patients with OSA suggests that the type of surgery is more important than the anesthetic (21). To the extent they are known, weighing these factors permits reasonable preoperative prediction of those patients who will require intensive monitoring and possible continued intubation into their recovery period.

Before extubation, an appropriate level of consciousness, respiratory rate, negative inspiratory force, head lift, oxygen saturation, and end-tidal CO_2 should be demonstrated (33). Obese patients and those who have chronic neurologic diseases should be fully awake before extubation (45). Raising the head of the bed removes the pressure of abdominal weight from the diaphragm, improving pulmonary excursion. Extubation is deferred if the patient had a difficult intubation or if airway edema is suspected (due to the nature of the surgery, large volume of crystalloid administration, or pronounced manipulation of the airway). Those patients who are hemodynamically unstable, have intraoperative complications, or come with a preoperative history of pulmonary hypertension will automatically require an intensive care unit (ICU) admission. In the recovery room, the patient should receive usual monitoring, which includes SaO_2, cardiac rhythm strip, and standard vital signs. If satisfactory oxygen saturation cannot be achieved due to a difficult balance between level of consciousness and adequacy of pain control, the patient will need admission to the hospital for additional management (33).

In the recovery room, oxygen therapy is widely used to prevent hypoxemia postoperatively. However, studies show that it does not affect the number or severity of the episodes of obstruction (23). Special monitoring or an ICU admission is warranted if, in addition to symptoms mentioned earlier, preoperative assessment of OSA reveals a severe level of obstruction, airway management was difficult in the operating room (OR), severe obesity exists, the patient is very sedated postoperatively, or pain cannot be managed without opioids (21). There is no evidence to support risk stratification or the necessity for a period of observation in the ICU based on whether the patient with OSA is having airway surgery (46,47). However, for those that do require it, the ICU combines oxygen therapy, airway clearance techniques, medications, incentive spirometry, and airway-pressure modalities, to provide much benefit (48).

What about the ambulatory setting: is it ever appropriate for the patient with OSA? There is no large body of data addressing the issue of whether preoperative testing of OSA should be required for the patient in the outpatient setting (33). For adults, an algorithm has been suggested to determine a means for perioperative triage of these patients, selecting which patients are appropriate for the outpatient setting (Fig. 6). While applicable to children, additional risk

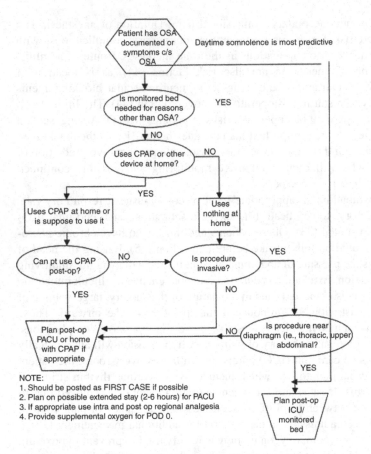

Figure 6 Proposed algorithm for the need for postoperative intensive care unit in the adult patient with obstructive sleep apnea undergoing surgery at The Johns Hopkins Hospital. *Abbreviations*: OSA, obstructive sleep apnea; CPAP, continuous positive airway pressure; ICU, intensive care unit. *Source*: From Ref. 33.

factors for respiratory compromise postoperatively include age younger than three years, neuromuscular disorders, chromosomal abnormalities, loud snoring with apnea, or respiratory tract infection within four weeks of surgery (49). In all patient populations, outpatient surgery is only appropriate when rapid and complete restoration of postoperative consciousness is possible, there is a limited need for narcotic analgesics, and the patient's OSA does not require continuous positive airway pressure (CPAP) (21).

CONSIDERATIONS IN THE OBESE PATIENT

As the incidence of OSA is increased in the obese patient, there are several anesthetic considerations specific for this population that shall be considered.

TIME TO HEMOGLOBIN DESATURATION WITH INITIAL F_AO_2 = 0.87

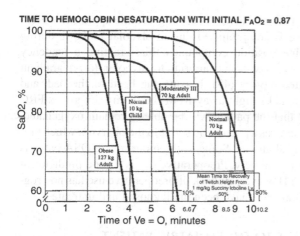

Figure 7 SaO_2 versus time of apnea for various types of patients. *Source*: From Ref. 66.

Pediatric growth charts for the U.S. population now include body mass index (BMI) for age and gender. BMI at or above the 95th percentile is considered overweight or obese. Data from 2000 cite the prevalence of overweight children at 16.5% (50,51). The obese patient has a reduced FRC and reduced pulmonary oxygen stores, leading to rapid desaturation when apnea occurs (Fig. 7). Their awake respiratory pattern involves rapid, shallow breaths, predisposing them to atelectasis, ventilation/perfusion mismatching, and increased degrees of airway closure. Positive-pressure ventilation is made more difficult because of decreased chest wall compliance. Their mask airway may be difficult due to redundant oropharyngeal tissue. Furthermore, their intubation may also be difficult for similar reasons (52). In one review of 18,500 patients, laryngoscopy in obese patients was described as "awkward" ($\leq$2 laryngoscopies) 4.9% of the time, and "difficult" ($>$2 laryngoscopies) 5.5% of the time, as compared to 1.8% and 2.5% of the total population (53). If a surgical airway is necessary, that too may be complicated by redundant soft tissue and poor landmarks (52). Finally, the increased risk of aspiration is also an important consideration (33).

Tools for managing the airway specific to this population include several special devices and techniques. The Datta laryngoscope handle is a shortened version of a standard laryngoscope handle. It improves the user's ability to maneuver the laryngoscope into the mouth when flexion and extension of the patient's neck are limited and a large chest restricts the placement of the blade. Positioning also plays a therapeutic role in these patients. While the obese patient with OSA is awakening, the natural airway will have a tendency to collapse. Change from supine to lateral position in patients with OSA has been shown endoscopically to enlarge retropalatal and retroglossal airways (54). This provides a useful technique for their airway management while the spontaneously breathing patient is recovering from anesthesia. Another positional component relates the effect of the obese abdomen on the patient's FRC. As closing volume approaches FRC, the degree of oxygen reserve is compromised due to alveolar collapse during normal breathing. The supine position compounds this, creating a tendency toward arterial hypoxemia and a widened arterial to alveolar (a-A) gradient within the first 48 hours after surgery (48). Raising the head of the bed, and thereby displacing the abdominal weight away from the thorax, improves FRC and increases the likelihood that the patient will be able to remain oxygenated. Finally, nasal CPAP therapy creates a pneumatic splint in the pharynx, which prevents collapse of the pharyngeal airway. Some of the more severe OSA patients will require this therapy postoperatively. Preoperative use is a good predictor of postoperative need for CPAP. However, the lack of preoperative use has no prognostic indication: many patients will have been undiagnosed and untreated.

CONSIDERATIONS UNIQUE TO THE PEDIATRIC PATIENT

The pediatric patient is another population that commonly presents to the otolaryngologist with symptoms of OSA. Children differ from adults in that adults tend to break the obstruction completely when they achieve arousal; children tend to have incomplete relief of the obstruction with arousal. There are dramatic differences in pediatric versus adult airways: these differences are most pronounced at birth and become less significant as the child grows. The larynx is located at the level of C3-4 in the infant and C4-5 in the adult. This makes the tongue situated more superiorly and more likely to oppose the palate. In addition, the infant tongue is larger in relation to the size of the mouth. An oral or nasal airway alleviates obstruction due to the tongue. To be effective, the nasal airway must be long enough to pass through the nasopharynx but short enough that it remains above the glottis. A large-sized head, and specifically the occiput, relative to the body alters the optimal positioning for both mask airway and intubation. Ideally, a roll placed under the shoulders compensates for this difference. Regarding the pediatric epiglottis, it is larger, narrower, and shorter (55), adding advantage to a straight blade when intubating. The narrowest part of the pediatric airway is at the level of the cricoid cartilage rather than the vocal cords. This obviates the need for a cuffed endotracheal tube. Using an uncuffed tube allows for the use of a tube with greater internal diameter. Immediately after intubation, a leak test should be performed to assess appropriate tube size: 10-25 cm of water pressure leak around the endotracheal tube is optimal to best ventilate while still avoiding tracheal trauma. Vocal-cord orientation is slanted with the posterior aspect more cephalad rather than perpendicular to the pharynx. This may increase the difficulty in achieving a good view, again lending itself to the choice of a straight blade. In addition, the likelihood of intubation trauma may be greater, as this position predisposes the endotracheal tube to being encumbered on the anterior tracheal rings. Twisting the endotracheal tube up to 360° can overcome this difficulty due to the bevel at the end of the tube. Although not unique to OSA, the risk for adverse events after anesthesia continues to be higher in infants and young children compared with older children and adults. In addition, pediatric patients have a higher incidence of respiratory events (laryngospasm and bronchospasm) than do adults (56). The highest risk OSA pediatric patients are those with cor pulmonale. They should have a hematocrit and an ECG performed preoperatively, as they are at risk for perioperative hypoxemia and acute right heart failure. Monitoring in the ICU should be available for them postoperatively, as the likelihood that they will have obstructive events actually may increase during the first 24 hours postoperatively (35,56).

The overwhelming majority of OSA cases in children are due to adenotonsillar hypertrophy. With oximetry or polysomnogram data available, the temptation to react to profound nocturnal desaturation with urgent adenotonsillectomy intervention arises. This should be balanced against the fact that when performed urgently, the surgery places these children at increased risk for postoperative complications as compared to routine surgery (42). Children who undergo tonsillectomy and adenoidectomy for OSA are at increased risk for airway obstruction postoperatively for two reasons. First, their obstructive sleep apnea is severe enough that it requires surgery. Second, there is sometimes an erroneous assumption that the obstruction should be resolved immediately after the surgery. This usually is not the case due to soft-tissue swelling, bleeding, and residual lymphoid tissue (39,57). Patients who are at the highest risk—those under age 3, documented severe OSA, preoperative sleep SaO_2 nadir of $<80\%$, neuromuscular disorders, chromosomal abnormalities, upper respiratory infection within four weeks of surgery, or an associated medical condition—should be monitored in an ICU postoperatively (42,43,49,56,57).

A number of childhood syndromes are well known to be associated with OSA due to craniofacial abnormalities included in the syndrome. An incomplete list includes Pierre Robin sequence, Goldenhar's syndrome, trisomy 21, Treacher-Collins syndrome, velocardiofacial syndrome, Carpenter syndrome, Crouzon disease, Freeman-Sheldon syndrome, and Beckwith–Wiedemann syndrome (57–59). Comorbid conditions in children that have an OSA association include severe scoliosis, cleft lip and palate, spinal cord injury, traumatic brain injury, cerebral palsy, hypothyroidism, mucopolysaccharidoses, and neuromuscular disorders (59). It may be difficult to intubate children with these syndromes and disorders; the use of laryngeal mask airways, light wands, fiberoptic bronchoscopes, retrograde intubation kits, and other difficult airway techniques and devices may be useful in the care of these children.

Unique to the pediatric patient population are the techniques used to induce anesthesia. Adults go to the operating room with an intravenous line already in place. For children, we must find a way to overcome their anxieties regarding being placed in the care of stranger and leaving the safety of their parents. To that end, the choices are to give the child a premedication prior to separation from their parent (oral, nasal, intravenous, or intramuscular), have their parent present for the induction of anesthesia, rely on behavioral techniques to ease the transition, or some combination of these. In the OSA population, anesthetic goals lead us to rely less heavily on premedication (see section on anesthetic drugs). Although they are not absolutely contraindicated, premedications should be given in moderate doses. In their place, a number of behavioral interventions have been utilized. Currently, most children's hospitals offer behavioral programs to children and their parents preoperatively, to help familiarize them with what to expect (60). In the 1990s, a trend existed in the United States to have parents be present for induction. The evidence to date does not depict a clear advantage in having parents present, and some data suggest a disadvantage (61,62). Nonetheless, anesthesiologists are continuing to address the issue of increased anxiety with increased utilization of all the interventions available. The trend is toward greater treatment with premedication and increased parent present inductions (63). The point in the setting of OSA is that premedication, although useful, should be dosed judiciously and anxiety allayed with the addition of other methods.

CONCLUSION

Management of patients with OSA requires a high index of suspicion that the syndrome is present to begin with. One should use sedatives judiciously. Short-acting anesthetic and neuromuscular blockade agents are preferred. Nonnarcotic analgesics should be employed as adjuncts to pain control. Difficult airway precautions should be taken. Appropriate triage relative to postoperative care needs strongly depends on thorough history taking. Clinical significance of polysomnography remains questionable: preoperative nighttime oxygen saturation testing may prove to be more clinically relevant. Finally, one must be ready to administer positive pressure to the airway postoperatively, in the event patients cannot maintain the airway on their own.

REFERENCES

1. Strollo P, Rogers R. Obstructive sleep apnea: current concepts. N Engl J Med 1996; 334:99–104.
2. Willett WC, Dietz WH, Colditz GA. Guidelines for healthy weight. N Engl J Med 1999; 341(6):427–434.
3. Gastaut H, Tassinari C, Duron B. Etude polygraphique des manifestations episodiques (hypniques et respiratoires) diurnes et nocturnes, du syndrome de Pickwick. Rev Neurol 1965; 112:568–579.
4. Guilleminault C, Eldridge F, Dement W. Insomnia with sleep apnea: a new syndrome. Science 1973; 181:856–858.
5. Veasey SC. Molecular and physiologic basis of obstructive sleep apnea. Clin Chest Med 2003; 24(2):179–193.
6. Eisele DW, Schwartz AR, Smith PL. Tongue neuromuscular and direct hypoglossal nerve stimulation for obstructive sleep apnea. Otolaryngol Clin North Am 2003; 36(3):501–510.

7. Benumof JL. Obstructive sleep apnea in the adult obese patient: implications for airway management. Anesthesiol Clin North Am 2002; 20(4):789–811.

8. Bowes G, Townsend ER, Bromley SM, Kozar LF, Phillipson EA. Role of the carotid body and of afferent vagal stimuli in the arousal response to airway occlusion in sleeping dogs. Am Rev Respir Dis 1981; 123(6):644–647.

9. Bowes G, Townsend ER, Kozar LF, Bromley SM, Phillipson EA. Effect of carotid body denervation on arousal response to hypoxia in sleeping dogs. J Appl Physiol 1981; 51(1):40–45.

10. Berthon-Jones M, Sullivan CE. Ventilation and arousal responses to hypercapnia in normal sleeping humans. J Appl Physiol 1984; 57(1):59–67.

11. Kimoff RJ, Cheong TH, Olha AE, et al. Mechanisms of apnea termination in obstructive sleep apnea. Role of chemoreceptor and mechanoreceptor stimuli. Am J Respir Crit Care Med 1994; 149(3 Pt 1):707–714.

12. Gleeson K, Zwillich CW, White DP. The influence of increasing ventilatory effort on arousal from sleep. Am Rev Respir Dis 1990; 142(2):295–300.

13. Issa FG, McNamara SG, Sullivan CE. Arousal responses to airway occlusion in sleeping dogs: comparison of nasal and tracheal occlusions. J Appl Physiol 1987; 62(5):1832–1836.

14. Guilleminault C, Connolly SJ, Winkle RA. Cardiac arrhythmia and conduction disturbances during sleep in 400 patients with sleep apnea syndrome. Am J Cardiol 1983; 52(5):490–494.

15. Capp PK, Pearl PL, Lewin D. Pediatric sleep disorders. Prim Care 2005; 32(2):549–562.

16. Otsuka N, Ohi M, Chin K, et al. Assessment of cardiac sympathetic function with iodine-123-MIBG imaging in obstructive sleep apnea syndrome. J Nucl Med 1997; 38(4):567–572.

17. Peppard PE, Young T, Palta M, Skatrud J. Prospective study of the association between sleep-disordered breathing and hypertension. N Engl J Med 2000; 342(19):1378–1384.

18. Man GC. Obstructive sleep apnea. Diagnosis and treatment. Med Clin North Am 1996; 80(4):803–820.

19. Lagasse RS. Anesthesia safety: model or myth? A review of the published literature and analysis of current original data. Anesthesiology 2002; 97(6):1609–1617.

20. Sprung J, Warner ME, Contreras MG, et al. Predictors of survival following cardiac arrest in patients undergoing noncardiac surgery: a study of 518,294 patients at a tertiary referral center. Anesthesiology 2003; 99(2):259–269.

21. Rock P, Passannante A. Preoperative assessment: pulmonary. Anesthesiol Clin North Am 2004; 22(1):77–91.

22. Evans RG, Crawford MW, Noseworthy MD, Yoo SJ. Effect of increasing depth of propofol anesthesia on upper airway configuration in children. Anesthesiology 2003; 99(3):596–602.

23. Drummond GB. Controlling the airway: skill and science. Anesthesiology 2002; 97(4):771–773.

24. Joshi GP. Multimodal analgesia techniques and postoperative rehabilitation. Anesthesiol Clin North Am 2005; 23(1):185–202.

25. Lang SA, Duncan PG, Shephard DA, Ha HC. Pulmonary oedema associated with airway obstruction. Can J Anaesth 1990; 37(2):210–218.

26. Guyton AC. Textbook of Medical Physiology. 7th ed. Philadelphia, PA: W.B. Saunders Company, 1986:353.

27. Stoelting R, Dierdorf S. Anesthesia and Co-existing Disease. New York, NY: Churchill Livingstone, Inc., 1993:162.
28. Moss IR, Laferriere A. Central neuropeptide systems and respiratory control during development. Respir Physiol Neurobiol 2002; 131(1–2):15–27.
29. Brown KA, Laferriere A, Moss IR. Recurrent hypoxemia in young children with obstructive sleep apnea is associated with reduced opioid requirement for analgesia. Anesthesiology 2004; 100(4):806–810; discussion 5A.
30. Grunstein R, Wilcox I, Yang TS, Gould Y, Hedner J. Snoring and sleep apnoea in men: association with central obesity and hypertension. Int J Obes Relat Metab Disord 1993; 17(9):533–540.
31. Wilson K, Stoohs RA, Mulrooney TF, Johnson LJ, Guilleminault C, Huang Z. The snoring spectrum: acoustic assessment of snoring sound intensity in 1,139 individuals undergoing polysomnography. Chest 1999; 115(3):762–770.
32. Guilleminault C, Tilkian A, Dement WC. The sleep apnea syndromes. Annu Rev Med 1976; 27:465–484.
33. Stierer T, Fleisher LA. Challenging patients in an ambulatory setting. Anesthesiol Clin North Am 2003; 21(2):243–261, viii.
34. Rama AN, Tekwani SH, Kushida CA. Sites of obstruction in obstructive sleep apnea. Chest 2002; 122(4):1139–1147.
35. Helfaer MA, Wilson MD. Obstructive sleep apnea, control of ventilation, and anesthesia in children. Pediatr Clin North Am 1994; 41(1):131–151.
36. Loadsman JA, Hillman DR. Anaesthesia and sleep apnoea. Br J Anaesth 2001; 86(2):254–266.
37. Mallampati SR, Gatt SP, Gugino LD, et al. A clinical sign to predict difficult tracheal intubation: a prospective study. Can Anaesth Soc J 1985; 32(4):429–434.
38. Qureshi A, Ballard RD, Nelson HS. Obstructive sleep apnea. J Allergy Clin Immunol 2003; 112(4):643–651.
39. Wilson K, Lakheeram I, Morielli A, Brouillette R, Brown K. Can assessment for obstructive sleep apnea help predict postadenotonsillectomy respiratory complications? Anesthesiology 2002; 96(2):313–322.
40. International Classification of Sleep Disorders: Diagnostic and Coding Manual. 2nd ed. Westchester, IL, 2005:56–59.
41. Schechter MS. Technical report: diagnosis and management of childhood obstructive sleep apnea syndrome. Pediatrics 2002; 109(4):e69.
42. Brown KA, Morin I, Hickey C, Manoukian JJ, Nixon GM, Brouillettte RT. Urgent adenotonsillectomy: an analysis of risk factors associated with postoperative respiratory morbidity. Anesthesiology 2003; 99(3):586–595.
43. Cote CJ, Sheldon SH. Obstructive sleep apnea and tonsillectomy: do we have a new indication for extended postoperative observation? Can J Anaesth 2004; 51(1):6–12.
44. Arozullah AM, Conde MV, Lawrence VA. Preoperative evaluation for postoperative pulmonary complications. Med Clin North Am 2003; 87(1):153–173.
45. Oliveira E, Michel A, Smolley L. The pulmonary consultation in the perioperative management of patients with neurologic diseases. Neurol Clin 2004; 22(2):277–291, v.
46. Ulnick KM, Debo RF. Postoperative treatment of the patient with obstructive sleep apnea. Otolaryngol Head Neck Surg 2000; 122(2):233–236.
47. Terris DJ, Fincher EF, Hanasono MM, Fee WE Jr, Adachi K. Conservation of resources: indications for intensive care monitoring after upper airway surgery on patients with obstructive sleep apnea. Laryngoscope 1998; 108(6):784–788.

48. Tamul PC, Peruzzi WT. Assessment and management of patients with pulmonary disease. Crit Care Med 2004; 32(suppl 4):S137–S145.
49. Fishkin S, Litman RS. Current issues in pediatric ambulatory anesthesia. Anesthesiol Clin North Am 2003; 21(2):305–311, ix.
50. Hedley AA, Ogden CL, Johnson CL, Carroll MD, Curtin LR, Flegal KM. Prevalence of overweight and obesity among US children, adolescents, and adults, 1999–2002. JAMA 2004; 291(23):2847–2850.
51. Ogden CL, Flegal KM, Carroll MD, Johnson CL. Prevalence and trends in overweight among US children and adolescents, 1999–2000. JAMA 2002; 288(14):1728–1732.
52. Doyle DJ, Arellano R. Upper airway diseases and airway management: a synopsis. Anesthesiol Clin North Am 2002; 20(4):767–787, vi.
53. Rose DK, Cohen MM. The airway: problems and predictions in 18,500 patients. Can J Anaesth 1994; 41(5 Pt 1):372–383.
54. Isono S, Tanaka A, Nishino T. Lateral position decreases collapsibility of the passive pharynx in patients with obstructive sleep apnea. Anesthesiology 2002; 97(4): 780–785.
55. Eckenhoff JE. Some anatomic considerations of the infant larynx influencing endotracheal anesthesia. Anesthesiology 1951; 12(4):401–410.
56. Maxwell LG. Age-associated issues in preoperative evaluation, testing, and planning: pediatrics. Anesthesiol Clin North Am 2004; 22(1):27–43.
57. Infosino A. Pediatric upper airway and congenital anomalies. Anesthesiol Clin North Am 2002; 20(4):747–766.
58. Bandla H, Splaingard M. Sleep problems in children with common medical disorders. Pediatr Clin North Am 2004; 51(1):203–227, viii.
59. Sterni LM, Tunkel DE. Obstructive sleep apnea in children: an update. Pediatr Clin North Am 2003; 50(2):427–443.
60. O'Byrne KK, Peterson L, Saldana L. Survey of pediatric hospitals' preparation programs: evidence of the impact of health psychology research. Health Psychol 1997; 16(2):147–154.
61. Bevan JC, Johnston C, Haig MJ, et al. Preoperative parental anxiety predicts behavioural and emotional responses to induction of anaesthesia in children. Can J Anaesth 1990; 37(2):177–182.
62. Kain ZN, Mayes LC, Wang SM, Caramico LA, Hofstadter MB. Parental presence during induction of anesthesia versus sedative premedication: which intervention is more effective? Anesthesiology 1998; 89(5):1147–1156; discussion 9A–10A.
63. Kain ZN, Caldwell-Andrews AA, Krivutza DM, Weinberg ME, Wang SM, Gaal D. Trends in the practice of parental presence during induction of anesthesia and the use of preoperative sedative premedication in the United States, 1995–2002: results of a follow-up national survey. Anesth Analg 2004; 98(5):1252–1259; table of contents.
64. Benumof JL. Obstructive sleep apnea in the adult obese patient: implications for airway management. J Clin Anesth 2001; 13(2):144–156.
65. American Society of Anesthesiologists Task Force on Management of the Difficult Airway. Practice guidelines for management of the difficult airway: an updated report by the American Society of Anesthesiologists Task Force on Management of the Difficult Airway. Anesthesiology 2003; 98(5):1269–1277.
66. Benumof JL, Dagg R, Benumof R. Critical hemoglobin desaturation will occur before return to an unparalyzed state following 1 mg/kg intravenous succinylcholine. Anesthesiology 1997; 87(4):979–982.

15

Cardiovascular Consequences of Sleep-Disordered Breathing

Gregory S. Montgomery

*Department of Pediatrics, Riley Hospital for Children, Indiana University,
Indianapolis, Indiana, U.S.A.*

Steven H. Abman

*Department of Pediatrics, The Children's Hospital, University of Colorado,
Denver, Colorado, U.S.A.*

CHAPTER HIGHLIGHTS

- Alterations in cardiovascular physiology during normal sleep are intuitive changes.
- Cardiovascular consequences of obstructive sleep apnea (OSA) may include hypertension, arrhythmias, heart failure, and pulmonary hypertension.
- Severe sleep-disordered breathing (SDB) warrants thorough physical and clinical evaluations to assess potential associated cardiovascular impairments.

INTRODUCTION

SDB may often be thought of as primarily a respiratory or neurological concern. However, the intricate interplay between the respiratory system and the cardiopulmonary circulation underlies the frequent and prevalent complications that may arise in the heart as a consequence of obstructive or central sleep disorders (Fig. 1). The vasoactive properties of oxygen and carbon dioxide, the swings in intrathoracic pressures, and the variations in sympathetic and

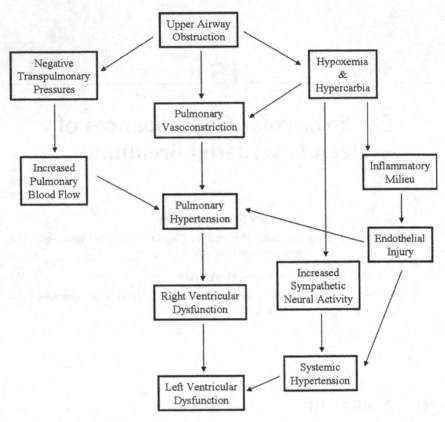

Figure 1 Sleep-related obstructive breathing may induce a number of cascading events, each of which may adversely affect the cardiovascular system. *Source*: Adapted from Ref. 30.

parasympathetic neural activity are some of the physiologic factors seen in SDB that can significantly influence the heart and circulatory systems.

NORMAL CARDIAC RESPONSE TO SLEEP

The typical cardiovascular system alterations seen in children during normal sleep are intuitive physiological changes that occur in the face of total-body muscular relaxation and parasympathetic neural activity prominence (Table 1). The observed vital signs of heart rate and blood pressure typically remain within normal age-appropriate parameters during sleep, but their fundamental alterations are important to appreciate while considering the extreme variations seen in children with SDB.

Table 1 Typical Alterations in Cardiopulmonary
Physiology with Sleep

Cardiac rhythm:	Sinus bradycardia
Heart rate:	Decreased
Stroke volume:	Unchanged
Cardiac output:	Decreased
Blood pressure:	Decreased in non-REM sleep
	Transient elevation in
	REM sleep

Abbreviation: REM, rapid eye movement.

Heart Rate and Rhythm

Metabolic demands are notably decreased during sleep, allowing a decrease in cardiac output through a reduction in heart rate. The mean decrease in heart rate during sleep may often be 10 to 15 beats/min. Although the mean heart rate is generally slower during sleep, the normal beat-to-beat variability seen while awake also continues during sleep. Short periods of tachycardia, occasionally followed by brief bradycardia, may be noted during active rapid eye movement (REM) sleep. Normal sinus variations in heart rate occur during sleep, which may be further modulated by the concurrent respiratory effort. This respiratory variation in heart rate during sleep may be less prominent in premature infants but typically becomes more evident with advancing age. In addition to sinus bradycardia, other variations in cardiac rhythm that may be commonly noted during sleep include brief sinus pauses and type 1, second-degree atrioventricular heart block. In most instances these rhythms are benign as they likely result from primary changes in autonomic tone during the transition between sleep stages or between sleep and wakefulness.

Blood Pressure

Like the heart rate, systemic blood pressure also decreases during sleep. Mean systolic and diastolic pressure values in healthy children may decline during sleep by as much as 13% and 23%, respectively, from wakeful measures (1). Sleep-associated decreases in systolic and diastolic blood pressures are mediated through a decrease in peripheral vascular tone associated with sleep. Parasympathetic neural activity predominance during nonREM sleep leads to diffuse vasodilation, modest reduction in peripheral vascular resistance, and subsequent reduction in systemic blood pressure measures. While the overall trend is a reduction in blood pressure with sleep, transient increase in blood pressure may also normally occur. Sympathetic neural tone briefly dominates during periods of REM sleep, causing an increase in vascular tone and periodic muscle twitches, both which may cause brief rises in systemic blood pressure. These short elevations in blood pressure may exceed wakeful measures, but usually still remain within the normal age-appropriate range.

Cardiac Output

As previously noted, there is a general decline in peripheral vascular tone with sleep, secondary to decreases in muscle tone and dominance of parasympathetic neural activity. This nocturnal decrease in peripheral vascular tone reduces the active return of venous blood to the heart. However, typical assumption of the recumbent position for sleep leads to greater thoracic pooling of blood, helping to maintain stroke volume. The combination of preserved stroke volume and slowing of the heart rate during sleep ultimately leads to a mild overall decline in cardiac output.

CARDIOVASCULAR CONSEQUENCES OF OBSTRUCTIVE SLEEP PATTERNS

Obstructive Sleep Apnea Syndrome

In the past, the severe cardiovascular morbidities of right ventricular dysfunction and failure were the hallmark of severe obstructive SDB. Earlier recognition and treatment of the signs and symptoms of obstructive sleep apnea (OSA) have fortunately led to a decline in the incidence of OSA-associated cardiac disease.

> Interplay between the respiratory and cardiac systems underlies the frequent and prevalent complications that may arise in the heart as a consequence of obstructive or central sleep disorders.

The incidence of OSA among children has remained relatively unchanged over time, occurring in nearly 2% of children (2). In children affected with even mild OSA symptoms, the presence of persistent nocturnal hypoxemia, frequent arousal from sleep, and chronic increases in the work of breathing places unwanted strain upon the cardiovascular system. The clinical manifestations of OSA-associated cardiac impairment in children may include elevations in systemic and pulmonary arterial blood pressures, cardiac arrhythmias, and even rarely "classic" ventricular dysfunction and failure.

Abnormalities of Systemic Blood Pressure

Children with chronic obstructed sleep patterns frequently do not manifest the subtle decline in systemic blood pressures seen in normal sleep. Affected children will often maintain systolic and diastolic blood pressure values similar to wakeful measures, with more severely affected individuals even showing a sleep-associated rise in systemic blood pressure. At least two studies of children with clinical evidence of OSA have demonstrated that systemic blood pressure elevations positively correlate with indices of OSA severity (3,4) and with frequency of nocturnal oxygen desaturation (4).

The etiology of OSA-associated blood pressure elevation is not well defined, although several hypotheses have been suggested. An exaggerated sleep-related sympathetic neural response may lead to nocturnal elevations in peripheral vascular tone, thus preventing the normal fall in peripheral vascular resistance with sleep (5). More recently, the systemic inflammatory markers, such as C-reactive protein (CRP), have been shown to be elevated in children with OSA (6), suggesting a state of chronic systemic inflammation. The CRP elevations were found to be correlated both with indices of OSA severity and with the degree of nocturnal hypoxemia. This heightened systemic inflammatory milieu in children with OSA may suggest some form of direct injury to the vascular endothelium, perhaps leading to chronically elevated vascular tone. Further molecular studies have demonstrated the importance of other vasoactive mediators such as endothelin and nitric oxide in vascular tone modulations with OSA (7,8).

Cardiac Arrhythmias

Infrequently, cardiac arrhythmias may be observed by rhythm strip or by formal electrocardiogram (EKG) evaluations in children with moderate to severe OSA. Exaggerated sinus bradycardia is the rhythm disturbance most commonly seen in children with OSA. These incidents of slowed heart rate may be associated with concomitant episodes of slowed or absent respiratory effort, particularly during REM sleep. This combination of decreased heart rate and apneic pause constitute the "classic" apnea and bradycardia "spells" often seen in premature infants. At the most extreme, this apneic bradycardia may become cyclic in nature, occurring with each breathing pause during sleep.

More rarely, ventricular ectopy may be observed on rhythm tracings in children with OSA. When seen, ventricular arrhythmias may suggest more advanced cardiac strain from the obstructive breathing or underappreciated intrinsic cardiac disease. If present, a more thorough cardiac evaluation by a cardiovascular specialist should be undertaken prior to any surgical intervention to address the OSA symptoms. This assessment should include a formal 12-lead EKG but may also incorporate, at the discretion of the specialist, a detailed echocardiogram to assess ventricular anatomy and function.

Finally, EKG assessments in patients with severe or long-standing obstructed breathing patterns may reveal evidence of right ventricular strain. Typical EKG findings include higher amplitude tracings in the precordial leads, suggesting either underlying right ventricular strain or blatant pulmonary hypertension.

No detailed explorations into the etiology of OSA-associated cardiac arrhythmias have been pursued in children. However, broad adult investigations in OSA have supported the proposal that worrisome cardiac arrhythmias are secondary to disease-related autonomic instability, rather than intrinsic abnormalities of cardiac conduction.

Heart Failure

The incidence of cardiac failure in children with OSA has declined significantly because early clinical signs of obstructed breathing patterns have become more readily recognized (9). However, more subtle evidence of undesired cardiac impairment can be observed in patients with even mild forms of obstructive sleep patterns (10,11). Because of the strong vasoactive properties of oxygen and carbon dioxide, OSA-associated chronic systemic hypercarbia and repeated episodes of nocturnal hypoxia combine to induce sustained elevations in peripheral and pulmonary vascular resistances. These changes place subsequent strain upon both the right and left cardiac ventricles. Further impairment of cardiac function may occur due to the wide swings in intrathoracic pressures seen in obstructive breathing patterns (12). The overall impact on the heart may include elevations in right and left ventricular afterload, increases in ejection time, and significant reductions in ventricular ejection fraction (13). While most evidence of cardiac dysfunction is fortunately reversible with elimination of the underlying airway obstruction, those children with evidence of cardiac impingement are at much greater risk for postoperative complications.

> The incidence of cardiac failure in children with OSA has declined as early clinical signs have become more readily recognized.

Pulmonary Hypertension

Nocturnal elevation of systemic carbon dioxide and reduction in oxygen saturation frequently occur in patients with chronic obstructive breathing patterns. The pulmonary vascular bed is exquisitely sensitive to sleep-related regional alveolar hypoxia, arterial hypercarbia, and associated acidosis. Each of these may induce episodes of pulmonary artery vasoconstriction (14). Prospective EKG and echocardiogram studies in children have demonstrated the presence of clinically significant elevation of pulmonary artery pressures in patients with OSA (15,16). Unlike the brisk improvement seen in right ventricular function following correction of upper airway obstruction, clinically important pulmonary artery pressure elevations may remain despite surgical or medical interventions (17). Persistence of pulmonary hypertension most likely suggests key structural remodeling of the pulmonary vasculature, often seen with long-standing elevated pulmonary artery pressures. Children with evidence of OSA-associated pulmonary hypertension are at increased risk for postsurgical complications.

> The pulmonary vascular bed is sensitive to sleep-related hypoxia, hypercarbia, and acidosis, each of which may induce pulmonary artery vasoconstriction.

Primary Snoring

While snoring is a typical clinical characteristic of OSA, it often must be differentiated from the more benign entity of primary snoring. The latter is defined as the presence of habitual snoring during sleep without the presence of apnea, hypoventilation, hypoxemia, hypercarbia, or associated daytime complications of OSA. Unlike the worrisome cardiovascular consequences seen with true OSA, prospective studies in children with simple primary snoring have not shown clinically significant deleterious changes in blood pressure, heart rhythms, or signs of ventricular impairment (18,19).

Down Syndrome and Obstructive Sleep Apnea

Compared to the general population, clinical findings of OSA occur much more frequently in children with Down syndrome (20). The clinical findings of midface hypoplasia, micrognathia, hypopharyngeal muscular hypotonia, and obesity commonly seen in this genetic syndrome certainly contribute to the frequency of obstructed breathing patterns in these patients. The complexity of OSA in children with Down syndrome is further enhanced by the increased incidence of both congenital heart disease and pulmonary hypertension (21,22). While neither of these clinical features directly correlate with the clinical appearance of OSA, the presence of either congenital heart disease or pulmonary hypertension places those patients at much greater risk for perioperative complications. Guidelines published by the American Academy of Pediatrics recommend prenatal and first-month-of-life cardiac evaluations in all children with Down syndrome (21). In those children with a previously documented history of congenital heart disease or pulmonary hypertension, further cardiac evaluation via EKG or echocardiogram is recommended prior to adenotonsillectomy or other surgical interventions for OSA.

CARDIOVASCULAR CONSEQUENCES OF CENTRAL HYPOVENTILATION

Central breathing disorders describe a sleep disturbance resulting from decreased ventilatory drive from the central nervous system (CNS). With reduced or absent stimulus to breathe, a relative decrease in alveolar minute ventilation leads to an elevation in arterial partial pressure of carbon dioxide. These findings often occur despite the presence of a patent upper airway, normal functioning chest wall structures, and competent lung parenchyma. Central breathing disorders may be associated with the congenital central hypoventilation syndrome (CCHS), Arnold-Chiari and spina bifida–spectrum malformations, intrinsic CNS lesions (tumor, infarction), elevated intracranial pressure, some metabolic disorders, and CNS pharmacological interactions. The clinician should consider potential associations between individual disorders and known associations with cardiac complications, regardless of the severity of the disordered breathing.

Congenital Central Hypoventilation Syndrome

Children with CCHS (Ondine's curse) have been noted to have reduced heart rate variability and an inability to elevate systemic blood pressures with standing, suggesting dysfunctional vagal tone (23). CCHS is associated with a decreased baseline heart rate, decreased heart rate variability, and an increased number of cardiac arrhythmias per 24-hour period (24). Sinus bradycardia, with occasional features of prolonged sinus pauses, are the most frequently observed cardiac arrhythmias in CCHS. Chronic episodes of hypoxemia and hypercarbia also place these children at increased risk for development of pulmonary hypertension and cor pulmonale.

THE HEART AND SUDDEN INFANT DEATH SYNDROME

Sudden infant death syndrome (SIDS) is the leading cause of death in infants during the first year of life in the United States. The peak incidence of SIDS deaths occurs between two and four months of age. Although temporal associations between SIDS deaths and sleep have long been suggested, no clear relationship between any specific clinical phenomena and SIDS deaths has been established. A large population study has suggested a relationship between prolongation of the QT interval on EKG subsequent SIDS events (25). Interestingly, lengthening of the QT interval may be a normally observed event during periods of quiet (nonREM) sleep in healthy infants (26). While these population data suggest an association between abnormal lengthening of the QT interval and SIDS deaths, no formal recommendations for EKG screening of infants are currently in place (27).

CARDIOVASCULAR EVALUATIONS IN SLEEP-DISORDERED BREATHING

Clinical evaluations of children with suspected SDB should include a thorough medical history. Particular focus should be given to a prior history or symptoms of congenital or acquired cardiovascular disease. A complete physical examination should assess for clinical signs of cardiovascular system involvement. Physical exam findings suggestive of cardiac dysfunction include hypertension, hypotension, jugular venous distension, hepatomegaly, and peripheral edema. Cardiac auscultation should evaluate for the presence of rhythm irregularities, valvular flow murmurs, as well as prominence of the second heart sound. This latter finding may suggest elevation of pulmonary artery pressures. Additional

> Cardiovascular changes seen in pediatric SDB will typically improve and often resolve following appropriate clinical intervention.

Table 2   Potential Clinical Evaluations of Cardiac Involvement in Children with Known or Suspected Sleep-Disordered Breathing

Assessment	Test	Special considerations
Severity of SDB	Oxygen saturation (intermittent or prolonged)	Clinical significance varies with method (awake, somnolent, or formal polysomnography)
	Arterial blood gas	Identifies presence of hypercarbia as well as oxygenation status
Evidence of cardiac involvement	Chest radiograph	Observe heart size and shape, prominence of pulmonary vasculature, evidence of pulmonary edema
	EKG (12-lead or Holter)	Note axis, voltage criteria, and T-wave morphology to assess ventricular dysfunction or strain
		Assess for arrhythmia
	Echocardiogram	Noninvasive visualization of congenital or acquired disease
		May detect ventricular dysfunction or pulmonary hypertension

Abbreviations: SDB, sleep-disordered breathing; EKG, electrocardiogram.

findings that may necessitate more through cardiac evaluations may include the presence of prominent developmental delay, failure to thrive, or complex genetic or neuromuscular conditions. Beyond the medical history and physical examination, assessments should be tailored to the individual patient and the index suspicion for cardiac involvement (Table 2)

Significant oxygen desaturation while somnolent may suggest more severe obstructive or central sleep disturbances and potential associated surgical complications. However, it is important to note that absence of oxygen desaturation does not exclude underlying severe disease. Arterial blood gas sampling remains the gold standard for determining both oxygen status and the presence of hypercarbia in the face of SDB. An important consideration in patients with long-standing hypercarbia is the careful addition of supplemental oxygen therapy. While oxygen may be clinically warranted, the initial administration typically should be done under close observation, given the risk of diminished hypoxic respiratory drive (28,29).

Plain chest radiographs may exhibit signs of enlarged cardiac silhouette, right ventricular enlargement, increased size or prominence of the pulmonary vasculature, or even overt pulmonary edema. While some case series reports have shown a high incidence of chest radiograph findings in patients with evidence of cardiovascular complications of OSA, routine radiographic screening of these patients is not generally recommended (30).

EKGs in at-risk SDB patients may demonstrate evidence of cardiac dysfunction or the presence of rhythm disturbances. Voltage, axis, and t-wave morphology may suggest right or left ventricular dysfunction as well as imply the presence of pulmonary hypertension. A single 12-lead EKG may not be sufficient to exclude cardiac arrhythmias. If clinical suspicion remains high, clinicians may consider more extensive Holter or event monitor recordings.

In patients with pre-existing cardiac histories, evidence of sustained sleep-related hypoxemia, or general elevated suspicion of cardiac involvement, formal evaluation with an echocardiogram may be prudent. This noninvasive assessment can estimate the quality of right and left ventricular function, as well as provide reasonable estimations of pulmonary vascular disease through calculations of estimated pulmonary artery pressure, ventricular septum morphology, and right ventricular dimensions.

The cardiovascular changes associated with SDB in children will typically improve following appropriate clinical intervention (13,15,31). Beneficial improvements may include attenuation of somnolent oxygen desaturation, mitigation of systemic hypertension, and diminution of right ventricular strain. However, because the cardiovascular disturbances associated with SDB may frequently persist (32), any decision to clinically intervene should be carefully considered in the context of each patient's underlying comorbidities and severity of cardiovascular disease.

REFERENCES

1. Soergel M, Kirschstein M, Busch C, et al. Oscillometric twenty-four-hour ambulatory blood pressure values in healthy children and adolescents: a multicenter trial including 1141 subjects. J Pediatr 1997; 130:178–184.
2. Redline S, Tishler PV, Schluchter M, et al. Risk factors for sleep-disordered breathing in children. Associations with obesity, race, and respiratory problems. Am J Respir Crit Care Med 1999; 159:1527–1532.
3. Kohyama J, Ohinata JS, Hasegawa T. Blood pressure in sleep disordered breathing. Arch Dis Child 2003; 88:139–142.
4. Enright PL, Goodwin JL, Sherrill DL, et al. Blood pressure elevation associated with sleep-related breathing disorder in a community sample of white and Hispanic children: the Tucson children's assessment of sleep apnea study. Arch Pediatr Adolesc Med 2003; 157:901–904.
5. Yonkers AJ, Spaur RC. Upper airway obstruction and the pharyngeal lymphoid tissue. Otolaryngol Clin North Am 1987; 20:235–239.

6. Tauman R, Ivanenko A, O'Brien LM, et al. Plasma C-reactive protein levels among children with sleep-disordered breathing. Pediatrics 2004; 113:e564–569.
7. Allahdadi KJ, Walker BR, Kanagy NL. Augmented endothelin vasoconstriction in intermittent hypoxia-induced hypertension. Hypertension 2005; 45:705–709.
8. Teramoto S, Kume H, Matsuse T, et al. Oxygen administration improves the serum level of nitric oxide metabolites in patients with obstructive sleep apnea syndrome. Sleep Med 2003; 4:403–407.
9. James AL, Runciman M, Burton MJ, et al. Investigation of cardiac function in children with suspected obstructive sleep apnea. J Otolaryngol 2003; 32:151–154.
10. Amin RS, Kimball TR, Kalra M, et al. Left ventricular function in children with sleep-disordered breathing. Am J Cardiol 2005; 95:801–804.
11. Tal A, Leiberman A, Margulis G, et al. Ventricular dysfunction in children with obstructive sleep apnea: radionuclide assessment. Pediatric Pulmonol 1988; 4:139–143.
12. Buda AJ, Pinsky MR, Ingels NB Jr, et al. Effect of intrathoracic pressure on left ventricular performance. N Engl J Med 1979; 301:453–459.
13. Sofer S, Weinhouse E, Tal A, et al. Cor pulmonale due to adenoidal or tonsillar hypertrophy or both in children. Noninvasive diagnosis and follow-up. Chest 1988; 93:119–122.
14. Meyrick BO, Perkett EA. The sequence of cellular and hemodynamic changes of chronic pulmonary hypertension induced by hypoxia and other stimuli. Am Rev Respir Dis 1989; 140:1486–1489.
15. Miman MC, Kirazli T, Ozyurek R. Doppler echocardiography in adenotonsillar hypertrophy. Int J Pediatr Otorhinolaryngol 2000; 54:21–26.
16. Wilkinson AR, McCormick MS, Freeland AP, et al. Electrocardiographic signs of pulmonary hypertension in children who snore. Br Med J (Clin Res Ed) 1981; 282:1579–1581.
17. Perkin RM, Anas NG. Pulmonary hypertension in pediatric patients. J Pediatr 1984; 105:511–522.
18. Amin RS, Carroll JL, Jeffries JL, et al. Twenty-four-hour ambulatory blood pressure in children with sleep-disordered breathing. Am J Respir Crit Care Med 2004; 169:950–956.
19. Kaditis AG, Alexopoulos EI, Kostadima E, et al. Comparison of blood pressure measurements in children with and without habitual snoring. Pediatr Pulmonol 2005; 39:408–414.
20. Marcus CL, Keens TG, Bautista DB, et al. Obstructive sleep apnea in children with Down syndrome. Pediatrics 1991; 88:132–139.
21. American Academy of Pediatrics. Health supervision for children with Down syndrome. Pediatrics 2001; 107:442–449.
22. Rowland TW, Nordstrom LG, Bean MS, et al. Chronic upper airway obstruction and pulmonary hypertension in Down's syndrome. Am J Dis Child 1981; 135:1050–1052.
23. Trang H, Girard A, Laude D, et al. Short-term blood pressure and heart rate variability in congenital central hypoventilation syndrome (Ondine's curse). Clin Sci (Lond) 2005; 108:225–230.
24. Silvestri JM, Hanna BD, Volgman AS, et al. Cardiac rhythm disturbances among children with idiopathic congenital central hypoventilation syndrome. Pediatr Pulmonol 2000; 29:351–358.
25. Schwartz PJ, Stramba-Badiale M, Segantini A, et al. Prolongation of the QT interval and the sudden infant death syndrome. N Engl J Med 1998; 338:1709–1714.

26. Haddad GG, Krongrad E, Epstein RA, et al. Effect of sleep state on the QT interval in normal infants. Pediatr Res 1979; 13:139–141.
27. Hodgman JE, Siassi B. Prolonged QTc as a risk factor for SIDS. Pediatrics 1999; 103:814–815.
28. Brown OE, Manning SC, Ridenour B. Cor pulmonale secondary to tonsillar and adenoidal hypertrophy: management considerations. Int J Pediatr Otorhinolaryngol 1988; 16:131–139.
29. Luke MJ, Mehrizi A, Folger GM Jr, et al. Chronic nasopharyngeal obstruction as a cause of cardiomegaly, cor pulmonale, and pulmonary edema. Pediatrics 1966; 37:762–768.
30. Blum RH, McGowan FX Jr. Chronic upper airway obstruction and cardiac dysfunction: anatomy, pathophysiology and anesthetic implications. Paediatr Anaesth 2004; 14:75–83.
31. Shintani T, Asakura K, Kataura A. The effect of adenotonsillectomy in children with OSA. Int J Pediatr Otorhinolaryngol 1998; 44:51–58.
32. Lipton AJ, Gozal D. Treatment of obstructive sleep apnea in children: do we really know how? Sleep Med Rev 2003; 7:61–80.

16

Congenital Central Hypoventilation Syndrome: Update, Diagnosis, and Management

Anna S. Kenny and Debra E. Weese-Mayer

Pediatric Respiratory Medicine, Rush University Medical Center, Chicago, Illinois, U.S.A.

CHAPTER HIGHLIGHTS

- Congenital central hypoventilation syndrome (CCHS) is one of a growing number of disorders within the rubric of autonomic nervous system dysregulation (ANSD).
- Children with CCHS typically present in the newborn period with cyanosis upon falling asleep. The classic presentation is characterized by adequate ventilation while awake but hypoventilation typically with normal rather monotonous respiratory rates and shallow breathing during sleep.
- Children with CCHS do not typically increase their respiratory rate or have dyspnea in response to pneumonia (or the resulting hypoxemia and hypercarbia). The absence of these symptoms does not preclude severe respiratory compromise. Likewise, children with CCHS do not typically develop a fever in spite of an infection.
- Recently, seemingly normal children and adults with the CCHS phenotype have been identified. These individuals typically present with profound hypercarbia after an intercurrent respiratory illness.

- After confirming the absence of primary lung, cardiac, neuromuscular, or focal brainstem pathology, the diagnosis of CCHS may be considered. If the clinician strongly suspects a diagnosis of CCHS, confirmation can be achieved quickly with the PCR-based *PHOX2B* gene testing.
- The expectation is that vigilant management of ventilation and rigorous efforts to support an age-appropriate and progressively independent life-style will maximize the quality of life for these special children.

INTRODUCTION

Congenital central hypoventilation syndrome was first described in 1970 by Mellins et al. (1). Although CCHS was long considered to be primarily a disorder of respiratory control, over the ensuing 35 years it has become apparent that CCHS is one of a growing number of disorders within the rubric of ANSD. With the discovery that individuals with CCHS are heterozygous for mutations in the *PHOX2B* gene, a gene that is manifest early in the embryologic origin of the autonomic nervous system (ANS), this relationship has been confirmed.

The term "Ondine's curse" is a literary misnomer that has been used in past literature to describe children with CCHS. A German folk epic (2) tells the story of a young nymph, Ondine, who falls in love with a mortal. When the mortal is unfaithful to Ondine, the king of the nymphs places a curse on the mortal. The curse makes the mortal responsible for remembering to perform all bodily functions, including breathing. When the mortal falls asleep, he "forgets" to breathe and dies. Because Ondine did not curse the mortal (the king of the nymphs did the deed) and the children affected with CCHS worldwide do not "forget" to breathe (the *PHOX2B* mutation disrupts the developing ANS), the term "Ondine's curse" should be avoided.

CLINICAL PRESENTATION IN INFANTS

Children with CCHS have a complex phenotype consistent with imbalance of the ANS, yet it has taken several years for acceptance that CCHS is a more global phenomenon than strictly an abnormality of control of breathing. Identified abnormalities are described subsequently and presented in Table 1.

Facial Dysmorphology

A characteristic boxy-shaped facies has recently been described in children and young adults with CCHS. Their faces are generally shorter relative to the width and flatter, and with an inferior inflection of the lateral segment of vermillion border on the upper lip (3). A representative photograph is provided in Figure 1.

Table 1   ANS Symptoms for Probands with CCHS, by Organ System

Cardiovascular
Decreased heart rate variability
Dysrhythmia
Loss of consciousness
Vasovagal syncope
Gastrointestinal
Constipation without Hirschsprung disease
Dysphagia
Gastroesophageal reflux
Neurological
Altered perception of pain
Ophthalmologic
Altered lacrimation
Anisocoria
Miosis
Nonreactive/sluggish pupils
Strabismus
Psychological
Altered perception of anxiety
Respiratory
Alveolar hypoventilation
Extreme breath-holding spells
Lack of respiratory distress despite hypoxemia and hypercarbia
Sudomotor
Altered sweating
Altered temperature regulation

Abbreviations: ANS, autonomic nervous system; CCHS, congenital central hypoventilation syndrome.

Respiratory Dysfunction

The most apparent aspect of CCHS is disordered respiratory control (1,4,5–9) without any apparent respiratory distress. Children with CCHS typically present in the newborn period with cyanosis upon falling asleep. The classic presentation is characterized by adequate ventilation while awake but hypoventilation typically with normal rather monotonous respiratory rates and shallow breathing during sleep (8). Occasionally, these patients will demonstrate apneic pauses after discontinuation of mechanical ventilation and before initiation of spontaneous breathing. While asleep, the children with CCHS experience progressive hypercapnia and hypoxemia (1,4,5,7,8,10–22), though their ventilation is "more normal" in rapid eye movement sleep than in non-rapid eye movement sleep (13). They have absent or negligible ventilatory sensitivity to hypercarbia

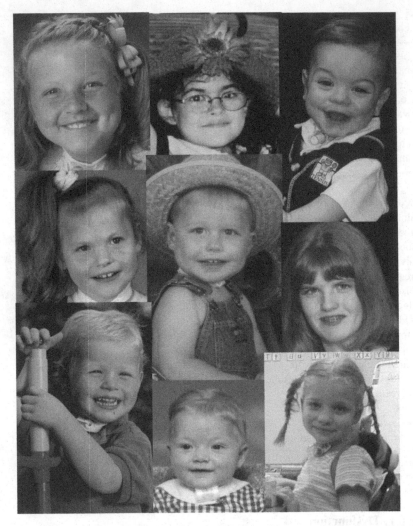

Figure 1 Composite of casual photographs from children with congenital central hypo-ventilation syndrome (CCHS). These casual photographs of children with CCHS are examples of the photos that prompted the authors to consider a characteristic facies in CCHS. *Source*: From Ref. 3.

and absent or variable ventilatory sensitivity to hypoxemia during sleep (1,4,5,7,8,10–17,20–22). They lack an arousal response to the endogenous challenges of isolated hypercarbia, hypoxemia, and to the combined stimulus of hypercarbia and hypoxemia (8). Awake ventilatory responsiveness to and perception of hypercarbia and hypoxemia are generally absent (6,8,13,20), even when awake minute ventilation is adequate.

Hirschsprung Disease and Tumors of Neural Crest Origin

CCHS occurs in association with Hirschsprung disease (4,5,8,10,18,23–28) in approximately 20% of the cases, and tumors of neural crest origin [neuroblastoma (10), ganglioneuroblastoma (29), ganglioneuroma (5,8,15)] in approximately 5% of the cases. The Hirschsprung disease is typically apparent in the newborn period and the tumors of neural crest origin present after the first year of life.

Diffuse Autonomic Nervous System Dysregulation

CCHS also occurs with symptoms of diffuse autonomic nervous system dysfunction/dysregulation (ANSD) (30), including decreased heart rate variability (31–34), an attenuated heart rate response to exercise (35), altered blood pressure homeostasis (33,36), severe constipation (8), esophageal dysmotility/dysphagia (37), decreased perception of discomfort, pupillary abnormalities (8,38), decreased perception of anxiety (39), sporadic profuse sweating, and decreased basal body temperature, among others. Interestingly, many of these characteristics and others were described in early case reports (decreased heart rate variability, diminished pupillary light response, feeding difficulty with esophageal dysmotility in infancy, breath-holding spells, poor temperature regulation with decreased basal body temperature, sporadic profuse sweating episodes with cool extremities), though not studied systematically until more recently. Yet, only in the recent past has methodological ANS testing progressed beyond heart rate variability assessment, with two recent important physiologic studies describing esophageal dysmotility (37) and blood pressure fluctuation (36). Development of proper laboratories to assess ANS function in children is essential to clearly characterize the phenotype of ANS imbalance in CCHS and other potentially related diseases (Table 1).

CLINICAL PRESENTATION IN CHILDREN AND ADULTS

Recently, several children and adults with the CCHS phenotype have been identified (40–42). These seemingly normal individuals typically present with profound hypercarbia after an intercurrent respiratory illness. Clinicians need to be aware that a subset, albeit small, of individuals will present beyond the newborn period. The hallmark of the presentation remains alveolar hypoventilation, but the diagnosis after infancy requires an exceedingly high index of suspicion.

DIFFERENTIAL DIAGNOSIS

CCHS mimics many treatable diseases; therefore, the disorders listed in Table 2 should be considered in the differential diagnosis.

Table 2   Differential Diagnosis in Congenital
Central Hypoventilation Syndrome

Altered airway or intrathoracic anatomy
Brainstem deformity or tumor
Confounding clinical conditions
   Asphyxia
   Infarction
   Infection
   Trauma
Congenital myasthenic syndrome
Diaphragm dysfunction
Metabolic diseases
Mobius syndrome
Multiminicore disease
X-linked myotubular myopathy

INITIAL EVALUATION

Initial evaluation of any child with a suspected diagnosis of CCHS should
include the recommended evaluations and tests provided in Table 3, in order to
confirm/refute the diagnosis of CCHS.

Table 3   Recommended Evaluations/Tests to Confirm/Refute the Diagnosis of
Congenital Central Hypoventilation Syndrome

Detailed chart review of prenatal, birth, infancy, and subsequent medical records
Meticulous physical exam, awake and asleep
Genetic testing for mutations in the *PHOX2B* gene
Awake and asleep physiologic in-laboratory attended recordings of respiratory inductance
   plethysmography of the chest/abdomen/sum, hemoglobin saturation, end tidal carbon
   dioxide, air flow, tidal volume, ECG, EEG, and EOG
MRI and/or CT images of the brain and brainstem
Bronchoscopy
Diaphragm fluoroscopy
Echocardiogram
Holter recording
Neurologic exam
Ophthalmologic exam
Potentially a muscle biopsy
Serum/carnitine concentration

Abbreviations: CT, computed tomography; ECG, electrocardiogram; EEG, electroencephalogram;
EOG, electro-oculogram; MRI, magnetic resonance imaging.

VENTILATORY SUPPORT

Several ventilatory support options are available for the infant and child with CCHS. Typically, the infant who requires ventilatory support 24 hr/day requires a tracheostomy and use of a home ventilator. As the infant becomes ambulatory, diaphragm pacing by phrenic nerve stimulation can be considered for use during wakefulness, allowing for increased mobility, and improved quality of life (QOL). Diaphragm pacers for the active child with CCHS should be implanted in the chest (43–46). Older infants and toddlers with diaphragm pacers may use a Passy–Muir one-way speaking valve while awake, allowing for vocalization and use of the upper airway on exhalation. Children with diaphragm pacers may also be assessed for capping of the tracheostomy tube during pacing while awake, thereby allowing for inspiration and exhalation via the upper airway. Nonetheless, these patients who require 24 hr/day support require a tracheostomy for mechanical ventilation during sleep. Although not yet accomplished, the older child with an entirely normal airway may be able to rely on diaphragm pacing while awake and on nasal mask ventilation while asleep, thus eliminating the need for a tracheostomy. However, in the event of severe illness requiring more aggressive ventilatory management, such a child may require interim endotracheal intubation to allow for adequate ventilation.

Those children who consistently require ventilatory support during sleep only (as opposed to sleep and wakefulness) and who are able to cooperate can be considered as candidates for noninvasive support with either nasal mask ventilation or negative-pressure ventilation. Implicit in noninvasive ventilation is recognition that in the event of severe illness the child may require interim endotracheal intubation. Likewise, the child who requires support only while asleep may also require ventilatory assistance while awake and asleep during an intercurrent illness.

Regardless of the method of support, the goal is to optimize the child's oxygenation and ventilation. Recommendations for hemoglobin saturation values are typically 95% or greater. An end tidal carbon dioxide level range from 30 to 50 mmHg allows for variation within sleep positions, though the target range is 35–40 mmHg. The goal for chronic care ventilation is to minimize exposure to hypoventilation and avoid exposure to hyperventilation.

Independent of the modality, the goal is to match the patient with the optimal technology for individual life style needs. Although diaphragm pacing is not typically recommended for the young child who requires only nighttime support (the benefits do not outweigh the risks), for the older adolescent and young adult, this might be an appropriate consideration.

LONG-TERM VENTILATOR MANAGEMENT

Meticulous follow-up and coordination of care by the family in conjunction with their local pulmonologist, pediatrician, and the physicians in a center with recognized expertise in CCHS are vital to achieve a successful outcome for each child. Infants and young children should be evaluated every one to two months by their pediatrician or pulmonologist. These local evaluations should include assessment of growth, speech, and mental and motor development. Every six months infants and young children should be evaluated by physicians at a center with recognized expertise in CCHS. These evaluations will include a four-to-five-day in-hospital evaluation with detailed recording during both sleep and wakefulness in a pediatric respiratory physiology laboratory to observe the adequacy of ventilation. Many infants appear to "acquire" awake hypoventilation at two to three years of age. This coincides with the natural occurrence of a decreased respiratory frequency. It is imperative for toddlers in this age group to be closely monitored to assure adequate ventilatory support. Physiologic evaluation of oxygenation and ventilation during exercise and recovery from exercise should be performed on a routine basis as advancing age permits. After about 3 years of age, the child may undergo detailed center evaluation on an annual basis. An echocardiogram should be performed every six months to assess for right-ventricular hypertrophy and pulmonary hypertension, occurring as a sign of unrecognized hypoxemia. A 72-hour Holter monitor should be performed annually to assess for transient asystole (32), especially in the event of dizziness or syncope. A bronchoscopy should be performed every 12 to 18 months to assess for suprastomal granulation tissue and/or adenotonsillar hypertrophy, which may interfere with successful use of the Passy–Muir one-way speaking valve or nocturnal mask ventilation. Detailed developmental and ophthalmologic assessments should be performed every 12 months to verify that the child is on track and/or to provide guidance for intervention. Pulmonary function testing should be performed as needed to identify and monitor the status of reactive airway disease.

GENETIC TESTING AND GENETIC COUNSELING

PCR-Based *PHOX2B* Testing in Congenital Central Hypoventilation Syndrome

After confirming the absence of primary lung, cardiac, neuromuscular, or focal brainstem pathology, the diagnosis of CCHS may be considered. If the clinician strongly suspects a diagnosis of CCHS, confirmation can be achieved quickly with the PCR-based *PHOX2B* gene testing. This is run on DNA from blood samples or other tissues (www.genetests.org). The normal *PHOX2B* allele size is 20 repeats and the affected allele size is 25 to 33 repeats. Although it is estimated that about 300 cases are known worldwide, molecular genetic testing in the United States has already identified more than 180 individuals with the CCHS phenotype and with the *PHOX2B* mutation (47, Weese-Mayer, Zhou, and Berry-Kravis, personal communication). If the test is negative and the physician is confident that the child has the phenotype for CCHS (especially, in the presence of severe Hirschsprung disease), then sequencing of the *PHOX2B* gene should be performed. Because of the autosomal dominant inheritance pattern, it would be advisable to perform the test on parents of CCHS probands and on probands with CCHS who are pregnant. Prenatal testing for CCHS can be done on cultured chorionic villus sampling (CVS) tissue or amniocytes if the *PHOX2B* mutation in the family is known.

The *PHOX2B* assay has identified the common polyalanine expansion mutation in 90% to 95% of the cases of CCHS (42,48–51). The remaining 5% to 10% of cases with the CCHS phenotype and severe Hirschsprung disease will have a unique mutation in the *PHOX2B* gene that will require sequencing for identification.

Mosaicism

Some individuals diagnosed with CCHS have an affected parent known to have CCHS. Approximately 10% of individuals with CCHS have an asymptomatic parent (non-CCHS) who has somatic mosaicism for a *PHOX2B* mutation (50). Recommendations for the evaluation of parents of a proband with an apparent *de novo* mutation include testing of both parents for the *PHOX2B* mutation. The possibility of a germline mosaicism situation cannot be excluded. If a parent of the proband has a somatic mosaic pattern for the *PHOX2B* repeat expansion, the recurrence risk to the sibs of the proband is 50% or less. When the parents are clinically unaffected, a risk to the sibs of a proband may still be present, as germline mosaicism (although not yet reported) remains a possibility (50).

Offspring of a Proband with Congenital Central Hypoventilation Syndrome

The autosomal dominant pattern of inheritance was identified in offspring of individuals with CCHS and the *PHOX2B* mutation (50). The mutation is stable from one generation to the next so that if a proband with CCHS has the genotype 20/25 and her infant is affected, then the infant will have the 20/25 genotype. Each child of an individual with CCHS has a 50% chance of inheriting the mutation.

Other Family Members

The risk to other family members depends upon the status of the proband's parents. If a parent is found to be affected, family members are at risk.

LONG-TERM OUTCOME

Children with CCHS experience an overall good QOL (20,45,52,53). Long-term follow-up and neurodevelopmental outcome demonstrate a broad range of results, with a great deal of variability. Unfortunately, it is difficult to determine whether neurodevelopmental outcome is related to ANSD specific to CCHS or is secondary to chronic/intermittent hypoxemia. Emphasis should be placed on the importance of early diagnosis with clinical assessment and *PHOX2B* testing, vigilant care in day-to-day management, communication between parents and local physicians, and collaboration between local physicians and centers with expertise in CCHS both from the diagnostic and treatment perspectives.

KEY TO SUCCESSFUL MANAGEMENT

Management of children with CCHS requires diligence and cooperation from all caregivers involved in their care. With the increased awareness of the disease process and the availability of genetic testing for the *PHOX2B* mutation, patients are being recognized much sooner. Early diagnosis and referral to a center with expertise in the management and research of CCHS are essential. The expectation is that vigilant management of ventilation and rigorous efforts to support an age-appropriate and progressively independent life-style will maximize the QOL for these special children.

Children with CCHS are very different from other ventilator-dependent children. Their lack of responsiveness to hypercarbia and hypoxemia requires extreme maintenance. They do not possess adequate responses to exercise and infection. Special consideration must be given in their management with regard to normal childhood activities and infections. Children with CCHS should be guided by conservative management; their sport activities should be non-contact with moderate levels of activity and frequent rest periods. Swimming should not be allowed, even in cases where no tracheostomy is present. Some physicians and caregivers will allow children with CCHS to swim, however, constant supervision by an adult caregiver and counting by the child to minimize the amount of time spent under the water is mandatory. Lacking the ability to sense their physiologic compromise (hypoxemia, hypercarbia, and acidosis), CCHS subjects will likely swim longer and farther than any of their friends. In the process, they will likely become severely physiologically compromised. Children with CCHS do not typically increase their respiratory rate or have dyspnea in response to pneumonia (or the resulting hypoxemia and hypercarbia). The absence of these symptoms does not preclude severe respiratory compromise. Likewise, children with CCHS do not typically develop a fever in spite of an infection. These limitations emphasize the importance of (*i*) the objective measures of hemoglobin saturation and end tidal carbon dioxide by noninvasive monitoring in the home, (*ii*) highly skilled and consistent nurses in the home, and (*iii*) the need for ongoing care by a center with known expertise in CCHS allowing for close supervision of each child. Early intervention is clearly in the best interest of the child, the family, and the healthcare provider with the goals of optimal neurodevelopmental outcome balanced with a satisfactory QOL.

REFERENCES

1. Mellins RB, Balfowr HH Jr, Turino GM, Winters RW. Failure of automatic control of ventilation (Ondine's curse). Report of an infant born with this syndrome and review of the literature. Medicine 1970; 49(6):487–504.
2. Sugar O. In search of Ondine's curse. JAMA 1978; 240(3):236–237.
3. Todd ES, Weinberg SM, Berry-Kravis EM, et al. Facial phenotype in children and young adults with *PHOX2B*—determined congenital central hypoventilation syndrome: quantitative pattern of dysmorphology. Pediatr Res 206(1):39–45.
4. Guilleminault C, McQuitty J, Ariagno RL, Challamel MJ, Korobkin R, McClead RE Jr. Congenital central alveolar hypoventilation syndrome in six infants. Pediatr 1982; 70(5):684–694.
5. Haddad GG, Mazza NM, Defendini R, et al. Congenital failure of automatic control of ventilation, gastrointestinal motility and heart rate. Medicine 1978; 57(6):517–526.
6. Paton JY, Swaminathan S, Sargent CW, Keens TG. Hypoxic and hypercapnic ventilatory responses in awake children with congenital central hypoventilation syndrome. Am Rev Respir Dis 1989; 140(2):368–372.
7. Shannon DC, Marsland DW, Gould JB, Callahan B, Todres ID, Dennis J. Central hypoventilation during quiet sleep in two infants. Pediatr 1976; 57(3):342–346.
8. Weese-Mayer DE, Hunt CE, Brouillette RT, Silvestri JM. Congenital central hypoventilation syndrome: diagnosis, management, and long-term outcome in thirty-two children. J Pediatr 1992; 120(3):381–387.
9. Weese-Mayer DE, Shannon DC, Keens TG, Silvestri JM. Idiopathic congenital central hypoventilation syndrome. Diagnosis and management. Am J Respir Crit Care Med 1999; 160:368–373.
10. Bower RJ, Adkins JC. Ondine's curse and neurocristopathy. Clin Pediatr 1980; 19(10):665–668.
11. Coleman M, Boros SJ, Huseby TL, Brennom WS. Congenital central hypoventilation syndrome: a report of successful experience with bilateral diaphragmatic pacing. Arch Dis Child 1980; 55(11): 901–903.
12. Deonna T, Arczynska W, Torrado A. Congenital failure of automatic ventilation (Ondine's curse): a case report. J Pediatr 1974; 84(5):710–714.
13. Fleming PJ, Cade D, Bryan MH, Bryan AC. Congenital central hypoventilation and sleep state. Pediatr 1980; 66(3):425–428.
14. Folgering H, Kuyper F, Kille JF. Primary alveolar hypoventilation (Ondine's curse syndrome) in an infant without external arcuate nucleus: case report. Bull Eur Physiopatholog Respir 1979; 15(4):659–665.
15. Hunt CE, Matalon SV, Thompson TR, et al. Central hypoventilation syndrome: experience with bilateral phrenic nerve pacing in 3 neonates. Am Rev Respir Dis 1978; 118(1):23–28.
16. Khalifa MM, Flavin MA, Wherrett BA. Congenital central hypoventilation syndrome in monozygotic twins. J Pediatr 1988; 113(5):853–855.
17. Liu HM, Loew JM, Hunt CE. Congenital central hypoventilation syndrome: a pathologic study of the neuromuscular system. Neurol 1978; 28(10):1013–1019.
18. Minutillo C, Pemberton PJ, Goldblatt J. Hirschsprung's disease and Ondine's curse: further evidence for a distinct syndrome. Clin Genet 1989; 36(3):200–203.

19. Nattie EE, Bartlett D, Rozycki AA. Central alveolar hypoventilation in a child: an evaluation using a whole body plethysmograph. Am Rev Respir Dis 1975; 112(2):259–266.

20. Oren J, Kelly DH, Shannon DC. Long-term follow-up of children with congenital central hypoventilation syndrome. Pediatr 1987; 80(3):375–380.

21. Ruth V, Pesonen E, Raivio KO. Congenital central hypoventilation syndrome treated with diaphragm pacing. Acta Paediatr Scandinavica 1983; 72(2):295–297.

22. Wells HH, Kattwinkel J, Morrow JD. Control of ventilation of Ondine's curse. J Pediatr 1980; 96(5):865–867.

23. Hamilton J, Bodurtha JN. Congenital central hypoventilation syndrome and Hirschsprung's disease in half sibs. J Med Genet 1989; 26(4):272–274.

24. Mukhopadhyay S, Wilkinson PW. Cerebral arteriovenous malformation, Ondine's curse and Hirschsprung's disease. Dev Med Child Neurol 1990; 32(12):1087–1089.

25. O'Dell K, Staren E, Bassuk A. Total colonic aganglionosis (Zuelzer–Wilson syndrome) and congenital failure of automatic control of ventilation (Ondine's curse). J Pediatr Surg 1987; 22(11):1019–1020.

26. Stern M, Erttmann R, Hellwege HH, Kuhn N. Total aganglionosis of the colon and Ondine's curse. Lancet 1980; 1(8173):877–878.

27. Verloes A, Elmer C, Lacombe D, et al. Ondine-Hirschsprung syndrome (Haddad syndrome). Further delineation in two cases and review of the literature. Euro J Pediatr 1993; 152(1):75–77.

28. Weese-Mayer DE, Brouillette RT, Naidich TP, McLone DG, Hunt CE. Magnetic resonance imaging and computerized tomography in central hypoventilation. Am Rev Respir Dis 1988; 137(2):393–398.

29. Swaminathan S, Gilsanz V, Atkinson J, Keens TG. Congenital central hypoventilation syndrome associated with multiple ganglioneuromas. Chest 1989; 96(2):423–424.

30. Weese-Mayer DE, Silvestri JM, Huffman AD, et al. Case/control family study of autonomic nervous system dysfunction in idiopathic congenital central hypoventilation syndrome. Am J Med Genet 2001; 100(3):237–245.

31. Ogawa T, Kojo M, Fukushima N, et al. Cardio-respiratory control in an infant with Ondine's curse: a multivariate autoregressive modelling approach. J Autonom Nerv Syst 1993; 42(1):41–52.

32. Silvestri JM, Hanna BD, Volgman AS, Jones PJ, Barnes SD, Weese-Mayer DE. Cardiac rhythm disturbances among children with idiopathic congenital central hypoventilation syndrome. Pediatr Pulmonol 2000; 29(5):351–358.

33. Trang H, Girard A, Laude D, Elghozi JL. Short-term blood pressure and heart rate variability in congenital central hypoventilation syndrome (Ondine's curse). [see comment]. Clin Sci 2005; 108(3):225–230.

34. Woo MS, Woo MA, Gozal D, Jansen MT, Keens TG, Harper RM. Heart rate variability in congenital central hypoventilation syndrome. Pediatr Res 1992; 31(3):291–296.

35. Silvestri JM, Weese-Mayer DE, Flanagan EA. Congenital central hypoventilation syndrome: cardiorespiratory responses to moderate exercise, simulating daily activity. Pediatr Pulmonol 1995; 20(2):89–93.

36. Trang H, Boureghda S, Denjoy I, Alia M, Kabaker M. 24-hour BP in children with congenital central hypoventilation syndrome. Chest 2003; 124(4):1393–1399.

37. Faure C, Viarme F, Cargill G, Navarro J, Gaultier C, Trang H. Abnormal esophageal motility in children with congenital central hypoventilation syndrome. Gastroenterol 2002; 122(5):1258–1263.
38. Goldberg DS, Ludwig IH. Congenital central hypoventilation syndrome: ocular findings in 37 children. J Pediatr Ophthalmol Strabismus 1996; 33(3):175–180.
39. Pine DS, Weese-Mayer DE, Silvestri JM, Davies M, Whitaker AH, Klein DF. Anxiety and congenital central hypoventilation syndrome. Am J Psychiatry 1994; 151(6):864–870.
40. Weese-Mayer DE, Berry-Kravis EM, Zhou L. Adult identified with congenital central hypoventilation syndrome—mutation in *PHOX2B* gene and late-onset CHS. (comment). Am J Respir Crit Care Med 2005; 171(1):88.
41. Trang H, Laudler B, Trochet D. *PHOX2B* gene mutation in a patient with late-onset central hypoventilation. Pediatr Pulmonol 2004; 38(4):349–351.
42. Matera I, Bachetti T, Puppo F, et al. *PHOX2B* mutations and polyalanine expansions correlate with the severity of the respiratory phenotype and associated symptoms in both congenital and late onset central hypoventilation syndrome. J Med Genet 2004; 41(5): 373–380.
43. Weese-Mayer DE, Silvestri JM, Kenny AS, et al. Diaphragm pacing with a quadripolar phrenic nerve electrode: an international study. Pacing Clin Electrophysiol 1996; 19(9):1311–1319.
44. Weese-Mayer DE, Morrow AS, Brouillette RT, Ilbawi MN, Hunt CE. Diaphragm pacing in infants and children. A life-table analysis of implanted components. Am Rev Respir Dis 1989; 139(4):974–979.
45. Weese-Mayer DE, Hunt CE, Brouillette RT, Silvestri JM. Diaphragm pacing in infants and children. J Pediatr 1992; 120(1):1–8.
46. Shaul DB, Danielson PD, McComb JG, Keens TG. Thoracoscopic placement of phrenic nerve electrodes for diaphragmatic pacing in children. J Pediatr Surg 2002; 37(7):974–978; discussion 974–978.
47. Weese-Mayer DE, Berry-Kravis EM. Genetics of congenital central hypoventilation syndrome: lessons from a seemingly orphan disease. (see comment). Am J Respir Crit Care Med 2004; 170(1):16–21.
48. Amiel J, Laudier B, Attie-Bitach T, et al. Polyalanine expansion and frameshift mutations of the paired-like homeobox gene *PHOX2B* in congenital central hypoventilation syndrome. [see comment]. Nat Genet 2003; 33(4):459–461.
49. Sasaki A, Kanai M, Kijima K, et al. Molecular analysis of congenital central hypoventilation syndrome. Hum Genet 2003; 114(1):22–26.
50. Weese-Mayer DE, Berry-Kravis EM, Zhou L, et al. Idiopathic congenital central hypoventilation syndrome: analysis of genes pertinent to early autonomic nervous system embryologic development and identification of mutations in *PHOX2B*. Am J Med Genet A 2003; 123(3):267–278.
51. Trochet DL, O'Brien D, Gozal H, et al. *PHOX2B* genotype allows for prediction of tumor risk in congenital central Hypoventilation syndrome. Am J Hum Genet 76(3):412–416.
52. Marcus CL, Jansen MT, Poulsen MK, et al. Medical and psychosocial outcome of children with congenital central hypoventilation syndrome. J Pediatr 1991; 119(6):888–895.
53. Silvestri JM, Weese-Mayer DE, Nelson MN. Neuropsychologic abnormalities in children with congenital central hypoventilation syndrome. J Pediatr 1992; 120(3):388–393.

17

Sudden Infant Death Syndrome and Apparent Life-Threatening Events

Ann C. Halbower

Pediatric Sleep Disorders Program, Division of Pediatric Pulmonology,
Johns Hopkins University School of Medicine,
Baltimore, Maryland, U.S.A.

CHAPTER HIGHLIGHTS

- Infants are vulnerable to death during sleep due to an immature autonomic nervous system and decreased arousal to abnormal blood gas values.
- Infants are vulnerable to death if they are overheated, if they sleep in the prone or side position, and if they are exposed to cigarette smoke.
- During rapid eye movement (REM) sleep, obstructions worsens due to loss of muscle tone. Decreased functional residual capacity (FRC) lowers lung volume which contributes to lower oxygen saturation. Neonates spend 50% of their time in REM sleep.
- Normal autonomic nervous system reflexes can cause apnea or bradycardia from vagal stimulation. These reflexes are exaggerated when infants are prone, sleeping, or sedated.
- Apnea monitors do not protect infants in unsafe sleep environments and do not guarantee survival.
- Apnea monitors do not detect obstructive breathing events, hypoxemia, gastroesophageal reflux, or seizure activity. Their use should be evidence-based.
- The physician prescribing the apnea monitor should be responsible for following the recorded events, determining whether increased diagnostic

evaluation is required, and discontinuing the monitor when clinically indicated.

- Modifiable risk factors for sudden infant death syndrom (SIDS) should be discussed with parents. The risk of SIDS is increased in infants under six months of age who sleep prone, are exposed to smoke, are over bundled, and are premature.

SUDDEN INFANT DEATH SYNDROME

Nothing could be more devastating for a parent than the sudden and unexpected death of an infant. SIDS is the number one killer of infants between one month and one year of age in the U.S.A. (1) and the third major cause of infant mortality. Infants suffer from a unique risk of sudden death during sleep that is not shared by toddlers, children, adolescents, or adults. Our lack of understanding of the mechanism for this mysterious risk extends from Biblical times to the present day. However, over the last decade and a half, epidemiological studies performed worldwide have identified environmental and physiological risk factors, which served as the basis for corrective actions that dramatically decreased the incidence of this disorder.

This chapter illustrates some of the various differences in sleep and respiratory control in infants compared with adults. A major focus of research is whether these age-related differences, in the right circumstance, could "set the infant up" for sudden death. Infants display various anatomical and physical differences that in themselves may not be pathologic; however, when added together, these physical differences create a vulnerable state for infants, especially during sleep, which could lead to a serious outcome.

An expert panel of the National Institute of Child Health and Human Development has defined SIDS as: "The sudden death of an infant under one year of age which remains unexplained after a thorough case investigation, including performance of a complete autopsy, examination of the death scene, and review of the clinical history" (2). Prior to the U.S. Back-to-Sleep campaign in 1991, SIDS, also known as crib death or cot death, had an estimated incidence of about two cases per 1000 live births, accounting for about 5000 deaths annually (3). This incidence dropped to 0.56 per 1000 in the year 2000 due to education campaigns focussing on modifiable risk factors, as will be discussed subsequently. SIDS occurs in sleep [often when the caretaker is asleep (4)], and the incidence peaks between the second and fourth month of life (5). According to epidemiological studies, SIDS victims are more likely to be premature, low birth weight, and born to young mothers or into crowded conditions. The incidence of SIDS is two to three times higher in the African American (1) and Native American populations.

Because the characteristics of the vast majority of SIDS victims are ubiquitous, for example, age less than one year and events occurring during sleep, and because events are rare in mathematical terms, some attempts to recognize SIDS victims prospectively have relied on research, searching for abnormal cardio-respiratory events before death. In England, Southall et al. (6) prospectively performed 24-hour recordings of respiration and heart rate on more than 6000 full-term infants, as well as premature or low birth weight infants before hospital discharge. Twenty-seven of these infants subsequently died from SIDS. Of these victims, 23 had no recognized abnormalities on the recordings. Thus, prospective recordings of heart rate and respiration did not identify infants at risk for SIDS. In another attempt to identify future SIDS victims, polygraphic sleep recordings of 30 infants who eventually died of SIDS were compared with normal controls (7). Subtle differences were noted; the infants who died demonstrated fewer body movements during sleep and had more frequent obstructive breathing efforts. Again, there was no way to prospectively identify the infants destined to die. More recently, the CHIME study of infant apnea indicates that apnea and brady-cardia are common in all infants, including healthy term infants of normal birth weight, supporting the notion that identification of future SIDS infants is not likely with cardiorespiratory monitoring (8).

In the mid 1980s, the low rate of SIDS in Hong Kong and certain Asian countries was noted. Speculations on the reasons for this low rate included environmental and social differences. Then, between 1987 and 1990, an associ-ation between SIDS and the prone (face down) sleeping position was discovered in the New Zealand Cot Death Study. This was a nationwide case-controlled study comparing 485 SIDS cases with 1800 controls (9). Other modifiable risk factors noted in the study were exposure to cigarette smoke, bottle-feeding, and excess thermal insulation. Enormous prevention campaigns were initiated in New Zealand, Austria, Finland, and the Netherlands, followed by campaigns in the U.K. These campaigns promoted the safe supine sleeping position, breast-feeding, education on parental smoking, and avoidance of over-bundling of the infant. Since 1990, a decline of more than 60% in the SIDS rate was reported in New Zealand (10), with similar results across Europe (11,12), even in areas with previously low SIDS rates (13). In 1992, on the basis of evidence accumu-lated from several studies performed worldwide, the American Academy of Pediatrics issued recommendations against prone positioning of infants. The concept was not initially received with enthusiasm in the U.S.A., and the more publicized "Back-to-Sleep" campaign was finally initiated in 1994, when the evidence from around the world about the safety of sleeping supine was very convincing. The Back-to-Sleep campaign promoted the supine position for sleep, as well as modification of other risk factors such as over-bundling of the infant and exposure to smoking. Now, since 1994, the SIDS rate in U.S.A. has dropped by about 50%.

Although risk factors for SIDS are recognized (Table 1), the underlying mechanism is still not understood. Infants with SIDS and infants dying unexpect-edly of known causes such as congenital abnormalities have been shown to share many of the same risk factors (14). These include low maternal age, race, early gestational age, and low birth weight. Additionally, environmental

Table 1 Risk Factors Associated with Sudden Infant Death
Syndrome

Premature birth	Cigarette smoke exposure
Low birth weight	Over-bundling
Young maternal age	Sleep in prone position
High maternal parity	Sleep on soft bedding or sofa
African-American race	Unemployment
Recent infection	Some co-sleep situations
Congenital abnormalities	Crowded conditions

situations increase unexpected deaths in infants, specifically sleep position, body temperature, cigarette smoke exposure, and socioeconomic factors such as unemployment (14).

Studies show that the prone position during infancy may contribute to decreased arousal from sleep (15–17). Indeed, many mothers report that their babies sleep better on their stomach, but arousal from sleep is decreased which could be potentially dangerous (18). The prone position causes decreased arousal to hypoxia and hypercapnia (19,20), and may cause re-breathing of exhaled gases (21), or changes in autonomic function and heart rate (5,22). There are decreased cough and swallow reflexes in the prone position (23). The prone position also has been shown to cause collapse of the pharynx in infants (24). In a large population study across the U.K., most recent evidence demonstrates that premature infants placed in the prone position have 80 times the risk of SIDS compared with controls, and side sleeping was found to have an increased risk for SIDS as well (25). These findings demonstrate that the combination of two risk factors can be more than additive, but also that there may be an environmental factor contributing to the increased incidence of SIDS in preterm infants or infants of low birth weight.

Overheating due to clothing, blankets, and ambient room temperature [often in association with soft bedding or the prone position (9,26)] is associated with increased infant death. In a large population in England, infants who died of SIDS were likely to be heavily bundled in quilts or over-wrapped with their heads covered. More than half the SIDS infants had slipped down underneath the covers (12). Franco et al. (27) have shown differences in heart rate, autonomic balance, and thermoregulation associated with head covering in sleeping infants.

Prenatal smoke exposure has been linked to a two-fold risk increase in SIDS, and a causal relationship is suggested (28). The mechanism for this relationship is not known. Infants dying of SIDS have been shown to have increased concentrations of nicotine, even when smoke exposure was denied, indicating a problem with parental reports at the time of death (29). There is an increased incidence of obstructive apnea and low birth weight in infants exposed to prenatal cigarette smoke (30). Arousal from sleep has been demonstrated to be affected by cigarette smoke (31–33). Smoke may alter the body's inflammatory response to viral illnesses (34,35). Actual physical differences in brain development, specifically of the serotinergic neurons of the brainstem, have been noted in infants who died of SIDS compared with controls, and this finding was increased in the face of prenatal smoke exposure (36). Although the majority of the research on smoke and SIDS focusses on prenatal exposure, there is evidence that postnatal environmental smoke may also contribute to increased risk (37,38), and there appears to be a dose–response increased risk with increasing postnatal exposure (39). Considered a modifiable risk factor, the danger of smoking and SIDS should be discussed with both parents of newborn infants. Infants should remain in a smoke-free zone.

Infants sleeping on surfaces not designed for them, such as couches or sofas, have an enormous (more than 50 times) increased risk for death (12). Factors implicated in infant sleep-related accidents (often in association with the prone position) have included placing infants on soft bedding such as water beds, adult beds with thick quilts, bean-bag pillows, or sheepskin rugs with a speculated disruption of airflow at the nose (10,19,21,40). Infants co-sleeping with others in the same bed are at increased risk if the parents drink, smoke, or take drugs, if the child is less than 14 weeks old, if the child is covered with adult quilts, and if there are multiple people in the bed (25,41,42). Infants sleeping in a separate room from the parents were at much higher risk of death than infants in the same room as found in a large population study in England (41), and the new AAP guidelines suggesting that infants sleep in their own bed in the parent's room reflect that. Likewise, pacifier use has been linked to protection from SIDS in multiple studies (43), perhaps by lowering the arousal threshold (44), and is also suggested by AAP guidelines in bottle-fed infants, or after breastfeeding is well established (45).

Although several metabolic (46) and anatomic (47) abnormalities with a possibility of genetic linkage have caused sudden infant death, a unifying "SIDS gene" has not been found (48). In contrast, given the evidence that many SIDS victims may indeed have demonstrable alterations of autonomic nervous system neurotransmitters (49,50), brain development (51), and cardiac abnormalities (52), a genetic link to infant death remains a question to be answered (53). There is no evidence that SIDS is genetically determined in the majority of families, although there is increased risk of SIDS in survivors of twins and in infants with two or more preceding siblings who died from SIDS. These old statistics do not take into account the obvious question of whether modifiable risk factors such as sleep position and smoke exposure are repeated in siblings of SIDS victims. Several families have been reported with three or more SIDS deaths, and in these circumstances, concern is raised about possible intentional suffocation by a caregiver. Healthcare workers have been shown to be severely handicapped in the ability to recognize this possibility (54). If child abuse is suspected, health providers are legally bound to report it.

Because adults and children do not die of SIDS, the mechanism of infant death may relate in some way to an immature central nervous system (55). Certainly, the immature nervous system has been associated with physiologic reflexes that can cause profound apnea and bradycardia in infants (56). The vagus nerve plays a major role in respiratory activity, and delayed maturation of the vagus has been implicated in SIDS cases (57). One could speculate that an infant sleeping prone, with an immature autonomic nervous system, in the face of decreased arousal would be a "set-up" for stress, hypoxia, cardiac arrhythmia, or SIDS. The evidence points to a relationship between immaturity, the prone position, sleep, smoke, and SIDS (9,10,14).

The postmortem pathologic findings of SIDS infants indicate possible increased respiratory effort or illness in many of the victims. Hyperplasia of brainstem astroglia and smooth muscle in the pulmonary arteries, mild inflammation of the respiratory tract, and intrathoracic petechiae have all been noted in a majority of SIDS cases. The first two findings suggest that hypoxia may have occurred before death. Intrathoracic petechiae have been associated with repeated obstructed breathing attempts (55,58). Evidence of infection and/or inflammation is common in cases (59). In fact, a previous infection was shown to be a dangerously high risk factor for SIDS, and especially alarming was the lack of recognition of the severity of illness in infants before death (14).

In the event of a SIDS death, the families of victims often require outside help to cope with their grief. Guilt and anger are common reactions to infant death, and depression is a possible result. Parent-support groups are now available on the worldwide web, as is information from the National Sudden Infant Death Foundation (http://www.sidscenter.org) or other grief resources (http://www.sids alliance.org). Although future SIDS victims cannot yet be predicted, the incidence of death is decreasing due to the modification of identifiable risk factors. The American Academy of Pediatrics has asked healthcare providers to educate parents about the risks associated with SIDS that are modifiable, such as the prone sleeping position, exposure to smoking, and over-bundling. Recent studies also indicate that infants co-sleeping in crowded beds are quite prevalent, an ongoing risk factor present in many low income families (42).

Parent Instructions for Reducing Sudden Infant Death Syndrome Risk (60–62)

1. Infants under six months of age should not leave the hospital or clinic setting without a review of SIDS risk factors. Babies should be placed on their backs to sleep with no head covering, very light covering (requires demonstration) with low room temperatures, and should not be exposed at all to smoke.

2. Feet-to-Foot: infants should lie at the foot of the bed on their back so that they cannot roll or crawl underneath the covers. Covers should be tucked in so the infants cannot pull the cover over their head. Head covering is a high risk. Tuck covers in at the sides so infant cannot roll.

3. Pillows increase risk. Infants should lie on a mattress designed for infant sleep.
4. Premature infants sleeping prone have 80 times the risk of SIDS. Many infants in hospital nurseries are still sleeping prone prior to discharge. Special counseling should be stressed for parents of premature infants and also for hospital healthcare workers who require education on changing old habits for premature infants.
5. Infants should live and sleep in a smoke-free zone.
6. Infants co-sleeping with others in the same bed are at increased risk of death if they sleep with parents who drink, smoke, or take drugs to sleep, sleep with multiple people, if they are covered with quilts or comforters, and if they are less than 14 weeks of age.
7. Infants should sleep in the same room with the parents in a safe infant bed or bassinet for the first few months of life.
8. Pacifiers (dummies, comforters) are protective against SIDS and should be used in bottle-fed infants or after breastfeeding is well established for the first year of life.

APPARENT LIFE-THREATENING EVENTS

SIDS is not known to occur in children or adults. Similarly, episodes of apparent life-threatening events (ALTEs), formerly termed "near-miss SIDS" or "aborted crib deaths," are unique to infants. ALTEs are characterized as events that are frightening to the observer and include some combination of obstructive or central apnea, color change (usually cyanosis and/or pallor), a marked change in muscle tone (usually extreme limpness), choking, or gagging. In some cases, the observer fears that the infant has died (4) or would have died without significant intervention. Infants who have experienced an ALTE are at increased risk for SIDS (14), but whether or not these infants would have progressed to death without intervention is not known. Kahn et al. (4) studied 3799 infants suffering from ALTE events and found that unlike children who died, 82% of the ALTE victims were found during the day while the caretaker was awake, and tended to be discovered sooner than those who died. ALTEs may be triggered by various underlying disorders (Table 2), but the response

Table 2 Disorders Frequently Associated with Apparent Life-Threatening Events

Sepsis
Respiratory infection
Gastroesophageal reflux
Hypoxemia
Metabolic disorder
Cardiac disease
Bowel obstruction
Seizure

to the trigger is unique to infants. The ALTE is thought to be in part related to normal autonomic nervous system reflexes that may trigger apnea, bradycardia, or hypotension in infants due to an immature nervous system (56).

Maturational Influence of Cardiorespiratory Risk

Breathing rhythms undergo maturational changes during the first year of life. In utero the fetus makes intermittent breathing movements necessary for lung development during active REM sleep (63). After birth, the respiratory system can be described as immature in the neonate, and only after several months will breathing patterns mature to adult patterns of respiration. For example, the neonate can demonstrate long periods of periodic breathing (63). Periodic breathing is commonly defined as an episode of three or more respiratory pauses of three seconds or greater with intervening periods of normal respiration of <20 seconds (64). Although associated with immaturity, periodic breathing is not in itself considered a pathologic form of apnea, and does not appear to be related to the development of severe apnea in infancy. However, periodic breathing is increased in some abnormal conditions such as hyperthermia, hypoxia, high altitude, premature birth, and viral illness (65,66). The mechanism for periodic breathing seems to be multifactorial, but immaturity of the central nervous system is postulated to be involved because the incidence diminishes with age.

There is an increased risk for obstructive apnea during REM sleep in infants due to the atonia of that sleep state. Atonia of pharyngeal muscles that would normally keep the airway patent results in an obstructed airflow and an increased effort of inspiration. Additionally, in REM sleep, there is a loss in FRC, the volume of the lung at end expiration, due to decreased chest muscle tone. Because oxygen saturation is in part dependent on oxygen reserves during FRC, low lung volume results in a drop in oxygen saturation during REM sleep, especially in premature infants with reduced pulmonary reserve. Short apneas may cause more pronounced decreases in oxygen saturation in infants with decreased pulmonary reserve.

Unlike adults, the neonate spends about 50% of its entire 16 to 18 hours of sleep time in REM sleep. It is at this time when periodic breathing, added to other factors mentioned above, can start to tip the balance toward sleep-disordered breathing unique to infants. Note that REM sleep is termed "active" sleep in infants. This term seems counterintuitive because REM sleep in adults is associated with atonia and a lack of body movement. In infants, however, not only are heart rate and breathing rate variable in REM sleep, but also the infant demonstrates intermittent body movements including jerks, kicks, smiles, grimaces, and sucks. These REM-related movements, now considered forms of subcortical arousal, decrease with maturation but may be protective for the infant, where arousal to stimuli such as hypoxemia, even an FiO_2 as low as 11% (67,68) is decreased compared with adults. This age-related susceptibility to hypoxemia without arousal may be one risk factor for sudden death in infants.

Immaturity of the autonomic nervous system can play a role in other infant-related risk factors for sleep and breathing disorders. There is an age-related risk for apnea, bradycardia, and cardiorespiratory instability in infants secondary to stimulation of the vagal sensory nerve endings in the pharynx or esophagus (56,69–75). The vagus nerve is responsible for transmitting afferent sensory information from the nasopharynx, esophagus, intestine, and lung and for delivering efferent motor responses to the same area. The vagus also innervates the aortic and carotid bodies which influence blood pressure or respond to hypoxemia and hypercapnia. Stimulation of the sensory limb of the vagus nerve (as may happen, for example, with severe vomiting or gastroesophageal reflux) may cause cardiovascular responses in infants, which are decreased with maturation. As noted in both animal and human studies, stimulation of the infant pharynx or esophagus with water, milk, acid, or even a suction catheter can cause profound autonomic changes (70–72) including apnea and bradycardia. An important study (73) confirmed the age-related susceptibility to apnea with distal esophageal stimulation in dogs. Puppies less than six weeks old and adult dogs had little or no response to acid stimulation of the esophagus, whereas puppies aged 8 to 19 weeks responded with profound changes in heart rate, respiratory rate, blood pressure, and a sustained obstructive breathing pattern with audible stridor. Interestingly, this age group corresponded to the human age group most at risk for sudden infant death. Studies have also demonstrated a more profound apnea when the vagus nerve was stimulated when the infant was sleeping, sedated, or in the prone position (on their stomach) (23,76,77). Thus, autonomic immaturity likely plays a part in sudden infant death, in part explaining why the youngest infants are at particular risk, especially during sleep.

Medical Evaluation of Apparent Life-Threatening Events

Because many underlying conditions may result in an ALTE in a young infant, each event deserves a careful but individual evaluation (Table 3). The physician should do a thorough medical history and physical examination, and almost all

Table 3 Evaluations Considered in an Infant with
Apparent Life-Threatening Event

Blood cultures
Arterial blood gas
Respiratory viral, pertussis, and chlamydia cultures
Upper GI series for anatomy, reflux, and swallow evaluation
Abdominal films
Chest X-ray for anatomy and signs of infection
Electroencephalogram
Electrocardiogram
Polysomnogram
Serum electrolytes, blood counts, liver and kidney panels

---

cases of ALTE warrant some laboratory and/or radiographic assessment. In the febrile infant with an ALTE, especially infants experiencing a change in behavior or feeding, a sepsis work-up should be considered. In the infant who demonstrated tonic/clonic or repetitive movements during the episode, an evaluation for seizure is warranted. Infants with significant central or obstructive apnea, periodic breathing, tachypnea, or CO_2 retention are often diagnosed using sleep studies, thus, a polysomnogram might be a helpful diagnostic tool in some cases. If the serum pH is low, a preceding severe hypoxic episode with lactic acidosis or a metabolic disturbance should be considered. An electrocardiogram may detect evidence of prolonged QT or cardiac arrhythmia which has been linked to some cases of SIDS (52). The vast majority of infants who have just suffered an ALTE should be hospitalized for further assessment and for monitoring to help detect additional episodes of apnea or bradycardia during their hospitalization. In infants with an ALTE and a history of frequent vomiting or choking when fed, a barium swallow should be included to rule out anatomical causes of the ALTE, such as vascular ring, and to assess the infant's swallowing ability, esophageal function, or the presence of excessive gastroesophageal reflux. Occasionally, a continuous recording of esophageal pH may be helpful to detect significant gastroesophageal reflux, although these tests can underestimate reflux episodes due to increased gastric pH in frequently feeding infants (78). Gastroesophageal reflux is often blamed for playing a causative role in ALTE events; however, it must be noted that reflux events, normal in all humans, may also be increased in infants who are otherwise at risk for cardiorespiratory events, such as premature infants (79) or infants with autonomic disorders (80), and therefore may be true but unrelated to the cardiorespiratory event.

In infants with repeated ALTEs, for which no cause is identified, referral to a pediatric center with special expertise in apnea is indicated. In addition to the work-up listed above, magnetic resonance imaging to assess the anatomy of the brainstem, direct visualization of the airway, or work-up for rare metabolic or autonomic disorders might be indicated. In a few infants, prolonged hospitalization with a 24-hour direct observation is suggested to rule out asphyxia inflicted by the caregiver (Münchausen's syndrome by proxy).

When an underlying condition is identified, specific therapy can be initiated. However, in about half of the cases of ALTE, no underlying disease or condition will be identified (4); these infants are referred to with the term "apnea of infancy." The management of children with apnea of infancy or ALTEs should always include education about the modifiable SIDS risk factors, because altering these has been shown to decrease the risk of SIDS. Occasionally, a center will initiate home electronic monitoring of respiration and heart rate after discharge. The purpose of the home apnea monitor is to provide information about whether infants are having continuing problems with episodes of central apnea or bradycardia. A loud alarm is emitted when the monitor senses cessation of chest wall motion, bradycardia, or tachycardia. The duration of acceptable pauses in respiration (usually 20 seconds), and the low heart rate limit (usually 60–80 beats/min) are specified individually for each infant. This individual set point is important, as some infants have severe hypoxia with short respiratory pauses based on decreased pulmonary reserve, and the therapist should set the alarms according to known clinical information.

Apnea Monitors: Myths and Facts

Home use of apnea monitors was initiated after a study of infant apnea by Steinschneider (81), where five infants suffering from recurrent apnea and cyanosis were sent home with an apnea monitor. The focus at that time, and for years to come, was the "apnea hypothesis," where prolonged apnea was hypothesized to be a cause of SIDS, and that apnea recordings might prospectively identify future SIDS victims, and monitors designed to detect the apneas might save lives. Apnea monitors were designed with the intent to protect infants from death by identifying episodes of breathing cessation or slow heart rate. The hypothesis assumed that if apnea and bradycardia were common in infants with apnea of prematurity, it logically followed that monitors might protect other infants with ALTEs. Unfortunately, there was no controlled study of efficacy of these devices for saving lives before they were unleashed to the public. In fact, two of the five infants in Steinschneider's study died despite home monitoring [many years later, those infants were actually found to have been murdered (54)], yet no red flag was raised as to the need for more study before the devices were made available by homecare companies. The National Institutes of Health Consensus Development Conference on Infantile Apnea and Home Monitoring recommended continuous home monitoring in some cases of infant apnea (82). However, even though home monitoring has escalated in the last 30 years, the incidence of SIDS did not decline with monitor use. Since that time, millions of apnea monitors have been sent to the home, at a cost of millions of dollars, regardless of lack of efficacy for what they were designed to do. Recent epidemiological data demonstrate that, although large numbers of infants who died were monitored, the monitors did not correlate with protection from SIDS (12,14). Finally, 30 years after worldwide use of cardiorespiratory monitoring in infants, the CHIME study indicated that infant apnea events are largely made up of obstructive apneas, which are not detected by home monitors (8). Furthermore, Poets (83) published evidence about the recordable events occurring during ALTEs. Using experimental equipment that included transcutaneous and pulse oximetry monitoring, 65% of events without a known cause were preceded by oxygen saturation abnormalities not picked up by the majority of home monitors. More importantly, monitors are now prescribed by any doctor or healthcare worker and are even available over the Internet. The physician who prescribes the monitor is often not the same person who discontinues use, which impairs the ability to track the use of the monitor, recognize abnormal recordings, take responsibility for outcome measurements, and limit the use of the machine to the time considered necessary. Parents are the ones often left with a monitor that alarms frequently, without a physician taking responsibility for oversight. Monitors have been used for reasons well beyond apnea of prematurity, where they have efficacy due to the type of apnea (central) being recorded. They are now anecdotally used for episodes of cyanosis, feeding and swallowing disorders, seizures, and obstructive apnea or lung disease. Even the most recent American Academy of Pediatrics Policy Statement (2002) recommends the use of apnea monitors for infants with oxygen requirements or tracheostomy tubes (84). These findings demonstrate a lack of understanding of device efficacy, device design, mechanism of disease, or a broader fear of liability. As mentioned earlier, most apnea monitors available to the public do not detect obstructive or struggled breathing efforts or oxygen saturation abnormalities. Therefore, if an infant with a tracheostomy tube in place for a subglottic stenosis becomes decannulated, the primary events will be obstructed breathing efforts and hypoxemia. Cardiorespiratory monitors would not be helpful in that case. The prescribing physician should (*i*) be aware of whether the device prescribed is designed to protect the infant in each individual case. (*ii*) The prescribing physician should be the one who follows the child during the use of the monitor, to collect data and determine length of use. (*iii*) Home apnea monitors are not treatment, nor are they diagnostic tools. Multiple alarms or abnormal downloads demonstrate the need for a diagnosis. The decision to eventually discontinue home monitoring is therefore based on clinical criteria. It is reasonable to stop monitoring when there have been two or three months free of serious events, but monitoring for as short as two weeks or less is appropriate in many cases, such as the premature infant reaching 45 weeks of postconceptual age where apnea is not more likely than in the full-term infant (8). Education of the parents about risk factors that can be modified is the one intervention that has been shown to be effective against sudden unexpected infant deaths. Caregivers sent home with a monitor must be trained in infant cardiopulmonary resistability (CPR) and must understand that cardiorespiratory monitoring does not guarantee survival. Apnea monitors do not protect infants sleeping in unsafe sleep environments such as exposure to smoke, prone positioning, and overwrapping.

REFERENCES

1. Mathews TJ, Menacker F, MacDorman MF. Infant mortality statistics from the 2001 period linked birth/infant death data set. Natl Vital Stat Rep 2003; 52:1–28.
2. Willinger M, James LS, Catz C. Defining the sudden infant death syndrome (SIDS): deliberations of an expert panel convened by the national institute of child health and human development. Pediatr Pathol 1991; 11:677–684.
3. MMWR. Sudden Infant Death Syndrome-United States, 1983–1994. MMWR 96 A.D.; 45:859–863.
4. Kahn A, Groswasser J, Sottiaux M, et al. Clinical problems in relation to apparent-life-threatening-events in infants. Acta Pediatr 1993; 82(suppl 389):107–110.
5. Harper RM, Bandler R. Finding the failure mechanism in sudden infant death syndrome. Nat Med 1998; 4:157–158.

6. Southall DP et al. Prospective Population Based Studies into Heart Rate and Breathing Patterns in Newborn Infants: Prediction of Infants at Risk of SIDS? In: Tilden JR, Roeder LM, Steinschneider A, eds. Sudden Infant Death Syndrome. Proceedings of the 1982 International Research Conference. Baltimode: Academic Press, 1983.

7. Kahn A, Groswasser J, Rebuffat E, et al. Sleep and cardiorespiratory characteristics of infant victims of sudden death: A prospective case-control study. Sleep 1992; 15:287–292.

8. Ramanathan R, Corwin MJ, Hunt CE, et al. Cardiorespiratory events recorded on home monitors: comparison of healthy infants with those at increased risk for SIDS. JAMA 2001; 285:2199–2207.

9. Mitchell EA, Taylor BJ, Ford RPK, et al. Four modifiable and other major risk factors for cot death: The New Zealand Study. J Paediatr Child Health 1992; 28:S3–S8.

10. Mitchell EA. The changing epidemiology of SIDS following the National Risk Reduction Campaigns. Pediatr Pulmonol 1997; 82(suppl 16):117–119.

11. Willinger M. SIDS Prevention. Pediatr Ann 1995; 24:358–364.

12. Leach CE, Blair PS, Fleming PJ, et al. Epidemiology of SIDS and explained sudden infant deaths. CESDI SUDI Research Group. Pediatrics 1999; 104:e43.

13. Wennergren G, Alm B, Oyen N, et al. The decline in the Incidence of SIDS in Scandinavia and its relation to risk-intervention campaigns. Nordic Epidemiological SIDS Study. Acta Paediatr 1997; 86:963–968.

14. Platt MW, Blair PS, Fleming PJ, et al. A clinical comparison of SIDS and explained sudden infant deaths: how healthy and how normal? CESDI SUDI Research Group. Confidential Inquiry into Stillbirths and Deaths in Infancy study. Arch Dis Child 2000; 82:98–106.

15. Franco P, Pardou A, Hassid S, Lurquin P, Groswasser J, Kahn A. Auditory arousal thresholds are higher when infants sleep in the prone position. J Pediatr 1998; 132:240–243.

16. Sawaguchi T, Franco P, Kato I, et al. From physiology to pathology: arousal deficiency theory in sudden infant death syndrome (SIDS)—with reference to apoptosis and neuronal plasticity. Forensic Sci Int 2002; 130:S37–S43.

17. Sawaguchi T, Franco P, Groswasser J, Kahn A. Relationship between arousal reaction and autonomic nervous system in the sudden infant death syndrome. Am J Forensic Med Pathol 2001; 22:213–214.

18. Horne RS, Franco P, Adamson TM, Groswasser J, Kahn A. Effects of body position on sleep and arousal characteristics in infants. Early Hum Dev 2002; 69:25–33.

19. Thach BT. How Does prone sleeping increase prevalence of sudden infant death syndrome. Pediatr Pulmonol 1997; 82(suppl 16):115–116.

20. Kahn A, Groswasser J, Sottiaux M, et al. Prone or supine body position and sleep characteristics in infants. Pediatrics 1993; 91:1112–1115.

21. Kemp JS, Livne M, White DK, et al. Softness and potential to cause rebreathing: differences in bedding used by infants at high and low risk for sudden infant death syndrome. J Pediatr 1998; 132:234–239.

22. Amemiya F, Vos JE, Prechtl HFr. Effects of prone and supine position on heart rate, respiratory rate and motor activity in fullterm newborn infants. Brain Dev 1991; 13:148–154.

23. Thach BT. Maturation and transformation of reflexes that protect the laryngeal airway from liquid aspiration from fetal to adult life. Am J Med 2001; 111:69–77.

24. Ishikawa T, Isono S, Aiba J, Tanaka A, Nishino T. Prone position increases collapsibility of the passive pharynx in infants and small children. Am J Respir Crit Care Med 2002; 166:760–764.

25. Blair P, Ward Platt MP, Smith IJ, Fleming PJ. Sudden infant death syndrome and sleeping position in pre-term and low birthweight infants: an opportunity for targeted intervention. Arch Dis Child 2005

26. Stanton AN. Overheating and cot death. Lancet 1984; 2:1199.

27. Franco P, Lipshutz W, Valente F, Adams S, Scaillet S, Kahn A. Decreased arousals in infants who sleep with the face covered by bedclothes. Pediatrics 2002; 109:1112–1117.

28. Anderson HR, Cook DG. Passive smoking and sudden infant death syndrome: review of the epidemiological evidence. Thorax 1997; 52:1003–1009.

29. McMartin KI, Platt MS, Hackman R, et al. Lung tissue concentrations of nicotine in sudden infant death syndrome. J Pediatr 2002; 140:205–209.

30. Kahn A, Groswasser J, Sottiaux M, et al. Prenatal exposure to cigarettes in infants with obstructive sleep apneas. Pediatrics 1994; 93:778–783.

31. Horne RS, Franco P, Adamson TM, Groswasser J, Kahn A. Influences of maternal cigarette smoking on infant arousability. Early Hum Dev 2004; 79:49–58.

32. Lewis KW, Bosque EM. Deficient hypoxia awakening response in infants of smoking mothers: possible relationship to sudden infant death syndrome. J Pediatr 1995; 127:691–699.

33. Chang AB, Wilson SJ, Masters IB, et al. Altered arousal response in infants exposed to cigarette smoke. Arch Dis Child 2003; 88:30–33.

34. Raza MW, Essery SD, Elton RA, Weir DM, Busuttil A, Blackwell C. Exposure to cigarette smoke, a major risk factor for sudden infant death syndrome: effects of cigarette smoke on inflammatory responses to viral infection and bacterial toxins. FEMS Immunol Med Microbiol 1999; 25:145–154.

35. Gordon AE, EI Ahmer OR, Chan R, et al. Why is smoking a risk factor for sudden infant death syndrome? Child Care Health Dev 2002; 28(suppl 1):23–25.

36. Kinney HC, Randall LL, Sleeper LA, et al. Serotonergic brainstem abnormalities in Northern Plains Indians with the sudden infant death syndrome. J Neuropathol Exp Neurol 2003; 62:1178–1191.

37. Machaalani R, Waters KA, Tinworth KD. Effects of postnatal nicotine exposure on apoptotic markers in the developing piglet brain. Neuroscience 2005; 132:325–333.

38. Rushton L, Courage C, Green E. Estimation of the impact on children's health of environmental tobacco smoke in England and Wales. J R Soc Health 2003; 123:175–180.

39. Blair PS, Fleming PJ, Bensley D, et al. Smoking and the sudden infant death syndrome: results from 1993–5 case-control study for confidential inquiry into stillbirths and deaths in infancy. Confidential Enquiry into Stillbirths and Deaths Regional Coordinators and Researchers. BMJ 1996; 313:195–198.

40. Gilbert-Barness E, Barness LA. Cause of Death: SIDS or Something Else? Contemp Pediatr 1992; 9:13.

41. Blair PS, Fleming PJ, Smith IJ, et al. Babies sleeping with parents: case-controlstudy of factors influencing the risk of the sudden infant death syndrome. CESDI SUDI Research Group. BMJ 1999; 319:1457–1461.

42. Hauck FR, Herman SM, Donovan M, et al. Sleep environment and the risk of sudden infant death syndrome in an urban population: The Chicago Infant Mortality Study. Pediatrics 2003; 111:1207–1214.
43. Hauck FR, Omojokun OO, Siadaty MS. Do Pacifiers reduce the risk of sudden infant death syndrome? a meta-analysis. Pediatrics 2005.
44. Franco P, Chabanski S, Scaillet S, Groswasser J, Kahn A. Pacifier use modifies infant's cardiac autonomic controls during sleep. Early Hum Dev 2004; 77:99–108.
45. The Changing Concept of Sudden Infant Death Syndrome: Diagnostic Coding Shifts, Controversies Regarding the Sleeping Environment, and New Variables to Consider in Reducing Risk. Pediatrics 2005.
46. Forsyth L, Hume R, Howatson A, Busuttil A, Burchell A. Identification of novel polymorphisms in the glucokinase and glucose-6-phosphatase genes in infants who died suddenly and unexpectedly. J Mol Med 2005; 83:610–618.
47. Obonai T, Yasuhara M, Nakamura T, Takashima S. Catecholamine neurons alteration in the brainstem of sudden infant death syndrome victims. Pediatrics 1998; 101:285–288.
48. Opdal SH, Rognum TO. The sudden infant death syndrome gene: does it exist? Pediatrics 2004; 114:e506–e512.
49. Weese-Mayer DE, Berry-Kravis EM, Maher BS, Silvestri JM, Curran ME, Marazita ML. Sudden infant death syndrome: association with a promoter polymorphism of the serotonin transporter gene. Am J Med Genet A 2003; 117:268–274.
50. Kinney HC, Filiano JJ, White WF. Medullary serotonergic network deficiency in the sudden infant death syndrome: review of a 15-year study of a single dataset. J Neuropathol Exp Neurol 2001; 60:228–247.
51. Lavezzi AM, Ottaviani G, Matturri L. Adverse effects of prenatal tobacco smoke exposure on biological parameters of the developing brainstem. Neurobiol Dis 2005.
52. Schwartz PJ, Stramba-Badiale M, Segantini A, et al. Prolongation of the QT interval and the sudden infant death syndrome. N Engl J Med 1998; 338:1709–1714.
53. Hunt CE. Gene-environment interactions: implications for sudden unexpected deaths in infancy. Arch Dis Child 2005; 90:48–53.
54. Firstman R, Talan J. The Death of Innocents. New York: Bantom Books, 1997:632.
55. Rambaud C. Pathology of SIDS and new understandings. Pediatr Pulmonol 1997; 82(suppl 16):120–122.
56. Halbower AC, Jones MD, Jr. Physiologic reflexes and their impact on resuscitation of the newborn. Clin Perinatol 1999; 26:621–627.
57. Becker LE, Zhang W. Vagal nerve complex in normal development and sudden infant death syndrome. Can J Neurol Sci 1996; 23:24–33.
58. Richardson MA, Adams J. Fatal apnea in piglets by way of laryngeal chemoreflex: postmortem findings as anatomic correlates of sudden infant death syndrome in the human infant. Laryngoscope 2005; 115:1163–1169.
59. Alexander RT, Radisch D. Sudden infant death syndrome risk factors with regards to sleep position, sleep surface, and co-sleeping. J Forensic Sci 2005; 50:147–151.
60. http://www.cdc.gov/reproductivehealth/SIDS/sleep_recommend.htm.
61. http://www.cps.ca/english/statements/CP/cp04-02.htm.
62. http://www.keepkidshealthy.com/welcome/safety/back._to_sleep.html
63. Rigatto H. Maturation of breathing. Clin Perinatol 1992; 19:739–756.
64. Glotzbach SF, et al. Periodic breathing in preterm infants: incidence and characteristics. Pediatrics 1989; 84:785–792.

65. Glotzbach SF, Ariagno RL. Periodic breathing. In: Beckerman RC, Brouillette RT, Hunt CE, eds. Respiratory Control Disorders in Infants and Children. Baltimore: Williams & Wilkins, 1992:142–160.

66. Gaultier CL. Apnea and sleep state in newborns and infants. Biol Neonate 1994; 65:231–234.

67. Davidson Ward S, Keens TG. Ventilatory and arousal responses. In: Beckerman RC, Brouillette RT, Hunt CE, eds. Respiratory Control Disorders in Infants and Children. 1st ed. Baltimore: Williams & Wilkins, 1992:112–124.

68. Davidson Ward SL, Bautista DB, Keens TG. Hypoxic arousal responses in normal infants. Am Rev Respir Dis 1990; 141:A908.

69. Perkett EA, Vaughan RL. Evidence for a laryngeal chemoreflex in some human preterm infants. Acta Paediatr Scand 1982; 71:969–972.

70. Davies AM, Koenig JS, Thach BT. Upper airway chemoreflex responses to saline and water in preterm infants. J Appl Physiol 1988; 64:1412–1420.

71. Pickens DL, Schefft G, Thach BT. Prolonged apnea associated with upper airway protective reflexes in apnea of prematuriy. Am Rev Respir Dis 1988; 137:113–118.

72. Lee JC, Stoll BJ, Downing SE. Properties of the laryngeal chemoreflex in neonatal piglets. Am J Physiol 1977; 233:R30–R36.

73. Bauman NM, Sandler AD, Schmidt C, et al. Reflex laryngospasm induced by stimulation of distal esophageal afferents. Laryngoscope 1994; 104:209–214.

74. Downing SE, Lee JC. Laryngeal chemosensitivity: a possible mechanism for sudden infant death. Pediatrics 1975; 55:640–649.

75. Rimell F, Goding GS, Johnson K. Cholinergic agents in the laryngeal chemoreflex model of sudden infant death syndrome. Laryngoscope 1993; 103:623–630.

76. Davies AM, Koenig JS, Thach BT. Characteristics of upper airway chemoreflex prolonged apnea in human infants. Am Rev Respir Dis 1989;139:668–673.

77. Jacobi MS, Gershan WM, Thach BT. Effect of pentobarbital on spontaneous-recovery from hypoxic apnea in mice. Respir Physiol 1991; 84:337–349.

78. Orenstein SR. Controversies in pediatric gastroesophageal reflux. J Pediatr Gastroenterol Nutr 1992; 14:338–348.

79. Poets CF. Gastroesophageal reflux: a critical review of its role in preterm infants. Pediatrics 2004; 113:e128–e132.

80. Manabe N, Haruma K, Hata J, Nakamura K, Tanaka S, Chayama K. Autonomic nerve dysfunction is closely associated with the abnormalities of esophageal motility in reflux esophagitis. Scand J Gastroenterol 2003; 38:159–163.

81. Steinschneider A. Prolonged apnea and sudden infant death syndrome—clinical and laboratory observations. Pediatrics 1972; 50:646.

82. National Institutes of Health Consensus Development Conference on Infantile Apnea and Home Monitoring, Sept 29 to Oct 1, 1986. Pediatrics 1987; 79:292–299.

83. Poets CF. Apparent life-threatening events and sudden infant death on a monitor. Paediatr Respir Rev 2004; 5(suppl A):S383–S386.

84. Apnea, sudden infant death syndrome, and home monitoring. Pediatrics 2003; 111:914–917.

18

Adolescent Sleepiness

Karen E. Murtagh

The Center for Sleep and Wake Disorders, Chevy Chase, Maryland, U.S.A.

Helene A. Emsellem

The Center for Sleep and Wake Disorders, Chevy Chase, Maryland, and George Washington School of Medicine, Washington, D.C., U.S.A.

CHAPTER HIGHLIGHTS

- Daytime sleepiness affects more than 50% of teenagers in the United States.
- Sleepiness is the most obvious manifestation of insufficient sleep.
- The consequences of insufficient sleep include poor academic performance, mood disorders, increased use of alcohol and stimulants such as caffeine and nicotine, increased risk-taking behaviors and risk of injury, as well as alterations in immune, endocrine, and metabolic function.
- The basic concept that governs the timing of sleep and wakefulness is determined by the two-process model. The two-process model of sleep regulation addresses the circadian day-night influences on sleep and wakefulness (Process C) and the concept of a homeostatic sleep drive (Process S).
- Developmental changes that occur in puberty with regard to sleep need and circadian pattern make it more likely for teenagers to sleep later into the morning. Subsequently, early school start times for secondary schools seem counterintuitive and counterproductive.
- Short sleep duration has been associated with increased hunger and increased risk of obesity in children.

OVERVIEW OF THE PROBLEM

Daytime sleepiness is an important issue in adolescent health, regularly affecting more than 50% of teenagers in the United States (1). Sleepiness can be a manifestation of a primary disorder of alertness such as narcolepsy, but more commonly occurs as a consequence of insufficient sleep, unrecognized by 90% of parents, with the majority of teens obtaining less than the 8.5 to 9.25 hours of sleep they need (1). The tendency toward obtaining an inadequate amount of sleep during adolescence has been well documented in the United States, as well as other developed countries (2–5).

Sleepiness is the most obvious manifestation of insufficient sleep and can be seen after even one night of partial sleep restriction. Sleepiness results in an increased risk of accidental injury, decreased focus and concentration, lapses in attention, decreased reaction time and memory, and even falling asleep during class. Insufficient sleep has been associated with lower school grades, increased daytime sleepiness, depressed mood, and a complaint of sleep or alertness difficulties (2,3,6). Teens report having difficulty waking up in the morning (5), an increased stress level, and they are more likely to smoke, use alcohol (7), and engage in risk-taking behaviors (8) when there is insufficient sleep.

A delay in circadian sleep phase is often the cause of insufficient adolescent sleep, although other primary or secondary sleep disorders should also be considered. Many of the primary sleep disorders contributing to sleep disruption and consequent sleepiness are covered elsewhere in this text and will not be reviewed here. This chapter will focus primarily on the delayed sleep-phase syndrome (DSPS) of adolescence, the factors that serve to promote and perpetuate it, treatment options, the consequences of insufficient sleep in this age group, and other diagnoses to consider.

DEVELOPMENTAL ASPECTS OF ADOLESCENT SLEEP AND SLEEPINESS

There are basic changes in sleep physiology that begin with the onset of puberty and evolve through adolescence, creating a unique pattern of sleep and wakefulness during the teenage years (2,9,10). These physiological changes result in the timing of optimal teen alertness being out of synchrony with that of younger siblings, parents, and the school schedule. In order to appreciate the changes in sleep and alertness during puberty, it is first necessary to understand the basic concepts that govern the timing of sleep and wakefulness. The two-process model of sleep regulation (11) addresses the circadian day-night influences on sleep and wakefulness (Process C) and the concept of a homeostatic sleep drive (Process S).

During the course of the day, there is a building sleep drive, or sleep debt, with increasing hours of alertness. The neurochemical underpinnings of this drive have not been defined; it is unclear whether there is a buildup of a compound that reaches critical levels and causes sleep, or whether an alerting compound is being depleted. The building sleep debt is offset by the alerting influence of the suprachiasmatic nucleus (SCN) of the hypothalamus, and therefore is not manifested as a progressive increase in sleepiness during the day. During the daylight hours, the retino-hypothalamic pathway is responsible for providing light cues to the SCN, a region presently thought of as our internal body clock. As long as the SCN is firing, we are able to maintain alertness. In the late afternoon, typically five to six hours prior to sleep initiation, the onset of melatonin secretion, termed the dim light melatonin onset (DLMO) occurs. Melatonin gradually suppresses the activity of the SCN, allowing for the manifestation of the building sleep debt and the onset of sleep. During sleep, the SCN is suppressed as melatonin secretion peaks and the sleep debt is satisfied. Toward the morning hours, melatonin secretion diminishes, the sun rises, and the activity of the SCN again reinforces alertness. Superimposed on this pattern is a basic circadian variation in daytime alertness with a dip in alertness in the late afternoon, typically between 2 p.m. and 5 p.m. at "siesta time."

This system operates in a similar fashion in children and adults, with a longer total sleep requirement in children than adults. With the onset of puberty, closely linked to the Tanner stages of development, there are basic changes in the system (10). First, there is a slowing of the rate of accumulation of sleepiness/sleep debt. Thus, an adolescent may feel alert later into the evening and teens may find it effortless to stay up later than they should, making it difficult to get sufficient sleep before their necessary weekday wake-up time. Secondly, adolescents are thought to have a longer internal day compared to adults. This, too, works to keep adolescents awake later in the evening. Lastly, there is a shift in the DLMO to a later clock time (12), delaying the onset of melatonin secretion and suppression of the alerting influence of the SCN. Together, these factors leave teens with a later onset of alertness in the morning and persistence of alertness later in the evening and night. This basic physiology puts teens at odds with their school start times and daily expectations, resulting in what some believe is an epidemic of teen sleepiness.

ADOLESCENT DELAYED SLEEP-PHASE SYNDROME

All of the physiological factors mentioned above contribute to the development of a DSPS, experienced to varying extents by the majority of adolescents. The concept of a DSPS is perhaps most easily illustrated by tracking typical teens in the fall as they transition from the freedom of a summer sleep schedule to the school year. At the end of the summer, the teens may be falling asleep between 11:30 p.m. and midnight, if not later, and sleeping the necessary 9.25 hours per night, having a wake-up time shortly after 8:30 a.m. Once school starts, students are required to wake up at 6:30 a.m., given early high school start times, and then sleep a maximum of seven hours per night. By Friday night, the accumulated sleep debt is at least 10 hours. Over the weekend, the sleep onset time may be later, because of social activity, and there is catch-up sleep late into the morning, with a total sleep time that may be extended up to 10 to 12 hours. Even if teens make up three hours of the sleep debt on each weekend night, they may still start the school week on Monday morning four hours sleep-deprived. By the end of the second week of school, the sleep debt may be as much as 14 hours, and a nonrelenting pattern of increasing sleep debt and daytime sleepiness ensues as the school year progresses.

Sleeping in late on weekend mornings helps to make up for some of the weekday-sleep restriction, but is not without repercussions. As the homeostatic sleep drive begins ticking off the hours of alertness and building sleep debt from the time of awakening, the later weekend wake-up time sets the overall internal clock schedule later. This results in alertness lasting later into the evening and even greater difficulty initiating sleep. Napping on weekday afternoons may be unavoidable as the teen becomes increasingly sleep-deprived later into the school year. Afternoon naps may enhance evening alertness, however, and further fuel the delay in sleep phase. This vicious cycle of late bedtimes, insufficient sleep during the school week, afternoon napping, and late weekend sleep-ins perpetuates the delay in sleep phase, leaving teens increasingly out of synchrony with their school schedules.

TREATMENT OF DELAYED SLEEP-PHASE SYNDROME

Managing the sleepiness and altered circadian rhythm of the average adolescent can be extremely challenging. Parents are often at loggerheads with their teens regarding their late bedtime and difficulty awakening in the morning. They may view the behavior as obstinate and defiant, rather than a physiological reality. Educating parents and teens about normal sleep requirements and the changes in sleep timing associated with puberty is a necessary first step in addressing this problem.

Critical to successful management of teen sleep-wake behaviors is limitation and regulation of the weekend wake-up time. This is difficult to accomplish in a sleep-deprived teen, but the later the weekend sleep-in, the harder it will be to fall asleep the next night. Generally, more than a two-hour difference between weekday and weekend wake-up times is discouraged, as it may aggravate an underlying sleep-phase delay.

Teens need to agree to limit their engagement in evening activities and set a reasonable lights-out time, ensuring that enough time is allocated for sleep. A relaxing wind down time in the evening before bed, when there is no longer any computer or phone use or homework being done, should be encouraged. Daily exercise, though not in the evening, and avoidance of caffeine from midafternoon onward should also be encouraged. Organization of homework and chores, and planning of attire for the next day help teens use their time well at night and minimize the amount of time it takes to get up and out in the morning. A mutually agreeable method of awakening the teen in the morning is often needed in order to prevent or minimize the aggressive and hostile interactions that may occur, and which may set a negative tone for the day for parents and teens alike, when the tired teen does not want to get out of bed.

In more severe cases, specific interventions to phase advance the teen's sleep-wake schedule may be required. These may include: strict regulation of the wake-up time on the weekends, as well as during the week; the use of bright light (13) to activate circadian driven alertness earlier in the day; and the use of low dose melatonin. Bright light can be delivered via a commercially available light box or light visor, and provides one of the most potent influences on the timing of the circadian sleep-wake rhythm. It is exposure to light in the morning that effectively "resets" the circadian clock on a daily basis, so that we are in synchrony with a 24-hour day, despite our inherent tendency for a day slightly longer than 24 hours. While light provides a powerful clock-resetting stimulus, it, and the behavioral interventions mentioned, may not be enough to re-entrain the desired sleep-wake pattern. In this case, the addition of melatonin to the treatment regimen may be needed. Low-dose melatonin (0.5–1 mg) is used to reinforce the desired DLMO (14), and is taken approximately six hours prior to sleep onset. It should be mentioned that melatonin is available without prescription but has not been studied extensively from a safety standpoint in adolescents, nor is there a guarantee of potency or purity with any given preparation. Recommendations for its use should be made with this in mind and a clear discussion of this issue with the teen and parent.

Alternatively, the DSPS of adolescence may be treated with chronotherapy (15) over a five-to-seven day period of time (ideal for school breaks) by delaying sleep onset and the morning wake-up time by three hours daily, until the bedtime is aligned with the school schedule. Strict behavioral reinforcement of the desired schedule is then required and light therapy and melatonin may be needed for success.

INFLUENCE OF SCHOOL START TIMES ON SLEEPINESS AND PERFORMANCE

Considering the developmental changes that occur in puberty with regard to sleep need, circadian pattern, and propensity to sleepiness, early school start times for secondary schools seem counterintuitive and counterproductive. An improvement in school performance was observed when school start times were delayed, from either 7:15 a.m. and or 7:25 a.m. to 8:30 a.m., in three school districts in Minnesota as detailed by Wahlstrom, et al. (16). The delay in start time resulted in students obtaining an additional hour of sleep on school nights. Students were more alert, less likely to miss school or be late, and more apt to complete assignments. Improvements in behavior were also noted. An increase in total sleep time when the school start time is delayed has also been noted by others (17,18) and results from sleeping longer in the morning as a consequence of the later school start time, with the time to bed remaining relatively unchanged.

Wolfson and Carskadon (19), in a review of a number of studies examining the relationships between adolescent sleep patterns and school performance, felt that all of the studies reviewed, despite differing methodologies and limitations, suggested that a reduced total sleep time, later weekend-rise times, longer sleep latencies, more erratic sleep schedules, and daytime sleepiness contribute to poor school performance. They also comment on two studies (20,21) that have associated ease of getting going in the morning and being rested with motivation and self-image, both critical in the journey through adolescence.

According to the National Sleep Foundation (22), schools or districts in 19 states have delayed their start times, with an additional 17 states considering doing the same. Congresswoman Zoe Lofgren has introduced resolutions to the House of Representatives, the most recent being House Congressional Resolution 200, in June 2005, expressing that the secondary schools should start after 9:00 a.m. The latest major action on this resolution occurred in July 2005, with referral to the Subcommittee on Education Reform (23). While a number of arguments against changing school start times have been made, for instance, the impact on timing of extracurricular activities, work schedules, transportation costs, darkness at the end of the school day, etc., it is clear from a physiological perspective as well as from a public health perspective that a later start time would provide the opportunity for more sleep and consequently, an improved level of alertness in the adolescent population.

SLEEPY ADOLESCENTS BEHIND THE WHEEL

The risk of motor vehicle accidents is increased in adolescents, and inexperienced driving is undoubtedly contributory. Couple this with sleepiness, and the inattention and decreased reaction time associated with it, and the risk is magnified. Driving to school in the morning when inadequate sleep is obtained, or returning from after school activities when the siesta time occurs, is a recipe for disaster. The effect of sleep deprivation on driving risk has been equated to driving under the influence of alcohol. On a simulated driving test, measuring the parameters of ability to maintain speed and road position, 18.5 hours of wakefulness was equivalent to a blood alcohol level of 0.05% and 21 hours of wakefulness with a 0.08% alcohol level (24).

The teen who experiments with alcohol and who is sleep-deprived can be even more at risk, depending on the amount of alcohol consumed. At legal blood levels (for adults), alcohol, when combined with partial sleep deprivation, has been shown to result in impairment of driving simulator performance, an increased incidence of microsleeps, and a diminution of the ability to assess crash risk (25,26). The danger of even one drink in a sleep-deprived teen, who may not manifest good judgment to begin with, is readily apparent.

According to statistics from the National Highway Traffic Safety Administration, car crashes are the leading cause of death for American teenagers. In 2003, there were 6002 fatalities in drivers aged 16 to 20, and 482,000 injuries.

This age group has the highest fatality rate of all drivers. Two-thirds of the fatalities occurred in males. Being drowsy, asleep, fatigued, ill, or blacking out were factors in 2.7% of all fatal crashes in 2003 though, unfortunately, this data point is not broken down by age group and it is not clear how many teen accidents had sleepiness as a causative factor compared to other age groups (27). In past years, it was estimated that drivers under 25 were responsible for greater than 50% of sleep-related crashes (28). These data, in addition to those presented earlier, are compelling for ensuring our youth be adequately rested to avoid unnecessary deaths and injury.

SLEEPY ADOLESCENTS AT WORK AND PLAY

An estimated 80% of youth work at some point during their high school years. Over 200,000 experience work-related injuries annually and at least 70 die as a result of them, with the risk of injury in a young worker almost twice that of an adult worker (29). It is not known how many of these injuries are attributable to sleepiness, given that sleep problems are not routinely assessed either in primary care (30) or emergent care settings. In one study of patients presenting with injury to an emergency department, it was found that there was a greater likelihood of acute sleep deprivation prior to injury, with 34% of patients at high risk of a sleep problem. It was also noted that inquiry about sleep by health providers in this environment usually did not occur as part of the initial evaluation (31). It is known that part-time work exceeding 20 hours per week is associated with a reduction in total sleep time, daytime sleepiness, and increased alcohol and caffeine use (29).

Injury in the setting of sleepiness can also occur on the sports field or during other recreational activities as a result of a decreased reaction time or misjudgment. In a study of 14 days of chronic partial sleep deprivation in subjects (age 21–38), Van Dongen, et al. (32) found significant deficits in neurobehavioral functioning tests of behavioral alertness (psychomotor vigilance test), working memory (digit symbol substitution task), and cognitive throughput (serial addition/subtraction task) in subjects restricted to four or six hours sleep per night versus eight hours. The deficits in the four and six hour sleep-restricted groups were comparable to those with one to two days of total sleep deprivation. Interestingly, subjective ratings of sleepiness in the chronically sleep-deprived groups did not continue to progressively increase significantly with time, suggesting that, despite worsening cognitive performance deficits, one's assessment of sleepiness becomes less reliable the longer the sleep-deprived state persists. This finding is similar to the reduction in the ability to assess crash risk when sleep deprivation is paired with alcohol, even at legal limits—the ability to be introspective with regard to one's state is impaired. Potentially dangerous recreational activities such as contact sports could obviously put a sleepy adolescent at greater risk of injury, as could any activity involving hazardous machinery or equipment.

SLEEP DEPRIVATION AND MOOD

Depressed mood has been found in teens with insufficient sleep (33), and it may be difficult to determine whether a mood disorder is primary and the sleep abnormality secondary, or vice versa. Given that suicide is one of the top three causes of death in adolescents in the United States, preventing sleep-related mood disorders and/or appropriately screening for them is extremely important. An increased suicide risk in rural Chinese adolescents was found to be associated with sleeping less than eight hours per night versus nine or more hours nightly in a recent study by Liu (34). The suicide risk was three times greater in the shorter sleepers. Those with frequent nightmares were also at an increased risk for suicidal ideation or attempts.

Roberts, et al. (35) looked at the issue of disordered sleep on teen functioning in a prospective study of a large community sample of adolescents of varying racial backgrounds in Texas. As part of the study, a number of questions relating to sleep were posed, yielding an insomnia score. They also asked questions about self-esteem, depression, perceived mental health, and life satisfaction as indicators of psychological functioning. They found that 17% of teens reported trouble falling asleep, 23% reported daytime tiredness, and 16% reported falling asleep during the day, "often" or "almost every day." The insomnia scores, which did not discriminate among causes of the sleep problem or total hours of sleep, were predictive of low self-esteem and symptoms of depression, supporting the important relationship between sleep and mental health.

PHYSIOLOGIC FUNCTION AND SLEEP DEPRIVATION

Some of the most revealing studies involving sleep deprivation are those that have been conducted in a rat model, using a disk-over-water method. In this scenario, a control rat and the experimental animal are at opposite sides of a divided horizontal disk that is suspended over water. Rotation of the disk, when the test animal appears sleepy, is a means of preventing sleep. Sleep deprivation in this model is associated with an increase in energy expenditure, weight loss despite increased food intake, ulcerative and keratotic skin lesions, debilitated scrawny appearance, decreased body temperature, increased plasma norepinephrine, decreased thyroxine levels, and an increase in the T_3/T_4 ratio (36). Sleep-deprived rats eventually die because of sepsis from opportunistic facultative anaerobes that exist in the gut (37). Recovery sleep can reverse the changes induced by sleep deprivation, though those rats with the greatest body temperature declines succumbed (36). Such extreme examples of sleep deprivation are impossible to simulate in the human. The role of sleep deprivation with regard to host defenses and endocrine and metabolic function has been explored and is an active area of research.

Sleep and immune function has been studied from a number of perspectives, including evaluating the circadian changes, as well as changes with sleep restriction in subsets of leukocytes, cellular adhesion molecule expression, cytokine levels, and the relationship between these, and hormonal factors involved in sleep regulation. While a number of relationships have been shown to exist, for instance, changes in cellular adhesion molecule expression with sleep deprivation that may reflect decreased immune activation, or changes in natural killer cell activity with sleep deprivation, it is not clear what the changes mean with regard to overall immune functioning on a day-to-day basis.

Several studies have suggested that sleep deprivation might play a positive role with regard to immune function. In one study, sleep-deprived rats manifested smaller tumors in response to a subdermal allogeneic carcinoma challenge compared to control animals (38). Another study looked at sleep deprivation and progression of influenza virus infection in the respiratory tract of immune versus nonimmune mice. Less progression of viral infection into the lung in the nonimmune group that was sleep-deprived versus the normal sleeping group was observed (39). These results are in contrast, however, to those of Brown et al. (40), who demonstrated a detrimental effect of sleep deprivation on ability to respond to influenza rechallenge in immunized mice.

In humans, the relationship between adequate sleep and humoral immunity has been studied by looking at antibody titers in response to hepatitis A vaccination. When subjects who were allowed to sleep normally the night after hepatitis A vaccination were compared with those who were sleep-restricted for the next 36 hours, titers at four weeks nearly two-fold higher were seen in the normal sleep group (41). Response to influenza vaccination after four nights partial sleep deprivation, followed by two more nights of sleep deprivation, and then seven days of recovery sleep, showed decreased titers at the ten-day post-immunization point versus controls, though the difference did not persist at three weeks (42).

Clearly, the relationship between sleep loss and immune function is complex and the functional correlates of the findings in research studies are yet to be elucidated. The rat model of sleep deprivation shows us the extreme to which sleep deprivation can impact morbidity and mortality. Whether there is any beneficial effect of mild, intermittent sleep restriction on immune function is not known. Certainly, it could be hypothesized that sleep restriction in adolescents, if ongoing, puts them at greater risk for infections commonly occurring in community settings.

One other important aspect of insufficient sleep and health that deserves to be mentioned is the relationship between obesity and sleep. Obesity has increased in prevalence in the past several decades and is becoming a significant public health issue. Short sleep duration has been associated with increased hunger and increased risk of obesity in children (43–46), adolescents (47,48), and adults (49–52), perhaps modulated by the decreased leptin levels and increased ghrelin levels that have been observed in the setting of insufficient sleep (53). Insulin resistance has also been observed as a consequence of sleep deprivation (54), an important finding given the increasing incidence of obesity-related diseases in youth.

CONCLUSION

Insufficient sleep and consequent daytime sleepiness are prevalent in youth in the United States and other developed nations. The maturational changes in sleep physiology during adolescence contribute to insufficient sleep, often as a result of a DSPS. The 24/7 nature of our society, availability of technologies that allow rapid communication and stimulating activity prior to bedtime, after school activities, including part-time work, and early secondary school start times may all contribute to a less than adequate amount of sleep in this age group. The consequences of insufficient sleep include poor academic performance, mood disorders, increased use of alcohol and stimulants, such as caffeine and nicotine, increased risk-taking behaviors and risk of injury, as well as alterations in immune, endocrine, and metabolic function. These all point to the need for regular assessments of sleep by pediatricians with appropriate interventions as needed, as well as family education on the importance of sleep, particularly as relates to physiologic and cognitive functioning and injury prevention.

APPENDIX

    I. Key Features of DSPS
       Difficulty initiating sleep
       Late timing of sleep onset
       Nonproblematic sleep maintenance
       Difficulty awakening on school mornings
       Preference for late bedtime and rise time
       Adequate quantity/quality of sleep when allowed to sleep in
    II. Treatment of DSPS
       Regulation of wake-up time
       Allocation of adequate sleep time
       Wind down time before bed
       No caffeine after mid-afternoon
       Organize homework/chores/attire
       Light treatment at desired wake-up time
       Possible melatonin 0.5 mg to 1 mg six hours
         prior to desired bedtime
   III. Differential Diagnosis of the Sleepy Teen
      A. Insufficient sleep
          a. inadequate sleep hygiene
          b. delayed sleep-phase syndrome of adolescence
          c. sleep onset insomnia
          d. sleep maintenance insomnia
          e. non-24 hour sleep-wake pattern/free running
          f. sleep state misperception

  B. Disorders of nocturnal sleep
    a. upper-airway resistance syndrome
    b. obstructive sleep apnea
    c. periodic limb movements of sleep
  C. Disorders of daytime alertness
    a. narcolepsy
    b. idiopathic daytime hypersomnia
    c. Kleine–Levin syndrome (periodic hypersomnia)
  D. Medical disorders
    a. asthma
    b. thyroid dysfunction
    c. anemia
    d. infection
    e. occult malignancy
    f. rheumatoid arthritis
    g. epilepsy
    h. reflux
  E. Psychiatric disorders
    a. anxiety
    b. depression
    c. bipolar disease, especially hypomania
  F. Disorders associated with chronic pain
  G. Medications
  H. Substance use/abuse
IV. Work-up of the Sleepy Adolescent
  A. Thorough history including amount of sleep obtained, sleep pattern during school and nonschool days, sleep environment, sleep problems, for example, snoring, limb movements, awakenings, daytime naps, medications, caffeine intake, illicit drug use, and so on.
  B. Physical exam
  C. Sleep logs
  D. Labwork
  E. Consider polysomnography and multiple sleep latency test or maintenance of wakefulness test if there is an adequate amount of sleep and no other explanation for sleepiness.

REFERENCES

1. National Sleep Foundation. 2006 Sleep in America Poll Results. 2006.
2. Wolfson AR, Carskadon MA. Sleep schedules and daytime functioning in adolescents. Child Dev 1998; 69(4):875–887.
3. Yang CK, Kim JK, Patel SR, Lee JH. Age-related changes in sleep/wake patterns among Korean teenagers. Pediatr 2005; 115(suppl 1):250–256.
4. Reid A, Maldonado CC, Baker FC. Sleep behavior of South African adolescents. Sleep 2002; 25(4):423–427.
5. Arakawa M, Taira K, Tanaka H, et al. A survey of junior high school students' sleep habit and lifestyle in Okinawa. Psychiatry Clin Neurosci 2001; 55(3):211–212.
6. Shin C, Kim J, Lee S, Ahn Y, Joo S. Sleep habits, excessive daytime sleepiness and school performance in high school students. Psychiatry Clin Neurosci 2003; 57(4):451–453.
7. Ohida T, Osaki Y, Doi Y, Tanihata T, et al. An epidemiologic study of self-reported sleep problems among Japanese adolescents. Sleep 2004; 27(5):978–985.
8. O'Brien EM, Mindell JA. Sleep and risk-taking behavior in adolescents. Behav Sleep Med 2005; 3(3):113–133.
9. Carskadon MA, Vieri C, Acebo C. Association between puberty and delayed phase preference. Sleep 1993; 16:258–262.
10. Carskadon MA, Harvey K, Duke P, Anders TF, Litt IF, Dement WC. Pubertal changes in daytime sleepiness. Sleep 1980; 2(4):453–460.
11. Borbely AA. A two-process model of sleep regulation. Hum Neurobiol 1982; 1:195–204.
12. Carskadon MA, Wolfson AR, Acebo C, et al. Adolescent sleep patterns, circadian timing and sleepiness at a transition to early school days. Sleep 1998; 21(8):871–881.
13. Chesson AL, Littner M, Davila D, et al. Practice parameters for the use of light therapy in the treatment of sleep disorders. Sleep 1999; 22(5):641–660.
14. Mundey K, Benloucif S, Harsanyi K, Dubocovich ML, Zee PC. Phase-dependent treatment of delayed sleep phase syndrome with melatonin. Sleep 2005; 28(10):1271–1278.
15. Czeisler CA, Richardson GS, Coleman RM, et al. Chronotherapy: resetting the circadian clocks of patients with delayed sleep phase insomnia. Sleep 1981; 4:1–21.
16. Wahlstrom KL, Freeman CM. School Start Time Study: Final Report Summary. The Center for Applied Research and Educational Improvement, College of Education and Human Development, University of Minnesota, 1997.
17. Epstein R, Chillag N, Lavie P. Starting times of school: effects of daytime functioning of fifth-grade children in Israel. Sleep 1998; 21:250–256.
18. Giannotti F, Cortesi F, Ottaiano S. Sleep pattern, daytime functioning and school performance in adolescence: preliminary data on an Italian representative sample. Sleep Res 1997; 26:196.
19. Wolfson AR, Carskadon MA. Understanding adolescents' sleep patterns and school performance: a critical appraisal. Sleep Med Rev 2003; 7(6):491–506.
20. Horn JL, Dollinger SJ. Effects of test anxiety, tests and sleep on children's performance. J School Psychol 1989; 27:373–382.
21. Meijer AM, Habekothe HT, Van Den Wittenboer GLH. Time in bed, quality of sleep and school functioning of children. J Sleep Res 2000; 9:145–153.

22. National Sleep Foundation website. www.sleepfoundation.org
23. Library of Congress website. www.thomas.loc.gov
24. Arnedt JT, Wilde GJ, Munt PW, MacLean AW. How do prolonged wakefulness and alcohol compare in the decrements they produce on a simulated driving task? Accid Anal Prev 2001; 33(3):337–344.
25. Banks S, Catchside P, Lack L, Grunstein RR, McEvoy RD. Low levels of alcohol impair driving simulator performance and reduce perception of crash risk in partially sleep deprived subjects. Sleep 2004; 27(6):1063–1067.
26. Horne JA, Reyner LA, Barrett PR. Driving impairment due to sleepiness is exacerbated by low alcohol intake. Occup Environ Med 2003; 60:689–692.
27. Traffic Safety Facts 2003: A compilation of motor vehicle crash data from the fatality analysis reporting system and the general estimates system. National Highway Traffic Safety Administration. National Center for Statistics and Analysis. US Department of Transportation. Washington, D.C. 20590.
28. National Highway Traffic Safety Administration, US Department of Transportation. Crashes and fatalities related to driver drowsiness/fatigue. Research Notes. 1994.
29. Protecting Youth at Work: Health, Safety, and Development of Working Children and Adolescents in the United States (1998). Commission on Behavioral and Social Sciences and Education, National Academies Press.
30. Owens JA. The practice of pediatric sleep medicine: results of a community survey. Pediatrics 2001; 108(3):e51.
31. Goldberg R, Shah SJ, Halstead J, McNamara RM. Sleep problems in emergency department patients with injuries. Acad Emerg Med 1999; 6(11):1134–1140.
32. Van Dongen HPA, Maislin G, Mullington JM, Dinges DF. The cumulative cost of additional wakefulness: dose-response effects on neurobehavioral functions and sleep physiology from chronic sleep restriction and total sleep deprivation. Sleep 2003; 26(2):117–126.
33. Dahl RE, Lewin DS. Pathways to adolescent health: Sleep regulation and behavior. J Adolesc Health 2002; 31:175–184.
34. Liu X. Sleep and adolescent suicidal behavior. Sleep 2004; 27(7):1351–1358.
35. Roberts RE, Roberts CR, Chen IG. Impact of insomnia on future functioning of adolescents. J Psychosom Res 2002; 53:561–569.
36. Rechtschaffen A, Bergmann BA, Everson CA, et al. Sleep deprivation in the rat: X. Integration and discussion of the findings. Sleep 1989; 12(1):68–87.
37. Everson CA. Sustained sleep deprivation impairs host defense. Am J Physiol 1993; 265:R1148–R1154.
38. Bergmann BM, Rechtschaffen A, Gilliland MA, et al. Effect of extended sleep deprivation on tumor growth in rats. Am J Physiol 1996; 271:R1460–R1464.
39. Renegar KB, Crouse D, Floyd RA, Krueger J. Progression of influenza viral infection through the murine respiratory tract: the protective role of sleep deprivation. Sleep 2000; 23(7):1–5.
40. Brown R, Pang G, Husband AJ, et al. Suppression of immunity to influenza virus infection in the respiratory tract following sleep disturbance. Reg Immunol 1989; 2:321–325.
41. Lange T, Perras B, Fehm HL, Born J. Sleep enhances the human antibody response to hepatitis A vaccination. Psychosom Med 2003; 65:831–835.
42. Spiegel K, Sheridan JF, Van Cauter E. Effect of sleep deprivation on responses to immunization. JAMA 2002; 288:1471–1472.

43. von Kries R, Toschke AM, Wurmser H, et al. Reduced risk for overweight and obesity in 5- and 6-y-old children by duration of sleep: a cross-sectional study. Int J Obes Relat Metab Dis 2002; 26(5):710–716.

44. Locard E, Mamelle N, Billette A, et al. Risk factors for obesity in a five year old population. Parental versus environmental factors. Int J Obes Relat Metab Dis 1992; 16(10):721–729.

45. Sekine M, Yamagami T, Handa K, et al. A dose-response relationship between short sleeping hours and childhood obesity: results of the Toyama Birth Cohort Study. Child Care Health Dev 2002; 28(2):163–170.

46. Agras WS, Hammer LD, McNicholas F, Kraemer HC. Risk factors for childhood overweight: a prospective study from birth to 9.5 years. J Pediatr 2004; 145:20–25.

47. Reilly JJ, Armstrong J, Dorosty AR, Emmett PM, et al. Early life risk factors for obesity in childhood: cohort study. BMJ 2005; 330:357.

48. Gupta NJ, Mueller WH, Chan W, Meininger JC. Is obesity associated with poor sleep quality in adolescents? Am J Human Biol 2002; 14:762–768.

49. Vioque J, Torres A, Quiles J. Time spent watching television, sleep duration and obesity in adults living in Valencia, Spain. Int J Obes Relat Metab Disord 2000; 24(12):1683–1688.

50. Gangwisch JE, Malaspina D, Boden-Albala B, Heymsfield SB. Inadequate sleep as a risk factor for obesity: analyses of the NHANES I. Sleep 2005; 28(10): 1289–1296.

51. Hasler G, Buysse DJ, Klaghofer R, et al. The association between short sleep duration and obesity in yound adults: a 13 year prospective study. Sleep 2004; 27(4):661–666.

52. Vorona RD, Winn MP, Babineau TW, Eng BP, Feldman HR, Ware JC. Overweight and obese patients in a primary care population report less sleep than patients with a normal body mass index. Arch Intern Med 2005; 165(1):25–30.

53. Agras G, Spiegel K, Tasali E, Penev P, Van Cauter E. Brief communication: Sleep curtailment in health young men is associated with decreased leptin levels, elevated ghrelin levels and increased hunger and appetite. Ann Intern Med 2004; 141:846–850.

54. Spiegel K, Knutson K, Leproult R, et al. Sleep loss: a novel risk factor for insulin resistance and Type 2 diabetes. J Appl Physiol 2005; 99:2008–2019.

19

Restless Legs Syndrome and Periodic Limb Movement Disorder in Children and Adolescents

Daniel Picchietti

University of Illinois and Carle Clinic Association, Urbana, Illinois, U.S.A.

Karla M. Dzienkowski

Restless Legs Syndrome Foundation, Rochester, Minnesota, U.S.A.

CHAPTER HIGHLIGHTS

- Symptoms of restless legs syndrome (RLS) often begin in childhood or adolescence, with about 35% reporting onset prior to age 20.
- A family history of RLS increases the probability that the child also has the condition since it has been linked to an autosomal-dominant pattern of inheritance.
- An association of RLS/PLMD and ADD/ADHD has been shown in several studies.
- Serum ferritin values <50 mcg/L, although within normal limits, may still be responsible for clinical symptoms.
- Taking an iron supplement with vitamin C enhances absorption of the iron. However, food and tea will interfere with absorption.
- When starting medications for RLS or PLMD, start at a lower dose and titrate upwards for effectiveness.

Restless legs syndrome is a neurological disorder characterized by a distressing urge to move the legs and sometimes other parts of the body, usually accompanied by a marked sense of discomfort in the legs or other affected body parts. RLS is triggered by rest or inactivity, and its symptoms are temporarily relieved by movement. In adults, it follows a circadian pattern, meaning that symptoms vary by time of day—being most common and intense during the evening and nighttime hours. The disorder can be relatively mild or have profound disruptive effects on a patient's sleep and daily life.

RLS is a common and treatable condition. RLS affects 5% to 10% of adults in some countries (1). In the United States alone, RLS is believed to afflict more than 10 million adults and an estimated 1.4 million children and adolescents. Although most research has focused on adults, RLS symptoms often begin during childhood or adolescence. About 35% of patients report RLS onset prior to age 20, and one in ten report that the syndrome appeared during the first decade of life (2,3). Multiple reports now document the occurrence of RLS, as well as of the related problem, periodic limb movement disorder (PLMD), during childhood and adolescence (4–12).

INTRODUCTION TO RESTLESS LEGS SYNDROME AND PERIODIC LIMB MOVEMENT DISORDER IN CHILDREN

Symptoms of both RLS and PLMD can range from mild to severe and can negatively impact a child's quality of life. Accurate diagnosis of RLS and PLMD in pediatric patients offers substantial benefits. First, understanding why a child is uncomfortable and irritable can be very important in engendering a supportive parental response. Second, there is reason to hope that early, specific treatment may reduce or eliminate RLS symptoms in children. Third, as larger numbers of children with RLS are identified, researchers can draw on this growing patient population to seek specific information and explore treatment options. Fourth, and most importantly, children who experience poor intellectual or emotional function due to these sleep disorders can have their problems addressed more directly.

Signs and Symptoms of Restless Legs Syndrome

Like their adult counterparts, children with RLS tend to seek relief from their discomfort by moving their legs—often by fidgeting, stretching, walking, running, rocking, or changing position in bed. Parents or healthcare providers may mistakenly attribute the child's discomfort to "growing pains" (13). In the classroom setting, attempts to relieve the uncomfortable feelings of RLS may be viewed as inattentiveness, hyperactivity, or disruptive behavior. RLS, however, is a real medical condition that calls for proper evaluation, diagnosis, and treatment. Unlike most adults with RLS, some children with RLS complain of the RLS sensations more during the day than at night.

Restless Legs Syndrome and Sleep

Sleep disturbance is common among children and adults with RLS. In children, the sleep disturbance may precede or overshadow the complaint of leg discomfort (12,14). The quality and quantity of a child's sleep are often diminished, and this sleep deprivation can result in moodiness, irritability, inattentiveness, fatigue, or hyperactivity.

Periodic Limb Movements in Sleep

Periodic limb movements in sleep (PLMS) are characterized by brief jerks (0.5 to 5.0 seconds in duration) of the limbs during sleep, typically recurring at 20- to 40-second intervals (Fig. 1) (15,16). PLMS are more common in the toes, feet, and legs than in the arms. An affected individual is usually not aware of the movements or of the associated transient arousals that disrupt sleep continuity. Among adults, PLMS are present in an estimated 80% to 90% of individuals with RLS. In children, documentation of PLMS exceeding norms for age supports a diagnosis of RLS (17). On the other hand, PLMS are not specific to RLS; they can occur in certain other sleep disorders, and can be induced or aggravated by certain medications, particularly selective serotonin reuptake inhibitor type antidepressants such as fluoxetine (Prozac®), sertraline (Zoloft®), and venlafaxine (Effexor®) (18–20).

Periodic Limb Movement Disorder

A diagnosis of PLMD is based on three criteria: (*i*) PLMS exceeding norms for age (≥5/hr for children), (*ii*) clinical sleep disturbance, and (*iii*) the absence of

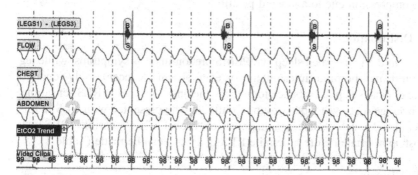

Figure 1 This sleep tracing demonstrates periodic limb movements in sleep (PLMS). PLMS are characterized by brief jerks (0.5 to 5.0 seconds in duration) of the limbs during sleep, typically recurring at 20- to 40-second intervals. To be considered periodic, there must be at least four leg movements in succession. The movements must be separated by at least five seconds but not more than 90 seconds. *Source*: Diagram courtesy of Norman R. Friedman, Director of Pulmonary Sleep Laboratory, The Children's Hospital, Denver.

another primary sleep disorder or underlying cause (including RLS) (16). In some children, a diagnosis of PLMD will evolve over time to a diagnosis of RLS with PLMS as the classic sensations of RLS develop. Current research suggests that PLMS are possibly due to underactive dopaminergic function in specific brain pathways, and are a marker of instability in the sleep system (21).

DIAGNOSIS OF RESTLESS LEGS SYNDROME AND PERIODIC LIMB MOVEMENT DISORDER IN CHILDREN AND ADOLESCENTS

Because children may experience and present symptoms of RLS differently than adults, establishing a diagnosis of RLS in a pediatric patient can be challenging. At this point, few physicians have had extensive experience in the diagnosis and treatment of RLS in children, since the childhood manifestations of RLS have been defined only recently. In a pediatric patient, the presenting complaint is usually either sensations of limb discomfort or disturbed sleep.

Restless Legs Syndrome Sensations in Children

For some children, the urge to move and uncomfortable leg sensations are the main concern. In the years past and even today, many children with these symptoms have been presumed to have "growing pains" (11,13)—vague, idiopathic episodes of leg pain. It is important to go beyond this and determine if the child truly has RLS. Further complicating the diagnostic picture, a child may describe these sensations with age-appropriate but nonspecific terms: "oowies," "boo-boos," "tickle," "bugs," "spiders," "ants," "want to run," or "a lot of energy in my legs." NonRLS childhood causes of lower limb extremity discomfort include joint pains, sore muscles, and cramps, as well as transient nerve compression due to awkward positions.

Sleep Disturbance

In other children, disturbed sleep and PLMS predominate as symptoms, while leg discomfort may be mild, intermittent, or even absent. A recent study reported chronic clinical sleep disturbance to precede the onset of specific RLS sensations by an average of 11 years in a group of children who presented with RLS in this manner (14). In such instances, a diagnosis of "probable" or "possible" RLS may be most appropriate before a definite RLS diagnosis can be made (Table 1).

Family History

A thorough family history is of great importance because an autosomal dominant pattern of inheritance is very common when RLS occurs at a young age (22–24). If a biological parent has RLS, for example, then there is an approximately 50:50 chance of passing the RLS trait on to each child. However, it is important to understand that a parent may receive the initial diagnosis of RLS in the course

Table 1   Criteria for the Diagnosis of Restless Legs Syndrome in Children: Definite, Probable, and Possible

---

Definite RLS

The child meets all four of the following adult criteria:
1. There is an urge to move the legs.
2. The urge to move begins or worsens with sitting or lying down.
3. The urge to move is partially or totally relieved by movement.
4. The urge to move is worse in the evening or night than during the day, or occurs exclusively in the evening or nighttime hours.

AND

The child describes leg discomfort using age-appropriate words. Examples of age-appropriate descriptors: oowies, tickle, tingle, static, bugs, spiders, ants, boo-boos, want to run, a lot of energy in my legs.

OR

The child meets criteria 1–4 above

AND

Two of the three following supportive criteria:
1. There is clinical sleep disturbance for age.
2. A biological parent or sibling has definite RLS.
3. A sleep study has documented a periodic limb movement index of 5 or more per hour of sleep.

Probable RLS

The child meets these three adult criteria:
1. There is an urge to move the legs.
2. The urge to move begins or worsens with sitting or lying down.
3. The urge to move is partially or totally relieved by movement.

AND

The child has a biological parent or sibling with definite RLS.

OR

The child shows signs of lower-extremity discomfort when sitting or lying down, with motor movement of the affected limbs. The discomfort has characteristics of adult criteria 2, 3, and 4: worsening with rest and inactivity, relief with movement, and worsening during evening and nighttime hours.

AND

The child has a biological parent or sibling with definite RLS.

Possible RLS

The child has PLMD.

AND

A biological parent or sibling has definite RLS, but the child does not meet the criteria for definite or probable childhood RLS.

Abbreviations: RLS, restless legs syndrome; PLMD, periodic limb movement disorder.
Source: From Ref. 17.

of medical attention for a child's symptoms. Thus, the child's evaluation should include an interview of the parents about RLS symptoms. The four essential criteria for adult RLS are listed in Table 1.

Physical Examination

In a child with RLS, the physical examination is typically normal. The finding of an associated underlying medical disorder in childhood RLS is unusual, except that a mild degree of iron deficiency may be present. An association between kidney failure, diabetes, or peripheral neuropathy and RLS is found more commonly in adults than in children.

Sleep Testing

Most children evaluated for RLS and PLMD are described as "restless" in their sleep. A sleep study (polysomnography) is often necessary to document the sleep disturbance and PLMS; simple observation of the sleeping child is not a reliable diagnostic tool for PLMD (9). The study should be carried out at a sleep center experienced in working with children, as proper technique and scoring are vital for accurate diagnosis (16).

RESTLESS LEGS SYNDROME DIAGNOSTIC CRITERIA

Medical professionals have developed special criteria for diagnosing RLS in children aged 2 through 12 years. Adolescents (13 years and older) are evaluated by means of standard adult criteria (17).

The criteria used to determine whether a child between the ages of 2 and 12 years can be given a diagnosis of definite, probable, or possible RLS are given in Table 1.

Keys to diagnosis
Does the child meet the four adult criteria?
Age-appropriate descriptors of RLS discomfort from the child.
A diagnosis of definite RLS does not require diagnostic polysomnography.
The diagnosis of probable or possible RLS requires a biological parent or sibling
   to have definite RLS.

Dilemma
Based on current criteria, a diagnosis for probable or possible RLS only exists
   for children less than 13 years of age. A child who is diagnosed with probable
   RLS at age 10 years will technically no longer have this diagnosis at age 13
   years without meeting all four of the adult diagnostic criteria. As more data
   on the natural history of this disorder become available, the diagnostic
   criteria will need to evolve.

CAUSES OF RESTLESS LEGS SYNDROME

Research into the causes of RLS is ongoing, and although answers are limited, three major themes have emerged. First, a strong genetic component is evident in early-onset RLS. Second, underactivity of the brain transmitter dopamine appears to be associated with both RLS and PLMD. Third, there is evidence for brain iron deficiency in early-onset RLS.

Genetic Component

Several family studies have demonstrated an autosomal-dominant hereditary pattern in primary RLS (RLS in which the onset of symptoms occurs before age 30) (22–26). The likelihood in primary RLS that any first-degree relative of an affected individual (i.e., parents, siblings, or children) will also have RLS is almost 50%. Researchers have identified chromosomes 9p, 12q, and 14q as possible genetic loci for the expression of RLS as an inherited trait (27–30). Future research will aim to more precisely locate RLS-specific gene sites and to determine the role of these genes.

Dopamine and Restless Legs Syndrome

The brain transmitter dopamine plays a role in several neural networks, including those that control muscle movements, sleep, and "executive functions" (e.g., attention span, advanced planning, and impulse control). Pharmacologic studies and some brain-imaging studies provide evidence for an underlying dopamine abnormality in RLS and PLMD.

Iron and Restless Legs Syndrome

Because iron is vital for brain dopamine function, the finding of iron deficiency as a causative or contributing factor for RLS begins to paint a more comprehensive picture of RLS pathophysiology (31).

ASSOCIATION OF RESTLESS LEGS SYNDROME AND PERIODIC LIMB MOVEMENT DISORDER WITH LEARNING AND EMOTIONAL PROBLEMS

Attention Deficit/Hyperactivity Disorder

Several studies have reported an association between attention deficit/hyperactivity disorder (ADD/ADHD), RLS, and PLMD in children (6–8,10,32). However, this appears to be a complex relationship. In some children, the sleep disturbance and/or restless legs sensations can induce or aggravate inattention and/or motor restlessness. Considerable evidence suggests that sleep deprivation in children can impair cognitive function, including attentiveness and memory (32–34). This is not to say that all children with ADD/ADHD have

RLS or PLMD, but rather that an RLS subgroup may exist within the larger group of ADD/ADHD children. Conversely, not all children with RLS have ADD/ADHD, perhaps because of other modulating factors (32). A recent study indicates that adults with RLS are also at increased risk for ADD (35). Underactivity of dopamine has been suggested to be the common factor between ADD/ADHD, RLS, and PLMD (36,37).

Regulation of Emotions

Less extensively studied is a possible association in some children between mood problems, RLS, and PLMD. As most parents will attest, a child in need of sleep is often moody or "cranky" rather than overtly sleepy. Irritability, easy frustration, negative affect, and poor control of impulses and emotions can be induced or aggravated in children by lack of sleep (38–40). Given the emerging association between RLS, depressive symptoms, and anxiety in some adults (41–43), further study in children of a possible relationship between these factors is indicated.

RESTLESS LEGS SYNDROME, PERIODIC LIMB MOVEMENTS IN SLEEP, AND THE CONNECTION WITH LOW IRON LEVELS

Iron and Ferritin

Studies in adults have found correlations between low serum ferritin levels (a marker of body iron stores) and increased RLS symptoms (31,37), probably because of iron's vital role in brain dopamine function. Similarly, systemic iron deficiency can induce or aggravate RLS in children, even when the deficiency is not severe enough to cause anemia. Serum ferritin is the best single measure of peripheral iron stores, much more accurate than hemoglobin or serum iron tests. A low ferritin level, even one in the low-normal range, indicates a potential problem. Although recognition of the association between low iron stores and RLS/PLMD in children is new (12,44,45), the fact that severe iron deficiency in children can affect brain development and function—likely via alterations in dopamine metabolism—has long been recognized (46–48). Infants, toddlers, and teenagers are at particular risk for iron deficiency. Several studies in adults and two studies in children have shown that replenishing diminished iron stores can reduce RLS and PLMS symptoms (44,45). ADD/ADHD—a comorbidity in some children with RLS and PLMD—has also been associated with low ferritin levels (49).

TREATMENT OPTIONS

Nonpharmacologic Treatment

Nonpharmacologic interventions should always be included in the treatment plan, and in some children will provide sufficient management of RLS. In general, medication should be considered only when nonpharmacologic interventions are insufficient and an RLS-related sleep disorder is affecting the child's daytime function. The goals of therapy, both pharmacologic and nonpharmacologic, are adequate sleep quantity, good sleep quality, and suppression of RLS sensations, with a resultant improvement in daytime function.

Good Sleep Habits for Children and Adolescents

All children and adolescents—especially those with sleep disorders—benefit significantly from establishing a routine of good sleep habits. Children and adolescents often test the limits of sleep, and for those with RLS the result can be sleep deprivation that significantly increases RLS symptoms and adversely affects daytime function. Parents should be made aware of the amount of sleep considered normal for each age, and advised to help the child get sufficient sleep on a regular basis. Typical sleep needs are as follows: age 2, 12 hours (including one nap); age 5, 11 hours; age 10, 10 hours; teen years, nine hours; and adulthood, seven to eight hours. A child or teenager should go to bed and awaken at about the same time every day, including weekends, avoid caffeine intake, especially late in the day or evening, get regular exercise, and maintain a comfortable, quiet bedroom environment, free of stimulating activities. Teens should avoid the use of tobacco and alcohol, which are known to disrupt sleep, confine any napping to the afternoon hours and nap no longer than 45 minutes, and avoid driving when tired (Appendix A).

Iron Supplementation

Treatment of Low Ferritin

Iron supplementation should be given if the child's serum ferritin level is low or in the low-normal range, below 35 mcg/L. While most labs have lower cut-off values than 35, it is clear that iron deficiency is common in the 10 to 35 range, as demonstrated by the "gold-standard" measure for iron deficiency—bone marrow testing (50). The dosage and course of therapeutic iron should be the same as that typically used to treat anemia in children. A multivitamin that includes iron does not have enough iron to replenish low iron stores. However, once full replenishment of iron stores is obtained, a daily multivitamin supplement with iron can be used to help maintain iron stores. Serum ferritin testing should be avoided when a child is ill, because the value can be falsely elevated by acute illness such as a cold and other infections. Studies in children and adults have shown decreased signs and symptoms of RLS and PLMS in association with serum ferritin concentrations rising to levels above 35 to 50 mcg/L (44,45,51–53). The results of iron therapy should be monitored by follow-up testing. Unless there is concern about possible hemochromatosis (a disorder of iron overload) or another reason for particular caution, a daily multivitamin with iron should be used to help prevent the body's iron from becoming depleted during the growth years (note: mcg/L equals ng/mL).

> Ferritin is a good measure of the body's iron stores but it is also an acute phase
> reactant.
> Do not obtain serum ferritin levels when a child has an acute illness.

Iron Absorption

Taking an iron supplement with vitamin C enhances absorption of the iron. Many beverages, such as orange juice and fruit drinks, contain vitamin C. Vitamin C tablets are also available. Ideally, food, calcium, and tea should not be taken within two hours of taking an iron supplement. These decrease iron absorption and will delay full replenishment of the body's iron stores.

Medication Options

The potential risks of medication must be balanced against the long-term consequences of poor intellectual and emotional function due to these sleep disorders. Two medications found particularly useful to treat children with RLS or PLMD are clonidine (Catapres®) and clonazepam (Klonopin®). Clonidine is the most commonly used medication for children's sleep (54–56), and is especially beneficial in children whose RLS results in severe sleep-onset problems. An occasional side effect of clonidine is the induction or aggravation of sleep terrors. Clonazepam is prescribed for children with RLS to improve sleep quality and to decrease RLS discomfort. In some children, clonazepam can have an activating effect (paradoxical activation); it should be discontinued if this occurs. Another option is gabapentin (Neurontin®), which has shown promise in reducing sensory and motor symptoms of RLS, resulting in improved sleep quality (57,58). Temazepam (Restoril®) and zolpidem (Ambien®) are helpful to some adults whose RLS is accompanied by severe, chronically disturbed sleep, and might be considered for use in older children and,teenagers with similar symptoms (53,59). As part of routine care, it is wise to remind families about the safe storage of all medications (including Tylenol®) in childproof containers, out of the reach of young children.

Medications that Increase Dopamine

Dopaminergics are the medications of choice for most adults with significant RLS, having been shown to suppress RLS sensations and PLMS more effectively and safely than medications in any other class (1,53,60). Dopaminergics commonly used to treat RLS in adults include levodopa (Sinemet®, others), pramipexole (Mirapex®), and ropinirole (Requip®). While the use of dopaminergics has not been studied extensively in children, the safe use in treating the rare neurologic movement disorder dopa-responsive dystonia suggests that they are well tolerated in pediatric patients (61). Although medications such as methylphenidate (Ritalin®) are not used to treat RLS or PLMS, they also raise dopamine levels and have a good long-term safety record in children (62). Dopaminergics that have been found to be effective in adult RLS may be tried with appropriate caution in children and teenagers who manifest severe RLS-related discomfort or significant PLMS (9,63,64).

Dopaminergic Medications and Augmentation

"More is not necessarily better." Augmentation—the worsening of RLS symptoms as the dosage of a dopaminergic medication is increased—is most commonly reported in patients taking levodopa, and is a less-frequent side effect of other dopaminergics (53). Augmentation is typically managed by dose reduction or by switching to another dopaminergic medication.

Does Treatment for Restless Legs Syndrome and Periodic Limb Movement Disorder Help Attention Deficit/Hyperactivity Disorder?

The relationship between RLS, PLMD, and ADD/ADHD is clearly a complex one. Considerable evidence suggests that the treatment of sleep disorders in children, including impaired sleep resulting from RLS, can reduce, or in some cases eliminate, symptoms of ADD/ADHD (32,63). Research in this area continues. In children who need medication to treat ADD/ADHD in addition to treatment for RLS or PLMD, the usual stimulant-type medications (Ritalin, Dexedrine®, others) have not been found to aggravate RLS or PLMD, as long as the stimulant effect has worn off by bedtime (7,65).

Importance of Monitoring

Any pharmacologic treatment prescribed for RLS must be closely monitored for safety and efficacy. The best treatment effectively addresses the individual patient's symptoms—there is no "one size fits all" in the treatment of RLS. Medication should be periodically reassessed, especially if the patient has been treated for iron deficiency.

Family Issues

A Family Affair

The effects of RLS can be felt by the whole family and not just the child with RLS. Parenting a child who does not sleep well can be a real challenge. Numerous, excellent resource materials are available for parents who have a difficult child (66–68). In some instances, working with a counselor may be valuable in helping both the child and the family develop methods for dealing with this chronic condition. If a parent has untreated RLS or PLMD, help for the child should include treatment for the parent also. Well-rested parents are typically more effective parents. Given the high prevalence of depression in adults with RLS, optimal treatment of depressive symptoms is important (42,43,69).

CONCLUSION

Research suggests that RLS affects an estimated 1.4 million children and adolescents in the United States, and confirms that RLS and PLMD are not unique to adulthood. Healthcare providers need to be alert to the signs and symptoms of these disorders, and be aware of ongoing research and treatment options.

Despite its high prevalence, RLS continues to be greatly underrecognized and undertreated. Many cases remain undiagnosed in patients of all ages. A child's complaints of leg pain or discomfort should not be dismissed as vaguely defined "growing pains" without consideration of a differential diagnosis that includes RLS. If a child has poor sleep, the specific cause should be sought.

The RLS Foundation leads the quest for better treatment options and, ultimately, a cure for RLS and related disorders. The Foundation provides starter funding for promising research projects, and in recent years several of these studies have progressed to qualify for National Institutes of Health-sponsored grants. Substantial advances have been made in the areas of diagnosis and treatment, and important research is ongoing on several fronts. Scientific studies continue to focus on causes and potential cures for RLS. For additional information, visit the Foundation's website at http://www.rls.org.

ACKNOWLEDGMENTS

This chapter is based on the Restless Legs Syndrome Foundation brochure *Restless Legs Syndrome and Periodic Limb Movement Disorder in Children*, copyright 2005, modified with permission. Besides the primary authors, other contributors include Anita Raj, Georgianna Bell, and Bruce L. Ehrenberg.

APPENDIX

The SANDMAN Chart gives several tips for a good night's rest

Sleep schedule: Go to bed and awaken at the same time daily. Even on the weekend, establish a bedtime routine.

Avoid caffeine-containing foods and drinks such as soda, iced tea, and chocolate, especially in the late afternoon and evening.

Naps for teens: Only in the early afternoon and no longer than 45 minutes. No driving if tired.

Do allow yourself a bedtime snack.

Make exercise a part of your daily routine.

A relaxing, quiet, comfortable bedroom. Use this room only for sleeping. This room is a no study, loud music, or TV zone. Find another room for time-out.

No use of tobacco, alcohol, or street drugs. All are known to cause sleep disruption.

Source: From Ref. 70.

Note: The "Sleep Well. Do Well. Star Sleeper Campaign" uses Garfield the Cat as its "spokescat" to encourage children ages 7 to 11 to get enough sleep. This is a free, fun, and interactive website for children. It is sponsored by the National Institutes of Health and the National Sleep Foundation. Garfield's key message is that adequate nighttime sleep is important for children to do their best at whatever they do (http://starsleep.nhlbi.nih.gov/).

REFERENCES

1. Earley CJ. Clinical practice. Restless legs syndrome. N Engl J Med 2003; 348:2103–2109.
2. Walters AS, Hickey K, Maltzman J, et al. A questionnaire study of 138 patients with restless legs syndrome: the 'Night-Walkers' survey. Neurology 1996; 46:92–95.
3. Montplaisir J, Boucher S, Poirier G, Lavigne G, Lapierre O, Lesperance P. Clinical, polysomnographic, and genetic characteristics of restless legs syndrome: a study of 133 patients diagnosed with new standard criteria. Mov Disord 1997; 12:61–65.
4. Walters AS, Picchietti DL, Ehrenberg BL, Wagner ML. Restless legs syndrome in childhood and adolescence. Pediatr Neurol 1994; 11:241–245.
5. Wilson VN, Buchholz D, Walters AS. Sleep Thief, Restless Legs Syndrome. Orange Park, FL: Galaxy Books, 1996:316.
6. Picchietti DL, Walters AS. Restless legs syndrome and periodic limb movement disorder in children and adolescents: comorbidity with attention-deficit hyperactivity disorder. Child Adolesc Psychiatr Clin North Am 1996; 5:729–740.
7. Picchietti DL, England SJ, Walters AS, Willis K, Verrico T. Periodic limb movement disorder and restless legs syndrome in children with attention-deficit hyperactivity disorder. J Child Neurol 1998; 13:588–594.
8. Picchietti DL, Underwood DJ, Farris WA, et al. Further studies on periodic limb movement disorder and restless legs syndrome in children with attention-deficit hyperactivity disorder. Mov Disord 1999; 14:1000–1007.
9. Picchietti DL, Walters AS. Moderate to severe periodic limb movement disorder in childhood and adolescence. Sleep 1999; 22:297–300.
10. Chervin RD, Archbold KH, Dillon JE, et al. Associations between symptoms of inattention, hyperactivity, restless legs, and periodic leg movements. Sleep 2002; 25:213–218.
11. Rajaram SS, Walters AS, England SJ, Mehta D, Nizam F. Some children with growing pains may actually have restless legs syndrome. Sleep 2004; 27:767–773.
12. Kotagal S, Silber MH. Childhood-onset restless legs syndrome. Ann Neurol 2004; 56:803–807.
13. Walters AS. Is there a subpopulation of children with growing pains who really have Restless Legs Syndrome? A review of the literature. Sleep Med 2002; 3:93–98.
14. Picchietti D, Stevens HE. Early manifestations of restless legs syndrome in childhood (abstract). Sleep 2005; 28:A74.
15. The Atlas Task Force. Recording and scoring leg movements. Sleep 1993; 16:748–759.
16. American Academy of Sleep Medicine. International Classification Of Sleep Disorders. Diagnostic and Coding Manual. 2nd ed. Westchester, IL: American Academy of Sleep Medicine, 2005.
17. Allen RP, Picchietti D, Hening WA, Trenkwalder C, Walters AS, Montplaisir J. Restless legs syndrome: diagnostic criteria, special considerations, and epidemiology. A report from the restless legs syndrome diagnosis and epidemiology workshop at the National Institutes of Health. Sleep Med 2003; 4:101–119.
18. Dorsey CM, Lukas SE, Cunningham SL. Fluoxetine-induced sleep disturbance in depressed patients. Neuropsychopharmacol 1996; 14:437–442.
19. Armitage R, Emslie G, Rintelmann J. The effect of fluoxetine on sleep EEG in childhood depression: a preliminary report. Neuropsychopharmacol 1997; 17:241–245.

20. Yang C, White DP, Winkelman JW. Antidepressants and periodic leg movements of sleep. Biol Psychiatry 2005; 58:510–514.
21. Silber MH. Commentary on controversies in sleep medicine. Montplaisir et al. Periodic leg movements are not more prevalent in insomnia or hypersomnia but are specifically associated with sleep disorders involving a dopaminergic mechanism. Sleep Med 2001; 2:367–369.
22. Trenkwalder C, Seidel VC, Gasser T, Oertel WH. Clinical symptoms and possible anticipation in a large kindred of familial restless legs syndrome. Mov Disord 1996; 11:389–394.
23. Lazzarini A, Walters AS, Hickey K, et al. Studies of penetrance and anticipation in five autosomal-dominant restless legs syndrome pedigrees. Mov Disord 1999; 14:111–116.
24. Winkelmann J, Muller-Myhsok B, Wittchen HU, et al. Complex segregation analysis of restless legs syndrome provides evidence for an autosomal dominant mode of inheritance in early age at onset families. Ann Neurol 2002; 52:297–302.
25. Walters AS, Picchietti D, Hening W, Lazzarini A. Variable expressivity in familial restless legs syndrome. Arch Neurol 1990; 47:1219–1220.
26. Ondo WG, Vuong KD, Wang Q. Restless legs syndrome in monozygotic twins: clinical correlates. Neurol 2000; 55:1404–1406.
27. Desautels A, Turecki G, Montplaisir J, Sequeira A, Verner A, Rouleau GA. Identification of a major susceptibility locus for restless legs syndrome on chromosome 12q. Am J Hum Genet 2001; 69:1266–1270.
28. Bonati MT, Ferini-Strambi L, Aridon P, Oldani A, Zucconi M, Casari G. Autosomal dominant restless legs syndrome maps on chromosome 14q. Brain 2003; 126:1485–1492.
29. Chen S, Ondo WG, Rao S, Li L, Chen Q, Wang Q. Genomewide linkage scan identifies a novel susceptibility locus for restless legs syndrome on chromosome 9p. Am J Hum Genet 2004; 74:876–885.
30. Desautels A, Turecki G, Montplaisir J, et al. Restless legs syndrome: confirmation of linkage to chromosome 12q, genetic heterogeneity, and evidence of complexity. Arch Neurol 2005; 62:591–596.
31. Earley CJ, Allen RP, Beard JL, Connor JR. Insight into the pathophysiology of restless legs syndrome. J Neurosci Res 2000; 62:623–628.
32. Lewin DS, Di Pinto M. Sleep disorders and ADHD: shared and common phenotypes. Sleep 2004; 27:188–189.
33. Sadeh A, Gruber R, Raviv A. The effects of sleep restriction and extension on school-age children: what a difference an hour makes. Child Dev 2003; 74:444–455.
34. Steenari MR, Vuontela V, Paavonen EJ, Carlson S, Fjallberg M, Aronen E. Working memory and sleep in 6- to 13-year-old schoolchildren. J Am Acad Child Adolesc Psychiatry 2003; 42:85–92.
35. Wagner ML, Walters AS, Fisher BC. Symptoms of Attention-Deficit/Hyperactivity Disorder in Adults with Restless Legs Syndrome. Sleep 2004; 27:1499–1504.
36. Roman T, Rohde LA, Hutz MH. Polymorphisms of the dopamine transporter gene: influence on response to methylphenidate in attention deficit-hyperactivity disorder. Am J Pharmacogenomics 2004; 4:83–92.
37. Allen R. Dopamine and iron in the pathophysiology of restless legs syndrome (RLS). Sleep Med 2004; 5:385–391.

38. Dahl RE. The impact of inadequate sleep on children's daytime cognitive function. Semin Pediatr Neurol 1996; 3:44–50.
39. Dahl RE, Lewin DS. Pathways to adolescent health sleep regulation and behavior. J Adolesc Health 2002; 31:175–184.
40. Chervin RD, Dillon JE, Archbold KH, Ruzicka DL. Conduct problems and symptoms of sleep disorders in children. J Am Acad Child Adolesc Psychiatry 2003; 42:201–208.
41. Winkelmann J, Prager M, Lieb R, et al. "Anxietas Tibiarum" Depression and anxiety disorders in patients with restless legs syndrome. J Neurol 2005; 252:67–71.
42. Depression and RLS: Restless Legs Syndrome Foundation, 2005. http://www.rls.org/publications/scientific.html.
43. Picchietti D, Winkelman JW. Restless legs syndrome, periodic limb movements in sleep, and depression. Sleep 2005; 28:891–898.
44. Kryger MH, Otake K, Foerster J. Low body stores of iron and restless legs syndrome: a correctable cause of insomnia in adolescents and teenagers. Sleep Med 2002; 3:127–132.
45. Simakajornboon N, Gozal D, Vlasic V, Mack C, Sharon D, McGinley BM. Periodic limb movements in sleep and iron status in children. Sleep 2003; 26:735–738.
46. Beard JL, Connor JR. Iron status and neural functioning. Annu Rev Nutr 2003; 23:41–58.
47. Grantham-McGregor S, Ani C. A review of studies on the effect of iron deficiency on cognitive development in children. J Nutr 2001; 131:649S–666S; discussion 666S–668S.
48. Halterman JS, Kaczorowski JM, Aligne CA, Auinger P, Szilagyi PG. Iron deficiency and cognitive achievement among school-aged children and adolescents in the United States. Pediatrics 2001; 107:1381–1386.
49. Konofal E, Lecendreux M, Arnulf I, Mouren MC. Iron Deficiency in Children With Attention-Deficit/Hyperactivity Disorder. Arch Pediatr Adolesc Med 2004; 158:1113–1115.
50. Guyatt GH, Oxman AD, Ali M, Willan A, McIlroy W, Patterson C. Laboratory diagnosis of iron-deficiency anemia: an overview. J Gen Intern Med 1992; 7:145–153.
51. Angulo-Kinzler RM, Peirano P, Lin E, Algarin C, Garrido M, Lozoff B. Twenty-four-hour motor activity in human infants with and without iron deficiency anemia. Early Hum Dev 2002; 70:85–101.
52. Beard JL. Iron status and periodic limb movements of sleep in children: a causal relationship? Sleep Med 2004; 5:89–90.
53. Silber MH, Ehrenberg BL, Allen RP, et al. An algorithm for the management of restless legs syndrome. Mayo Clin Proc 2004; 79:916–922.
54. Newcorn JH, Schulz K, Harrison M, DeBellis MD, Udarbe JK, Halperin JM. Alpha 2 adrenergic agonists. Neurochemistry, efficacy, and clinical guidelines for use in children. Pediatr Clin North Am 1998; 45:1099–1122, viii.
55. Owens JA, Rosen CL, Mindell JA. Medication use in the treatment of pediatric insomnia: results of a survey of community-based pediatricians. Pediatr 2003; 111:e628–e635.
56. Prince JB, Wilens TE, Biederman J, Spencer TJ, Wozniak JR. Clonidine for sleep disturbances associated with attention-deficit hyperactivity disorder: a systematic chart review of 62 cases. J Am Acad Child Adolesc Psychiatry 1996; 35:599–605.
57. Garcia-Borreguero D, Larrosa O, de la Llave Y, Verger K, Masramon X, Hernandez G. Treatment of restless legs syndrome with gabapentin: a double-blind, cross-over study. Neurol 2002; 59:1573–1579.

58. Happe S, Sauter C, Klosch G, Saletu B, Zeitlhofer J. Gabapentin versus ropinirole in the treatment of idiopathic restless legs syndrome. Neuropsychobiology 2003; 48:82–86.

59. Hening W, Allen R, Earley C, Kushida C, Picchietti D, Silber M. The treatment of restless legs syndrome and periodic limb movement disorder. An American Academy of Sleep Medicine Review. Sleep 1999; 22:970–999.

60. Hening WA, Allen RP, Earley CJ, Picchietti DL, Silber MH. An update on the dopaminergic treatment of restless legs syndrome and periodic limb movement disorder. Sleep 2004; 27:560–583.

61. Mink JW. Dopa-responsive dystonia in children. Curr Treat Options Neurol 2003; 5:279–282.

62. Hechtman L, Greenfield B. Long-term use of stimulants in children with attention deficit hyperactivity disorder: safety, efficacy, and long-term outcome. Paediatr Drugs 2003; 5:787–794.

63. Walters AS, Mandelbaum DE, Lewin DS, Kugler S, England SJ, Miller M. Dopaminergic therapy in children with restless legs/periodic limb movements in sleep and ADHD. Dopaminergic Therapy Study Group. Pediatr Neurol 2000; 22:182–186.

64. Konofal E, Arnulf I, Lecendreux M, Mouren MC. Ropinirole in a child with attention-deficit hyperactivity disorder and restless legs syndrome. Pediatr Neurol 2005; 32:350–351.

65. O'Brien LM, Ivanenko A, Crabtree VM, et al. The effect of stimulants on sleep characteristics in children with attention deficit/hyperactivity disorder. Sleep Med 2003; 4:309–316.

66. Turecki S, Tonner L. The Difficult Child. New York, NY: Bantam, 2000:302.

67. Phelan TW. 1-2-3 Magic: Effective Discipline for Children 2–12. Glen Ellyn, IL: ParentMagic, 2003:212.

68. Phelan TW. Surviving Your Adolescents: How to Manage and Let Go of Your 13–18 Year Olds. Glen Ellyn, IL: ParentMagic, 1998:176.

69. Burke L. The impact of maternal depression on familial relationships. Int Rev Psychiatry 2003; 15:243–255.

70. Mindell JA, Owens JA. A Clinical Guide to Pediatric Sleep: Diagnosis and Management of Sleep Problems. Philadelphia: Lippincott Williams & Wilkins, 2003: 284–286.

20

Narcolepsy in Children

Rafael Pelayo

Stanford Sleep Disorders Clinic, Stanford University, Palo Alto, California, U.S.A.

Maria Cecilia Lopes

*Stanford Sleep Disorders Clinic, Stanford University, Palo Alto, California, U.S.A.,
and Department of Psychobiology, Federal University of Sao Paulo, Sao Paulo, Brazil*

CHAPTER HIGHLIGHTS

- The symptoms of narcolepsy can be conceptualized as a blurring of the boundaries between the awake, sleeping, and dreaming brain.
- The mnemonic aide CHESS may help the reader remember the five symptoms of narcolepsy: **C**ataplexy, **H**ypnagogic hallucinations, **E**xcessive daytime sleepiness, **S**leep paralysis, and **S**leep disruption.
- To distinguish cataplexy from other clinical phenomena, a history of the episode being triggered by laughter and the patient being able to hear during the episode may be helpful.
- The incidence rate for narcolepsy is highest in the second decade.
- Within the context of the appropriate clinical history, one makes a clinical diagnosis of narcolepsy after a normal overnight polysomnogram is followed by a multiple sleep latency test (MSLT) with a short mean sleep latency of 8 minutes and two or more sleep onset rapid eye movement periods (SOREMs).
- If an experienced clinician observes unequivocal cataplexy the overnight polysomnogram and MSLT are not required to establish the diagnosis.
- Since narcolepsy is a chronic condition, the healthcare provider must not only be a source of medical care but must also be able to serve as an advocate for the patient.

INTRODUCTION

Narcolepsy is a chronic neurological disorder of excessive daytime sleepiness (EDS), which characteristically has a childhood onset and is associated with a hypocretin deficiency (1–4). Historically, the word "narcolepsy" was first coined by Gélineau in 1880 to designate a pathological condition characterized by irresistible episodes of sleep of short duration recurring at close intervals. The symptoms of narcolepsy can be conceptualized as a blurring of the boundaries between the awake, sleeping, and dreaming brain. The awake narcoleptic may feel sleepy. The sleeping narcoleptic may have disturbed sleep due to arousals. Dreaming phenomena may occur while the patient is awake. The onset of narcolepsy is typically in the second decade of life but may begin at a younger age or as an adult. Narcolepsy may have an abrupt or insidious onset. In the latter situation, the full syndrome may take 12 years to develop. During this time, patients may be misdiagnosed or simply labeled as lazy or depressed. It may not be until after the child is an adult that the correct diagnosis is made (5). It is therefore important for healthcare providers to consider narcolepsy as a possibility in any young person with an unexplained EDS.

CLINICAL SYMPTOMS

The cardinal features of narcolepsy are daytime somnolence, cataplexy, sleep paralysis and hypnagogic hallucinations. These symptoms were called the "tetrad" of narcolepsy by Yoss and Daly (6). Rechtschaffen et al. (7) reported presence of abnormal sleep onset rapid eye movement (REM) sleep periods in narcolepsy which allowed for objective physiological measurements. The disturbed nocturnal sleep has been described as an important complaint and may compose a fifth symptom associated with narcoleptic syndrome. The mnemonic aide CHESS may help the reader remember the five symptoms of narcoplesy: Cataplexy, Hypnagogic hallucinations, Excessive daytime sleepiness, Sleep paralysis, and Sleep disruption.

Cataplexy is characterized by the sudden, generally bilateral, loss of muscle tone while awake, typically triggered by a strong positive emotion such as laughter or surprise. It can also be triggered less commonly by anger or fear. Cataplexy is virtually a pathognomonic symptom of narcolepsy. When an experienced clinician witnesses a cataleptic attack, confirmatory sleep laboratory testing for narcolepsy might not be necessary (8). Narcoleptic patients remain conscious during the attack and are able to remember the details of the event afterwards. The episodes are typically brief and may last only a few seconds. Some patients can have other narcoleptic symptoms manifested during an episode of cataplexy such as hypnagogic hallucinations, sleep paralysis, or simply fall asleep. Cataplexy may involve only certain muscles or the entire voluntary musculature. Most typically, the jaw sags, the head falls forward, the arms drop to the sides, and the knees buckle. The severity and extent of cataplexy can range from a state of absolute powerlessness, which seems to involve the entire body, to no more than a fleeting sensation of weakness. Although the extraocular muscles are supposedly not involved, the patient may complain of blurred vision. Respiration may become irregular during an attack, which may be related to weakness of the abdominal or intracostal muscles. Complete loss of muscle tone that results in a fall with risk of serious injuries might occur during a cataplectic attack. The attacks may also be subtle and not noticed by nearby individuals. An attack may consist only of a slight buckling of the knees. Patients may perceive this abrupt and short-lasting weakness and may simply sit or stand against a wall. Speech may be slurred. If the attack involves the upper limbs, the individual may be described as clumsy due to dropping cups or spilling liquids when surprised or laughing. A patient may present with repetitive falls that cannot be easily explained. This may result in a misdiagnosis of atonic seizures (5). The duration of each cataplectic attack, partial or total, is highly variable. They usually range from a few seconds to two minutes and rarely up to 30 minutes. The term *status cataplecticus* can be applied to prolonged attacks. Attacks can be elicited by emotion, stress, fatigue, or heavy meals. Laughter and anger seem to be the most common triggers, but a feeling of elation while listening to music, reading a book, or watching a movie can also induce the attacks. Merely remembering a funny situation may induce cataplexy, and it may also occur without obvious precipitating acts or emotions. In children it often occurs while playing with others. The potential emotional impact of cataplexy cannot be overstated (9). Individuals may be misdiagnosed with a psychiatric disorder before recognition of narcolepsy. To distinguish cataplexy from other clinical phenomena, a history of the episode being triggered by laughter and the patient being able to hear during the episode may be helpful (10).

Hypnagogic hallucinations are fragments of auditory or dream-like imagery that occur at sleep onset. Similar episodes upon awakening are called hypnopompic hallucinations. This is a nonspecific symptom of narcolepsy. It probably occurs clinically more frequently in any sleep-deprived individual. Hypnagogic hallucinations should not be confused with psychosis. Auditory hallucinations are common. The patient may be frightened by the imagery.

Sleep paralysis is a self-descriptive term that can be a terrifying experience. It is a transient inability to move, usually upon awakening. Patients find themselves suddenly unable to move the limbs, to speak, or even to breathe deeply. This state is frequently accompanied by hallucinations. During episodes of sleep paralysis, particularly the first occurrence, the patient may have extreme anxiety associated with fear of dying. This anxiety is often greatly intensified by the hallucinations, sometimes terrifying, that may accompany the sleep paralysis. Patients may be reluctant to talk about these events, and these experiences can be so frightening that the patient may resist going to bed to sleep. Sleep paralysis, like hypnagogic hallucinations, may occur in any sleep-deprived individual in the absence of narcolepsy. They do not occur in all narcoleptics and may be transitory. Patients with narcolepsy may, with time, learn to recognize hypnagogic hallucinations and sleep paralysis as frightening but otherwise essentially benign phenomena and be better able to tolerate them.

The most common complaint in narcoleptic patients is daytime sleepiness or an inability to maintain wakefulness in daytime. In young children, this may not be quickly recognized as abnormal. The parents may not complain if their children sleep more than usual or may view the sleepiness as a normal phase of development. Certainly, most adolescents falling asleep in the classroom do not have narcolepsy. Delays in diagnosis are usually related to an absence of clinical suspicion for narcolepsy. In the 24-hour cycle, established narcolepsy patients do not sleep more than average. The increased daytime sleep is countered by impaired nighttime sleep.

School impairment is not unusual in children with narcoleptic syndrome. Children and adolescents with narcolepsy may report embarrassment, academic decline, and loss of self-esteem. Patients may be misdiagnosed with attention-deficit disorder (5,11). Psychosocial problems are not uncommon. The differences in clinical manifestations between children and adults are summarized in the Table 1. It can be difficult to recognize daytime sleepiness in very young children, but cataplexy is a more obvious symptom in the young. A potential need for supportive psychotherapy or counseling should be anticipated when developing a therapeutic plan (9).

Although narcolepsy is reported as usually developing either in late adolescence or young adulthood, patients may report substantial delays prior to diagnosis. A retrospective review of adults with narcolepsy suggests that over 50% believed their symptoms emerged before the age of 15 years, with 4.5% claiming the disorder occurred before they were five years of age (12). Hood and Harbord (13) published a report of a possible case of narcolepsy beginning in infancy. Hypersomnolence is the primary characteristic of adult narcolepsy but the evaluation of hypersomnia in early childhood is difficult. In a case series of 51 prepubertal narcoleptics, there were no parental reports of EDS for children under five years of age, although, when asked, parents reported children requiring several daily naps, difficulty awakening, and the propensity of the children to sleep in unusual settings (5). Not only is hypersomnolence in childhood difficult to define, but children may deny their sleepiness. Attempts by children to either hide or manage daytime sleepiness may lead them to substitute behavioral symptoms such as hyperactivity, aggression, impulsiveness, irritability, and restlessness for sleepiness (5).

EPIDEMIOLOGY

Narcolepsy is not a rare disorder. A survey in the United States found an incidence rate per 1,00,000 persons per year of 1.37. The incidence rate was highest in the second decade, followed in descending order by the third, fourth, and first decades. The prevalence was estimated at 56.3 per 1,00,000 persons. Approximately 36% of prevalence cases did not have cataplexy (14). These results are consistent with

Table 1 Differences in Clinical Manifestations Between Children and Adults

Symptom	Children	Adults
Cataplexy	Seen in most narcoleptic children, because is easy to recognize. Often occurs while playing with other children, frequently the first symptom recognized. Differential diagnosis with other causes of drop attacks in children.	Around 70% of narcoleptic patients. Usually, occurs associated with laugher, and is the first symptom in 5–8%. Can be described similar to drop attacks. It may appear on average 6 yr after the onset of EDS.
Hypnagogic hallucination	Symptoms such as nightmares and hypnagogic hallucinations were considered as part of normal childhood. These facts may be difficult to diagnose.	Present in 30% of adults. Visual hallucinations usually consist of simple forms. Auditory hallucinations are also common.
EDS	Sometimes may be difficult to recognize. More usual symptom is falling asleep in class. Sleepiness can be hidden behind other abnormal behaviors such as hyperactivity.	Easier to recognize than in children. Difficult to concentrate in slow activities. Problems in work that lead to sleep episodes in monotonous situations.
Sleep paralysis	Frequently accompanied by hallucinations. Children dislike to talk about these events.	Sometimes can be a terrifying experience. May occur in healthy subjects. Symptoms decrease with age.
Sleep disruption	This symptom may not affect children. Sometimes is a transitory complaint.	Worse during adulthood. May have influence in the treatment response.

Abbreviation: EDS, excessive daytime sleepiness.

previous narcolepsy prevalence estimates of 1 out of 2000 in the general population. Onset as young as two years of age has been reported (5).

PATHOPHYSIOLOGY

An animal model for narcolepsy was developed using dogs. Using positional cloning, an autosomal recessive mutation responsible for narcolepsy was discovered in this canine model (15). Independent work using a gene knock-out mouse model confirmed the role of hypocretin in narcolepsy (16). The hypocretins, which are also called orexins, are neuropeptides. Two novel neuropeptides have been described (Hcrt-1 and Hcrt-2), derived from the same precursor genes that are synthesized by neurons located exclusively in the lateral, posterior, and perifornical hypothalamus. Hypocretin-containing neurons have widespread projections throughout the central nervous system (CNS), with particularly dense excitatory projections to monoaminergic centers such as the noradrenergic locus coeruleus, histaminergic tuberomammillary nucleus, serotoninergic raphe nucleus, and dopaminergic ventral tegmental area. The hypocretins were originally believed to be primarily important in the regulation of appetite; however, a major function emerging from research on these neuropeptides is the regulation of sleep and wakefulness. Deficiency in hypocretin neurotransmission results in the sleep disorder narcolepsy in mice, dogs, and humans.

Hypocretins or orexins are a pair of neuropeptides expressed by a population of neurons located in the lateral hypothalamic area. Orexin receptor type 2-deficient animals exhibit a phenotype remarkably similar to the human sleep disorder, narcolepsy, which is characterized by sleep/wakefulness fragmentation. Human narcolepsy is known to be associated with metabolic abnormalities, including an increased frequency of obesity and noninsulin-dependent diabetes mellitus. Complex disruption of energy homeostasis in hypocretin/orexin neuron-deficient transgenic mice is also manifested as late-onset obesity despite eating less (17).

Canine narcolepsy is an autosomal recessive disease caused by disruption of the hypocretin receptor 2 gene (Hcrtr2). In most humans with narcolepsy, the Hcrtr receptor is intact but the actual peptide may be deficient or absent. This difference may account for genetic transmission differences between the canine model and humans. In humans, hypocretin levels can be measured in the cerebrospinal fluid (CSF) and have been found to be either very low or absent in most narcoleptics with cataplexy (3,18). In the canine model, narcolepsy can be predicted through breeding. In humans this is not the case. Although familial studies indicate a 20- to 40-fold increased risk of narcolepsy in first-degree relatives, only 25% to 31% of the monozygotic twins are concordant for narcolepsy (2,19,20).

Since most identical human twins are discordant for narcolepsy, an additional pathophysiological mechanism has been sought to explain the development of narcolepsy. The possibility that an autoimmune mechanism is damaging the hypocretin-producing cells in the hypothalamus has been raised (16,21). This is supported by the tight linkage of a subtype of human leukocyte antigen (HLA) DQ1 to humans with narcolepsy and cataplexy together. Similar linkages have been found in other autoimmune disorders such as multiple sclerosis (22,23). However, extensive searches for physical evidence of an autoimmune process has been inconclusive or negative (24).

The mechanisms through which hypocretin deficiency results in narcolepsy are unknown. A cholinergic/monoaminergic imbalance underlying the symptomatology of narcolepsy has been established, and is most likely caused by an absence of hypocretin signaling (Fig. 1). The widespread projections of hypocretin neurons make it difficult to elucidate hypocretin's exact functional importance (25,26).

Activity in the hypothalamic branch of the ascending arousal system and sleep regulation.

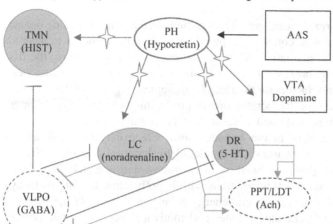

Figure 1 The ascending arousal system (AAS) sends projections from the brainstem and posterior hypothalamus (PH) (open oval) throughout the forebrain. Neurons of the latero-dorsal tegmental (LDT) nucleus and pedunculopontine tegmental (PPT) nucleus (dotted oval) send cholinergic fibers (Ach) to many forebrain targets, including the thalamus, which then regulate cortical activity. Aminergic nuclei (shaded circles and oval) diffusely project throughout much of the forebrain, regulating the activity of cortical and hypothalamic targets directly. Neurons of the tuberomammillary nucleus (TMN) contain histamine (HIST), neurons of the raphé nuclei contain 5-HT (serotoninergic neurons), neurons of the locus coeruleus (LC) contain noradrenaline (NA), and neurons of the ventral tegmental area (VTA) contain dopamine. Sleep-promoting neurons of the ventrolateral preoptic nucleus (VLPO, dotted circle) contain GABA. This figure represents the hypocretin deficiency, and increased Gabaergic system and cholinergic connections in PPT and LDT may explain several symptoms in narcolepsy syndrome. (→) activation; (⊣) inhibition; (⟨⟩) hypocretin deficiency.

More recent work detailing the synaptic input of the hypocretin/orexin-producing neurons has been reported by Sakuri et al. (27). These authors used a transgenic animal model to map upstream neuronal populations that have synaptic connections to hypocretin/orexin neurons, and revealed these neurons receive input from several brain areas. These include the amygdala, basal fore-brain cholinergic neurons, GABAergic neurons in the preoptic area, and serotonergic neurons in the median/paramedian raphe nuclei. Monoamine-containing groups that are innervated by orexin neurons do not receive reciprocal connections, while cholinergic neurons in the basal forebrain have reciprocal connections. The authors concluded this might be important for consolidating wakefulness.

The hypocretin system is consistently involved in the vast majority of patients with primary narcolepsy and cataplexy together. There have been reports of secondary narcolepsy, particularly associated with head injuries and neoplasms (28,29).

Hypocretin/orexins were initially identified as endogenous peptide ligands for two orphan G-protein coupled receptors. They have been shown to have an important role in the regulation of energy homeostasis. Furthermore, the discovery of hypocretin/orexin deficiency in narcolepsy patients indicates these peptides are important factors for the sleep/wakefulness regulation. The efferent and afferent systems of hypocretin/orexin-producing neurons suggest interactions between these cells and arousal centers in the brainstem as well as important feeding centers in the hypothalamus. Electrophysiological studies have shown that orexin neurons are regulated by humoral factors, including leptin, glucose, and ghrelin as well as monoamines and acetylcholine. Thus, these neurons have functional interactions with hypothalamic feeding pathways and provide a link between peripheral energy balance and the CNS mechanisms that coordinate sleep/wakefulness states and motivated behavior such as food seeking (30).

The pathophysiology of narcolepsy has been studied traditionally using animal models and with polysomnogram data from humans. These methods may not provide information regarding function in human brain structures that may be abnormal in narcolepsy. Functional neuroimaging methods may provide information regarding changes in brain function across the sleep–wake cycle in these patients. Functional neuroimaging methods have the potential to not only clarify the pathophysiology of narcolepsy but perhaps also to guide treatment strategies (31). Transcranial magnetic stimulation has also been studied in narcolepsy (32). Oliviero and colleagues used this technique to study the excitability of the motor cortex in patients with narcolepsy. They found resting and active motor thresholds were higher in narcoleptic patients than in controls and intracortical inhibition was more pronounced in narcoleptic patients. They hypothesized that the deficiency of the excitatory hypocretin/ orexin neurotransmitter system in narcolepsy is reflected in changes of cortical excitability, since circuits originating in the lateral hypothalamus and in the basal forebrain project widely to the neocortex, including motor cortex. This abnormal excitability of cortical networks could be the physiological correlate of EDS and it could be the substrate for allowing dissociated states of wakefulness and sleep to emerge suddenly while patients are awake, which constitute the symptoms of narcolepsy (32).

Immunity and Narcolepsy

The hypothesis that narcolepsy may be of autoimmune origin is primarily based on its tight association with HLA DQB1*0602. The peripubertal onset of narcolepsy, together with the reported low concordance rate in monozygotic twins and the complex genetic susceptibility in family studies, also argues in favor of this hypothesis. Narcolepsy shares many features with multiple sclerosis (HLA

DQB1*0602; disease of the central nervous system), however hypocretin level is usually normal in multiple sclerosis (18). The association of narcolepsy and multiple sclerosis suggest a HLA correlation with a different mechanism of action in both diseases.

Based on the striking association with a specific HLA subtype, narcolepsy is a good candidate to be an autoimmune disease. An autoimmune attack toward the hypocretin neurons would fit with this hypothesis. The attractiveness of this hypothesis has led to a fruitless search for serological evidence of autoimmunity. Perhaps the transient nature of such a putative process, together with the small number of hypocretin neurons and their presence in only a small part of the brain, could explain why direct evidence of autoimmunity has not been found to date. Possibly, the lack of evidence is secondary to the typical delay between onset of symptoms and clinical diagnosis (33). The putative auto-immune insult and any concomitant degeneration may have occurred years before the clinical diagnosis (33). However, unlike well-established autoimmune disorders, narcolepsy is not more frequent in women and is not associated with other autoimmune diseases.

Narcolepsy's pathophysiology may involve a combination of specific HLA alleles and environmental factors. Like many autoimmune disorders, these alleles have been sequenced in a large number of patients and shown to be identical to normal subjects with DQB1*0602 that have subclinical abnormalities indicative of narcolepsy (34,35). Human narcolepsy is a genetically complex disorder. Family studies indicate a 20- to 40-fold increased risk of narcolepsy in first-degree relatives, and twin studies suggest that nongenetic factors also play a role (33). The onset of narcolepsy–cataplexy may be associated with diffuse increased microglial HLA Class II expression in the white matter (36).

Although only a strong association is found with the HLA DQB1*0602 gene, other genetic susceptibility factors might be involved. Among these, the functional polymorphism of the catechol-O-methyltransferase gene is critically involved in the severity of narcolepsy and in the response to the stimulant modafinil. Other pharmacogenetic targets include the orexinergic, noradrenergic, and possibly the serotonergic pathways (36).

The strong association with HLA DQB1*0602 lends credence to the concept that the mechanism may be autoimmune, but there is no direct proof of this yet. The peripubertal onset of narcolepsy, together with the reported low concordance rate in monozygotic twins and the complex genetic suscepti-bility in family studies, also argues in favor of this hypothesis (20). Whether or not narcolepsy is an autoimmune disorder, a large portion of the normal population carry the exact HLA susceptibility alleles as narcoleptic patients. Additional support for the autoimmune hypothesis is that a substantial portion of healthy subjects with the corresponding susceptibility antigens have been found to display subclinical abnormalities: HLA B27-associated spondyloarthro-pathies with radiological sacroiliac joint abnormalities and HLA DQ2-associated celiac disease with increased mucosal gluten sensitivity (37,38).

There is no evidence for humoral autoimmunity in narcolepsy (39). In the CSF, no specific IgG oligoclonal bands have been observed in narcolepsy. Evidence for cellular autoimmunity in narcolepsy is also lacking. Blood levels and monolymphocyte secretion of tumor necrosis factor (TNF-α) and other proinflammatory cytokines such as interleukin (IL1-β), IL1-ra, IL-2, and TNF-β are not different between HLA DR2-positive narcoleptic patients and controls (40). Only IL-6 secretion was higher in narcoleptic patients. T-cell subsets and natural killer activity were identical in both populations, which do not support the hypothesis of a major peripheral proinflammatory cellular activation in narcolepsy, but does not exclude a local activation within the central nervous system. An autoimmune reaction without inflammation may also be possible with mainly neutralizing antibodies difficult to detect in situ, as in myasthenia gravis. The autoimmune reaction may take place initially earlier in the development of the disease during the asymptomatic phase (3).

Diagnosis

The American Academy of Sleep Medicine has recently released updated diagnostic criteria for narcolepsy in the *The International Classification of Sleep Disorders* (1). This diagnostic and coding manual describes three variants of narcolepsy. The first two are idiopathic variants of narcolepsy either with or without cataplexy. The former variant is very closely linked with a subtype of HLA DQ1 (33). The third variant is narcolepsy due to a medical condition. The diagnostic criteria for narcolepsy in children are the same as in adults (1).

Narcolepsy with cataplexy can be diagnosed solely on clinical grounds. Given the lifelong nature of this condition, obtaining collaborating sleep studies is reasonable. Narcolepsy without cataplexy may perhaps represent a continuum with the cataplexy variant. It is unknown if they have a common pathophysiology. The diagnosis of narcolepsy due to a medical condition requires either the unequivocal presence of cataplexy or supportive sleep studies. Disorders that have produced narcolepsy with cataplexy include: tumors, head trauma, sarcoidosis of the hypothalamus, multiple sclerosis, paraneoplastic syndrome with anti-Ma antibodies, and Nieman-Pick type C disease (1,41).

Within the context of the appropriate clinical history, a physician will request an overnight polysomnogram to be followed by an MSLT the morning after the polysomnogram. The MSLT measures the physiological tendency to fall asleep in quiet situations when the subject is instructed to try to fall asleep. The MSLT is a well-validated and standardized procedure (42). The presence of SOREMs has been considered diagnostic for narcolepsy (42–44). These MSLT criteria are constant for all narcolepsy variants. An MSLT should not be considered valid unless polysomnogram is done the night previous to this daytime test. If in the course of an evaluation for narcolepsy, the overnight polysomnogram demonstrates significant evidence of sleep-disordered breathing or the total sleep time is less than usual for the patient, then the results of the MSLT may be difficult to interpret. Given the potential lifelong consequences of a narcolepsy diagnosis, ideally it may be necessary to cancel the MSLT and reschedule the study after complicating factors such as sleep-disordered breathing are corrected. It is not uncommon for narcoleptics to have periodic limb movements (PLM) on an overnight polysomnogram. The presence of PLM alone would not require canceling the MSLT; however, the PLM should be taken into consideration in the clinical management of the individual patient after the diagnostic MSLT. The MSLT consists of five separate 20-minute napping opportunities every two hours after a documented full night of sleep. If the patient falls asleep within the 20-minute time frame, the nap is extended an additional 15 minutes to monitor for possible SOREMs. The MSLT final report will provide the mean sleep latency across five naps as well as the total number of SOREMs. The presence of two or more SOREMs is a very specific finding, whereas a mean sleep latency of less than eight minutes can be found in up to 30% of the general (perhaps sleep-deprived) population (1). Modifications to these diagnostic criteria have not been standardized or validated for preadolescents suspected of having narcolepsy. A urine toxicology screen is typically performed at some point during the MSLT.

If an experienced clinician observes unequivocal cataplexy, the overnight polysomnogram and MSLT are not required to establish the diagnosis. During an unequivocal bout of cataplexy, the deep tendon reflexes would be expected to be absent and not brisk when elicited with a reflex hammer.

The established diagnostic criteria may not always be applicable to children, since the MSLT was not validated for children younger than 8 years. If a person is taking medication that suppresses REM sleep, such as most antidepressants, the MSLT results may not be reliable. If a patient abruptly stops such antidepressants, a phenomenon of REM rebound may occur, giving a false-positive study for narcolepsy. A similar situation can occur if the MSLT is started at a time in the morning that a person usually sleeps; this scenario may occur in the context of an adolescent with a delayed sleep phase pattern. A false-positive MSLT for narcolepsy can occur if the subject is jet lagged, sleep-deprived or has subtle sleep-disordered breathing. Other techniques such as electroencephalogram (EEG) mapping are being studied as tools for measuring vigilance decrements in narcolepsy and their improvement under treatment (45).

Narcolepsy with cataplexy is rare prior to adolescence and extremely rare prior to the age of four years. Obesity may develop with narcolepsy when the onset is abrupt (1). If a child younger than eight years is suspected of having narcolepsy, the initial diagnostic question should be to determine if clear-cut cataplexy is present. If the presence of cataplexy is undisputable, then the diagnosis of narcolepsy can be made. However, in these young children the presence of cataplexy may be ambiguous. Measuring the CSF hypocretin level may help clarify the diagnosis (discussed later). In the absence of cataplexy and with normal or unavailable CSF hypocretin levels, the diagnosis is much harder to make in this age group. It is important to view narcolepsy as a potentially evolving disorder with the possibility that with time, the child will develop typical narcolepsy with cataplexy. An MSLT could be done in children less than eight years of age but may be difficult to interpret and may require repeating when the child is older. Diagnostic uncertainty requires clinical decision with close follow-up. If in this younger child the MSLT showed short sleep latency with four or five clear SOREMs, then the suspected diagnosis of narcolepsy is confirmed. If only two or three SOREMs are present, then the diagnosis will remain unclear, particularly, in a very young child that habitually naps. Children with narcolepsy without cataplexy may have a reappearance of regular daytime napping after having previously given up napping (1).

As our understanding of the pathophysiology of narcolepsy improves, modifications to the diagnostic criteria would be expected. Direct assays of hypocretin levels are more specific for the diagnosis of narcolepsy. Hypocretin can be measured in CSF. The absence of hypocretin in CSF is diagnostic of narcolepsy (3,41). CSF hypocretin level measurements may be particularly useful in complex or ambiguous clinical situations. However, the presence of normal CSF levels of hypocretin does not exclude the possibility of narcolepsy. A reliable blood serum equivalent test is not yet available. Its future development would be expected to change dramatically the diagnostic approach for narcolepsy. This would potentially decrease the delays between the onset of symptoms and conclusive diagnosis, which currently characterize the diagnosis. Hecht et al. reported on a child with evolving narcolepsy with a pathologically low CSF hypocretin level prior to the subsequent development of cataplexy (21). Perhaps, aggressive treatment prior to development of cataplexy could forestall or diminish any subsequent cataplexy.

Narcolepsy may be mistaken for epilepsy (46). Differentiating an epileptic seizure from some other paroxysmal event is a common challenge in clinical practice. A misdiagnosis can have serious consequences. Macleod and colleagues recently reported five patients referred for investigation of events initially suspected of being epileptic seizures. All five patients were subsequently diagnosed as having narcolepsy. Suspected diagnoses were absence of epilepsy (four patients), generalized epilepsy with astatic seizures (two patients), and focal epileptic seizures (two patients). Diagnostic confusion reportedly arose because lack of responsiveness due to excessive sleepiness was mistaken for epileptic absences, and cataplexy was confused with a variety of seizure types. Video/EEG monitoring during the episodes helped clarify the diagnosis (46). The importance of narcolepsy being considered in the differential diagnoses of paroxysmal events cannot be overemphasized.

TREATMENT

Successful treatment of narcolepsy includes both behavioral and pharmacological treatments (4,47). The situation is analogous to juvenile diabetes mellitus where a combination of diet with medication can control the condition.

Behavioral treatment begins with patients having as thorough an understanding of their condition as possible. Having the patient and family members meet other people with narcolepsy may be helpful. Volunteer support organizations such as the Narcolepsy Network have been established. Patients need to understand that developing healthy sleep habits is important for the rest of their lives. Two brief naps a day of about 20 minutes each should be strongly encouraged, if not required. For school-aged children, the healthcare provider should serve as an advocate on behalf of the patient to encourage the school to allow the child to nap in a safe and comfortable environment. Failure to consider or properly apply nondrug treatments as part of the comprehensive management may lead to unsatisfactory results for the patient and the family. These factors can result in patients with narcolepsy that are not properly managed due to either underdosing or overdosing of medication or incorrect medication selection.

Drug therapy must take into account possible side effects, with the fact kept in mind that narcolepsy is a lifelong illness and patients will have to receive medication for years. Tolerance or addiction may be seen with some compounds. Treatment of narcolepsy thus balances avoidance of side effects, including tolerance, with maintenance of an active life. There are no double-blind placebo-controlled trials of medication specifically for children with narcolepsy. The medications that are commonly prescribed are not specifically FDA-approved for narcolepsy in children.

The prescription drugs most widely used to treat EDS are the central nervous system stimulants. However, a number of side effects including irritability, anxiety, nervousness, headache, psychosis, tachycardia, hypertension, nocturnal sleep disturbances, tolerance, and drug dependence, may arise.

Traditionally, amphetamines and other stimulants such as methylphenidate were used as first-line treatment for the EDS of narcolepsy. This changed with the availability of a novel agent, modafinil. Modafinil may perhaps be better referred to as a "somnolytic" or as an atypical wakefulness-promoting agent in order to distinguish it from traditional stimulants (36,48,49).

The actual mechanism of action for modafinil is not entirely clear (50). Adrenergic signaling regulates the timing of sleep states and sleep state-dependent changes in muscle tone. Recent studies indicate a possible role for noradrenergic transmission in the wake-promoting action of modafinil. Wisor et al. recently reported that noradrenergic projections from the locus coeruleus to the forebrain are not necessary for the wake-promoting action of modafinil. The efficacy of modafinil was maintained after treatment of mice with *N*-(2-chloroethyl)-*N*-ethyl 2-bromobenzylamine (DSP-4), which eliminates all noradrenaline transporter-bearing forebrain noradrenergic projections. However, the necessity for adrenergic receptors in the wake-promoting action of modafinil was demonstrated by the observation that the adrenergic antagonist terazosin suppressed the response to modafinil in DSP-4-treated mice. The wake-promoting efficacy of modafinil was also blunted by the dopamine autoreceptor agonist quinpirole. The authors concluded these findings implicate nonnoradrenergic, dopamine-dependent adrenergic signaling in the wake-promoting mechanism of modafinil. The anatomical specificity of these dopaminergic–adrenergic interactions, which are present in forebrain areas that regulate sleep timing but not in brain stem areas that regulate sleep state-dependent changes in muscle tone, may explain why modafinil effectively treats EDS in narcolepsy but fails to prevent the loss of muscle tone that occurs in narcoleptic patients during cataplexy (51).

The initial dose should be relatively low to avoid headaches. Headaches are the most common side effects of modafinil and may be avoided or minimized by gradually increasing the dose. If the child can swallow the medication, low-dose modafinil should be considered the initial pharmacological agent used to treat the EDS of narcolepsy in children. Modafinil is specifically FDA-approved for narcolepsy, however dosing guidelines for very young children are not provided (47).

Potential abuse of any stimulant or wake-promoting agent may be a concern. Modafinil, however, does not have the euphoric properties of traditional stimulants. An assay to test for modafinil in plasma and urine has been developed (52). The assay can be used for therapeutic drug monitoring, pharmacokinetic studies, and drug abuse screening.

Gamma-hydroxybutyrate (GHB) is the first substance ever approved specifically in the United States for cataplexy (53,54). The drug's generic name is sodium oxybate. In the popular media, it has the infamous name of the "date rape drug." Illegal use of this substance for recreational purposes has been of great concern. Important CNS adverse events associated with abuse of GHB include seizure, respiratory depression, and profound decreases in level of consciousness, with instances of coma and death. Sodium oxybate has powerful central nervous system depressant effects. GHB can increase slow wave sleep. This medication, when given at bedtime, maybe of value to reduce cataplexy. Unlike most other medications discussed, sodium oxybate is available as a liquid. This is an obvious advantage for some children. Patients may prefer this medication to other medications used for cataplexy, particularly if insomnia is also present. Dosing guidelines for patients younger than 16 years old are not established. Analogs of GHB are being studied to further refine the treatment of narcolepsy (55). Animal research to elucidate the GHB mechanism of action have been carried out but are not conclusive (56).

Cataplexy seems to respond best to medications with noradrenergic reuptake blocking properties. There are no systematic trials of anticataplexy drugs on children. Postpubertal teenagers are usually treated as young adults. In this group, two medications have been more commonly used—clomipramine and fluoxetine. Both of these drugs have active noradrenergic reuptake blocking metabolites (desmethylclomipramine and norfluoxetine). It is through these metabolites that the therapeutic effect may be mediated. New medications with noradrenergic reuptake blocking are promising.

Given the putative autoimmune pathophysiology for narcolepsy, the possibility of using immunosuppressive therapy has been considered (21,57–59). Immunosuppressive treatment could, in theory, minimize or reverse the development of narcolepsy if initiated very early in the disease process. Dauvilliers and colleagues have reported on three patients who received high-dose intravenous immunoglobulins within a few months after acute onset of narcolepsy (58,59). A clear improvement in the frequency and severity of cataplexy was obtained up to seven months without any anticataplectic drugs at follow-up. The authors concluded that early diagnosis and treatment of narcolepsy may modify its long-term outlook. This potential therapy underscores the importance of healthcare providers have a high index of suspicion for narcolepsy when a patient presents with EDS.

With the recent discovery of a neuropeptide responsible for narcolepsy, novel, potential therapeutic approaches may be discovered. Hypocretin analogs may be potentially useful to treat narcolepsy (60). A further theoretic treatment possibility would be transplantation of hypocretin-producing cells.

CONCLUSIONS

It is imperative for children newly diagnosed with narcolepsy to understand they can lead very productive and fulfilling lives. Narcolepsy patients have a normal life span. Adolescents can obtain drivers' licenses as long as they are stable and compliant with their treatment. They can start families of their own someday, and their future children will not necessarily have narcolepsy. Children with narcolepsy should realize they are fortunate to be diagnosed at an early age and can avoid the difficulties that narcoleptic adults suffer due to the lack of proper diagnosis. If they undergo surgery for any reason, it is usually not necessary to stop their narcolepsy medications (61). It is important for young patients and their families to understand the rapid progress that has been made in understanding narcolepsy and the improvements in treatment options that have occurred in a relatively short period of time.

Since narcolepsy is a chronic condition, the healthcare provider must not only be a source of medical care but must also be able to serve as an advocate for the patient. This role may require the provider to help educate the child's teachers. Teachers should know that the child may suppress laughter to avoid cataplexy or that other students may purposefully try to trigger cataplexy episodes in the child. The child may need to take medication during the school day. The provider may need to aggressively demand that the school allow the child to briefly nap in a safe, quiet, and comfortable place. In older adolescents or college-age students, depending on the individual situation, specific accommodations may be reasonable such as allowing the patient to have a private dorm room if they have very disrupted sleep, or early registration of classes in specific time slots. Helping these children become responsible adults is professionally and personally very rewarding.

REFERENCES

1. American Academy of Sleep Medicine. International Classification of Sleep Disorders. 2nd ed. Westchester, Illinois: American Academy of Sleep Medicine, 2005.
2. Melberg A, Ripley B, Lin L, Hetta J, Mignot E, Nishino S. Hypocretin deficiency in familial symptomatic narcolepsy. Ann Neurol 2001; 49(1):136–137.
3. Mignot E, Chen W, Black J. On the value of measuring CSF hypocretin-1 in diagnosing narcolepsy. Sleep 2003; 26(6):646–649.
4. Mignot E. An update on the pharmacotherapy of excessive daytime sleepiness and cataplexy. Sleep Med Rev 2004; 8(5):333–338.
5. Guilleminault C, Pelayo R. Narcolepsy in prepubertal children. Ann Neurol 1998; 43(1):135–142.
6. Yoss RE, Daly DD. On the treatment of narcolepsy. Med Clin North Am 1968; 52(4):781–787.
7. Rechtschaffen A, Dement W. Studies on the relation of narcolepsy, cataplexy, and sleep with low voltage random EEG activity. Res Public Assoc Res Nerv Ment Dis 1967; 45:488–505.
8. Thorpy M. International Classification of Sleep Disorders: Diagnostic and Coding Manual. Rochester, MN: American Sleep Disorders Association, 1990.
9. Dahl RE, Holttum J, Trubnick L. A clinical picture of child and adolescent narcolepsy. J Am Acad Child Adolesc Psychiatry 1994; 33(6):834–841.
10. Krahn LE, Lymp JF, Moore WR, Slocumb N, Silber MH. Characterizing the emotions that trigger cataplexy. J Neuropsychiatry Clin Neurosci 2005; 17(1):45–50.
11. Guilleminault C, Pelayo R. Narcolepsy in children: a practical guide to its diagnosis, treatment and follow-up. Paediatr Drugs 2000; 2(1):1–9.
12. Challamel MJ, Mazzola ME, Nevsimalova S, Cannard C, Louis J, Revol M. Narcolepsy in children. Sleep 1994; 17(suppl 8):S17–S20.
13. Hood BM, Harbord MG. Paediatric narcolepsy: complexities of diagnosis. J Paediatr Child Health 2002; 38(6):618–621.
14. Silber MH, Krahn LE, Olson EJ, Pankratz VS. The epidemiology of narcolepsy in Olmsted County, Minnesota: a population-based study. Sleep 2002; 25(2):197–202.
15. Lin L, Faraco J, Li R, et al. The sleep disorder canine narcolepsy is caused by a mutation in the hypocretin (orexin) receptor 2 gene. Cell 1999; 98(3):365–376.
16. Taheri S, Zeitzer JM, Mignot E. The role of hypocretins (orexins) in sleep regulation and narcolepsy. Annu Rev Neurosci 2002; 25:283–313.
17. Hara J, Yanagisawa M, Sakurai T. Difference in obesity phenotype between orexin-knockout mice and orexin neuron-deficient mice with same genetic background and environmental conditions. Neurosci Lett 2005; 380(3):239–242.
18. Ripley B, Overeem S, Fujiki N, et al. CSF hypocretin/orexin levels in narcolepsy and other neurological conditions. Neurol 2001; 57(12):2253–2258.
19. Khatami R, Maret S, Werth E, et al. Monozygotic twins concordant for narcolepsy-cataplexy without any detectable abnormality in the hypocretin (orexin) pathway. Lancet 2004; 363(9416):1199–1200.
20. Dauvilliers Y, Maret S, Bassetti C, et al. A monozygotic twin pair discordant for narcolepsy and CSF hypocretin-1. Neurol 2004; 62(11):2137–2138.
21. Hecht M, Lin L, Kushida CA, et al. Report of a case of immunosuppression with prednisone in an 8-year-old boy with an acute onset of hypocretin-deficiency narcolepsy. Sleep 2003; 26(7):809–810.

22. Krahn LE, Pankratz VS, Oliver L, Boeve BF, Silber MH. Hypocretin (orexin) levels in cerebrospinal fluid of patients with narcolepsy: relationship to cataplexy and HLA DQB1*0602 status. Sleep 2002; 25(7):733–736.

23. Ebrahim IO, Sharief MK, De Lacy S, et al. Hypocretin (orexin) deficiency in narcolepsy and primary hypersomnia. J Neurol Neurosurg Psychiatry 2003; 74(1):127–130.

24. Overeem S, Steens SC, Good CD, et al. Voxel-based morphometry in hypocretin deficient narcolepsy. Sleep 2003; 26(1):44–46.

25. Fujiki N, Morris L, Mignot E, Nishino S. Analysis of onset location, laterality and propagation of cataplexy in canine narcolepsy. Psychiatry Clin Neurosci 2002; 56(3):275–276.

26. Kilduff TS, Peyron C. The hypocretin/orexin ligand-receptor system: implications for sleep and sleep disorders. Trends Neurosci 2000; 23(8):359–365.

27. Sakurai T, Nagata R, Yamanaka A, et al. Input of orexin/hypocretin neurons revealed by a genetically encoded tracer in mice. Neuron 2005; 46(2):297–308.

28. Rosen GM, Bendel AE, Neglia JP, Moertel CL, Mahowald M. Sleep in children with neoplasms of the central nervous system: case review of 14 children. Pediatr 2003; 112(1 Pt 1):e46–e54.

29. Marcus CL, Trescher WH, Halbower AC, Lutz J. Secondary narcolepsy in children with brain tumors. Sleep 2002; 25(4):435–439.

30. Sakurai T. Reverse pharmacology of orexin: from an orphan GPCR to integrative physiology. Regul Pept 2005; 126(1–2):3–10.

31. Nofzinger EA. Functional neuroimaging of sleep. Semin Neurol 2005; 25(1):9–18.

32. Oliviero A, Della Marca G, Tonali PA, et al. Functional involvement of cerebral cortex in human narcolepsy. J Neurol 2005; 252(1):56–61.

33. Chabas D, Taheri S, Renier C, Mignot E. The genetics of narcolepsy. Annu Rev Genomics Hum Genet 2003; 4:459–483.

34. Mignot E, Thorsby E. Narcolepsy and the HLA system. N Engl J Med 2001; 344(9):692.

35. Mignot E, Young T, Lin L, Finn L. Nocturnal sleep and daytime sleepiness in normal subjects with HLA-DQB1*0602. Sleep 1999; 22(3):347–352.

36. Tafti M, Dauvilliers Y. Pharmacogenomics in the treatment of narcolepsy. Pharmacogenomics 2003; 4(1):23–33.

37. Braun J, Bollow M, Remlinger G, et al. Prevalence of spondylarthropathies in HLA-B27 positive and negative blood donors. Arthritis Rheum 1998; 41(1): 58–67.

38. Dezi R, Niveloni S, Sugai E, et al. Gluten sensitivity in the rectal mucosa of first-degree relatives of celiac disease patients. Am J Gastroenterol 1997; 92(8): 1326–1330.

39. Mignot E. Sleep, sleep disorders and hypocretin (orexin). Sleep Med 2004; 5(suppl 1): S2–S8.

40. Fredrikson S, Carlander B, Billiard M, Link H. CSF immune variables in patients with narcolepsy. Acta Neurol Scand 1990; 81(3):253–254.

41. Mignot E, Lammers GJ, Ripley B, et al. The role of cerebrospinal fluid hypocretin measurement in the diagnosis of narcolepsy and other hypersomnias. Arch Neurol 2002; 59(10):1553–1562.

42. Arand D, Bonnet M, Hurwitz T, Mitler M, Rosa R, Sangal RB. The clinical use of the MSLT and MWT. Sleep 2005; 28(1):123–144.

43. Littner MR, Kushida C, Wise M, et al. Practice parameters for clinical use of the multiple sleep latency test and the maintenance of wakefulness test. Sleep 2005; 28(1):113–121.
44. Chesson AL, Jr. What do objective measures of daytime sleepiness measure? Sleep 2005; 28(1):14–15.
45. Saletu MT, Anderer P, Saletu-Zyhlarz GM, et al. EEG-mapping differences between narcolepsy patients and controls and subsequent double-blind, placebo-controlled studies with modafinil. Eur Arch Psychiatry Clin Neurosci 2005; 255(1):20–32.
46. Macleod S, Ferrie C, Zuberi SM. Symptoms of narcolepsy in children misinterpreted as epilepsy. Epileptic Disord 2005; 7(1):13–17.
47. Pelayo R, Chen W, Monzon S, Guilleminault C. Pediatric sleep pharmacology: you want to give my kid sleeping pills? Pediatr Clin North Am 2004; 51(1):117–134.
48. Littner M, Johnson SF, McCall WV, et al. Practice parameters for the treatment of narcolepsy: an update for 2000. Sleep 2001; 24(4):451–466.
49. Schwartz JR. Modafinil: new indications for wake promotion. Expert Opin Pharmacother 2005; 6(1):115–129.
50. Willie JT, Renthal W, Chemelli RM, et al. Modafinil more effectively induces wakefulness in orexin-null mice than in wild-type littermates. Neurosci 2005; 130(4):983–995.
51. Wisor JP, Eriksson KS. Dopaminergic-adrenergic interactions in the wake promoting mechanism of modafinil. Neurosci 2005; 132(4):1027–1034.
52. Schwertner HA, Kong SB. Determination of modafinil in plasma and urine by reversed phase high-performance liquid-chromatography. J Pharm Biomed Anal 2005; 37(3):475–479.
53. Borgen LA, Cook HN, Hornfeldt CS, Fuller DE. Sodium oxybate (GHB) for treatment of cataplexy. Pharmacotherapy 2002; 22(6):798–799; discussion 9.
54. Thorpy MJ. Sodium oxybate for the treatment of narcolepsy. Expert Opin Pharmacother 2005; 6(2):329–335.
55. Carter LP, Wu H, Chen W, et al. Novel {gamma}-hydroxybutyric acid (GHB) analogs share some, but not all, of the behavioral effects of GHB and GABAB receptor agonists. J Pharmacol Exp Ther 2005; 313(3):1314–1323.
56. Goodwin AK, Froestl W, Weerts EM. Involvement of gamma-hydroxybutyrate (GHB) and GABA-B receptors in the acute behavioral effects of GHB in baboons. Psychopharmacol (Berl) 2005; 180(2): 342–351.
57. Boehmer LN, Wu MF, John J, Siegel JM. Treatment with immunosuppressive and anti-inflammatory agents delays onset of canine genetic narcolepsy and reduces symptom severity. Exp Neurol 2004; 188(2):292–299.
58. Dauvilliers Y, Carlander B, Rivier F, Touchon J, Tafti M. Successful management of cataplexy with intravenous immunoglobulins at narcolepsy onset. Ann Neurol 2004; 56(6):905–908.
59. Lecendreux M, Maret S, Bassetti C, Mouren MC, Tafti M. Clinical efficacy of high-dose intravenous immunoglobulins near the onset of narcolepsy in a 10-year-old boy. J Sleep Res 2003; 12(4):347–348.
60. Schatzberg SJ, Cutter-Schatzberg K, Nydam D, et al. The effect of hypocretin replacement therapy in a 3-year-old Weimaraner with narcolepsy. J Vet Intern Med 2004; 18(4):586–288.
61. Burrow B, Burkle C, Warner DO, Chini EN. Postoperative outcome of patients with narcolepsy. A retrospective analysis. J Clin Anesth 2005; 17(1):21–25.

Index

Printed in the United States
by Baker & Taylor Publisher Services

Printed in the United States
by Baker & Taylor Publisher Services